Cystic Fibrosis

A Guide for Patient and Family

Second Edition

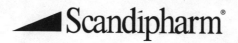

Cystic Fibrosis
A Guide for Patient and Family

Second Edition

David M. Orenstein, M.D.

Professor of Pediatrics
University of Pittsburgh School of Medicine
Professor of Health, Physical and Recreation Education
University of Pittsburgh School of Education
Director, Cystic Fibrosis Center and Pediatric Pulmonology Department
Children's Hospital of Pittsburgh
Pittsburgh, Pennsylvania

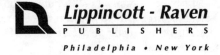

Lippincott - Raven
PUBLISHERS
Philadelphia • New York

Printed in the United States of America

9 8 7 6 5 4

Library of Congress Cataloging-in-Publication Data
Orenstein, David M., 1945-
    Cystic fibrosis : a guide for patient and family / David M. Orenstein.—2nd ed.
      p. cm.
    Includes bibliographical references and index.
    ISBN 0-397-51653-3
    1. Cystic fibrosis in children—Popular works. 2. Cystic fibrosis—Popular works.
    3. Patient education. I. Title.
RJ456.C9074   1996   96-27001
616.3'7—dc20   CIP

*To all those patients and families who have so enriched my life,
and have taught me so well,*

> *"it's not just what you're given,
> but what you do with what you've got."*
> *Si Kahn*

Contents

Contributors   ix

Introduction   xi
David M. Orenstein

Preface   xvii

Acknowledgments   xviii

1. The Basic Defect   1
   David M. Orenstein and Raymond A. Frizzell

2. Making the Diagnosis   13
   David M. Orenstein

3. The Respiratory System   19
   David M. Orenstein

4. The Gastrointestinal Tract   75
   Susan R. Orenstein and David M. Orenstein

5. Other Systems   93
   David M. Orenstein

6. Nutrition   101
   Judith A. Fulton, Susan R. Orenstein, and David M. Orenstein

7. Hospitalization and Other Special Treatments   121
   David M. Orenstein and Louise T. Bauer

8. Transplantation   141
   Geoffrey Kurland and David M. Orenstein

9. Daily Life   179
   David M. Orenstein

10. Exercise   187
    David M. Orenstein

11. Genetics   203
David M. Orenstein and Francis S. Collins

12. The Family   217
Jean Homrighausen Zander and David M. Orenstein

13. The Teenage Years   225
David M. Orenstein

14. Cystic Fibrosis and Adulthood   243
David M. Orenstein and Michael R. Knowles

15. Death and Cystic Fibrosis   261
David M. Orenstein

16. Research and Future Treatments   269
David M. Orenstein

17. The Cystic Fibrosis Foundation   281
Robert J. Beall

Appendices

A. Glossary of Terms   289

B. Medications (includes Glossary of Drugs)   293

C. Airway Clearance Techniques   321

D. Some High-Calorie Recipes   335

E. The History of Cystic Fibrosis   343

F. Cystic Fibrosis Care Centers and Chapters in the United States   345

G. Cystic Fibrosis Care Centers Worldwide   391

H. Cystic Fibrosis Associations Worldwide   429

I. Bibliography   435

Subject Index   437

Contributors

Louise T. Bauer, R.N. *Nurse Coordinator, Cystic Fibrosis Center and Pediatric Pulmonology Department, Children's Hospital of Pittsburgh, One Children's Place, 3705 Fifth Avenue at DeSoto Street, Pittsburgh, Pennsylvania 15213*

Robert J. Beall, Ph.D. *President and Chief Executive Officer, Cystic Fibrosis Foundation, 6931 Arlington Road, Bethesda, Maryland 20814*

Francis S. Collins, M.D., Ph.D. *Director, National Center for Human Genome Research, National Institutes of Health, Building 38A, Room 605, 9000 Rockville Pike, Bethesda, Maryland 20892*

Raymond A. Frizzell, Ph.D. *Chairman and Richard B. Mellon Professor of Cell Biology and Physiology, University of Pittsburgh School of Medicine, 818A Scaife Hall, 3550 Terrace Street, Pittsburgh, Pennsylvania 15261*

Judith A. Fulton, M.S., R.D. *Nutritionist, Cystic Fibrosis Center, Children's Hospital of Pittsburgh, One Children's Place, 3705 Fifth Avenue at DeSoto Street, Pittsburgh, Pennsylvania 15213*

Michael R. Knowles, M.D. *Professor of Medicine, University of North Carolina, Director, Adult Cystic Fibrosis Center, Chapel Hill, North Carolina 27599*

Geoffrey Kurland, M.D. *Associate Professor, Department of Pediatrics, University of Pittsburgh School of Medicine, Medical Director of Lung Transplant Program, Children's Hospital of Pittsburgh, One Children's Place, 3705 Fifth Avenue at DeSoto Street, Pittsburgh, Pennsylvania 15213*

David M. Orenstein, M.D. *Professor, Department of Pediatrics, School of Medicine; Professor of Health, Physical and Recreation Education, School of Education, University of Pittsburgh; and Director, Cystic Fibrosis Center and Pediatric Pulmonology Department, Children's Hospital of Pittsburgh, One Children's Place, 3705 Fifth Avenue at DeSoto Street, Pittsburgh, Pennsylvania 15213*

Susan R. Orenstein, M.D.   *Associate Professor, Division of Gastroenterology, Department of Pediatrics, University of Pittsburgh School of Medicine, Children's Hospital of Pittsburgh, One Children's Place, 3705 Fifth Avenue at DeSoto Street, Pittsburgh, Pennsylvania 15213*

Jean Homrighausen Zander, R.N., M.S.N.   *Nurse Specialist and Staff Nurse, Pediatric Intensive Care Unit, Pediatric Pulmonary Section, Room 293, Riley Children's Hospital, 702 Barnhill Drive, Indianapolis, Indiana 46223*

Introduction

David M. Orenstein

WHAT IS CYSTIC FIBROSIS?

CF is a life-shortening, inherited disorder that affects the way salt and water move into and out of the body's cells. The most important effects of this problem are in the lungs and the digestive system (especially the pancreas), where thick mucus blocks the small tubes and ducts. The lung problem can lead to progressive blockage, infection, and lung damage, and even death if there is too much damage, while the pancreatic blockage causes poor digestion and poor absorption of food, leading to poor growth and undernutrition. The sweat glands are also affected, in that they make a much saltier sweat than normal. Anyone reading this book has probably heard about the sweat test used to diagnose CF. Most parts of the body that make mucus are also affected, including the reproductive tract in men and women with CF.

ARE ANY PARTS OF THE BODY *NOT* AFFECTED BY CYSTIC FIBROSIS?

The list of body parts affected by CF can seem overwhelmingly long. But CF does *not* affect the brain and nervous system (it does *not* cause mental retardation); it does *not* affect the kidneys; it does *not* directly affect the heart; it does *not* affect the muscles; it does *not* affect the blood; and, except in the lungs, it does *not* interfere with the immune system (the body's ability to fight infection).

WHAT CAUSES CYSTIC FIBROSIS?

Cystic fibrosis is an inherited disorder that is present from birth, although signs and symptoms of it may not show up for weeks, months, or even years after birth. Although it is inherited, the parents of a child with CF do not have CF, and most often there is no history of it in the family. We all have two CF genes that determine whether or not we have CF. Both of these CF genes need to be abnormal for us to have CF, and CF is inherited by receiving one abnormal CF gene from each parent. Each parent usually has only one abnormal CF gene, and therefore has no sign of CF at all. Cystic fibrosis is very common among white people, and is *the most* commonly inherited life-shortening disease, affecting 1 in every 2,500 live babies born; 1 in 25 people carry the CF gene. CF is *not* caused by anything the parents did—or did not do—during the pregnancy. *The only way to get CF is to inherit one abnormal CF gene from each parent.* You cannot "catch" CF; it is not contagious.

HOW LONG DO PEOPLE WITH CYSTIC FIBROSIS LIVE?

It is impossible to predict how long a single patient will live. It *is* possible to give some overall stat stics. Just a few decades ago, nearly all children with CF died before they reacned 2 years of age. By 1995, the average survival had improved to nearly 30 years, with many people surviving into their 30s and 40s. A recent analysis predicted that for someone born today with CF, the average survival would be closer to 40 years. Some children do still die with CF, but this is much less common than in years gone by. For 1994, the death rate among CF patients under one year old was 0.007 (meaning a rate of 7 babies dying out of every 1,000), for children aged 6 to 7 years, it was 0.004 (a rate of 4 children dying out of every 1,000), for 14- to 15-year olds, it was 0.015 (15 of 1,000), and for 23-year-olds, it was 0.048.

There are several important factors that explain the tremendous improvement, and that explain why the outlook continues to improve almost year by year. First, CF is a newly recognized disease. (It is not a *new* disease, as is related in Appendix E, but a *newly recognized* disease.) It was not until 1938 that Dr. Dorothy Andersen wrote the first medical paper describing a number of children who had died with digestive problems and lung problems. She was the first to recognize that this was not just a coincidence, but represented a single disease, which she called "cystic fibrosis of the pancreas," because the children she examined after they died all had *cysts* (fluid-filled sacs) and scar tissue (*fibrosis*) replacing almost all the normal tissue of their pancreas. The name has been shortened to cystic fibrosis, but her description helped to lay the foundation for recognizing the disease, and therefore treating children who had it. Around this time, antibiotics were becoming available, and lung infections could be treated to a degree. In 1964, Dr. Doershuk and Dr. Matthews and their colleagues in Cleveland reported the results of 5 years of a comprehensive treatment program. These results were very much improved over previous results, and most modern treatment programs use the same basic principles these pioneers used.

In the last 30 years, many new antibiotics have become available, making treatment more effective. Further, knowledge of CF has spread widely, so that now most pediatricians and family doctors are able to recognize the signs and symptoms of CF and are able to give children treatment while it can still be helpful, that is, before there is too much irreversible lung damage. Very importantly, a nationwide network of CF centers has grown up, where CF experts deliver state-of-the-art care.

The point here is that the medical world has had good comprehensive treatment programs for patients with CF for only a little more than 30 years. This means that there are virtually no patients with CF who are 40 years old *and* were started on a treatment program in the first year of life. There are more and more teenagers and people in their 20s who were started on treatment programs early in life, before their lungs were in bad shape, and many of these young adults are doing extremely well. Therefore, there is every reason to be very optimistic about the future of a youngster diagnosed and started on treatment today. Certainly, while an average survival to age 30 years reflects a tremendous improvement, it is not something to be satisfied with; but this is a situation that is continually improving.

CYSTIC FIBROSIS CARE

Medical care of patients with CF is best carried out at one of the 112 CF centers accredited by the Cystic Fibrosis Foundation, in conjunction with your own pediatrician, family doctor, or internist. Doctors are becoming better informed about CF, but it is important to be in touch with the CF experts who stay up to date with the quickly changing field that CF has become. These experts are found in CF centers, and there are also many specially trained professionals (nutritionists, social workers, nurses, respiratory therapists) at these centers with extensive knowledge and experience taking care of people with CF. The record is fairly clear that CF patients whose care is coordinated by a CF center live longer than those who do not attend a center. With the health care system changing, it may be more difficult to get a referral to a CF center, but it is important to insist on it.

It is also important to continue to have care from a general pediatrician or family doctor, who can be very helpful with the non-CF health issues that arise in everyone's life.

RESEARCH AND THE BASIC DEFECT

When the first edition of this book was published just a few years ago, the basic defect in CF was not known. Much was understood about the kind of problems people with CF have, how to prevent many of those problems, and how to treat the problems that can't be prevented. But at a very basic chemical level, no one knew what exactly goes wrong within the cells of the body to cause the problems that occur. What this meant for treatment was that the medications and therapies were all directed at *secondary* problems (problems that are themselves caused by the basic defect) and not at the underlying problem itself. Another way of putting it is that there was no *cure* for CF.

Much has changed in the past few years, and our understanding of what goes wrong within and outside the cells of people with CF has increased tremendously. The gene for CF has been found and cloned (produced in the laboratory); there is now a "CF mouse," created through genetic engineering, while, previously, no nonhuman animal had CF, and we know infinitely more about the alterations of cell functioning caused by CF (the basic defect is discussed in Chapter 1). There are even some experimental treatments that have been designed to try to get around the basic problem with the abnormally functioning cells, and gene therapy trials are under way in centers around the world. However, there still is not a treatment that successfully (and safely) undoes the basic defect, and therefore, there is still no cure for CF.

The situation is similar to that of diabetes. It is known that people get sick with diabetes because they don't have enough insulin to control their blood sugar. These people can lead normal lives by taking daily insulin shots, but they still have diabetes and will have it until scientists discover and eliminate the cause of inadequate insulin production.

Tremendous progress has been made in the search for the ways to undo or get around the basic defect in CF. This is a very exciting time in CF research, because nearly every month an important piece of the puzzle is discovered and new experimental treatments come to light. The prospects for ever better treatment in the upcoming months and years are very bright.

A WORD TO NEWLY DIAGNOSED PATIENTS AND FAMILIES

If you are reading this book because you (or, more likely, your child) have (has) just been diagnosed with cystic fibrosis (CF), this is a hard time for you. Many people in your situation feel panicked, or numb, or "spacey." You may be angry, frightened, disbelieving. For some of you, along with the bad feelings, there may also be a sense of relief at having a diagnosis, particularly if you've known *something* was wrong, but couldn't get your fears taken seriously, or couldn't get your questions answered. This may be a time when you don't want to hear any more information, or it may be a time when you want to learn absolutely *everything* there is to know about CF. However you are feeling, it may be a little hard to take in a lot of new information. However you are feeling, you can be certain that there have been many, many people who have experienced these same feelings. It may be helpful to talk about how you're feeling with people in the CF center, and in some cases with other families who have been through what you're going through now. The people in the center can help you find such people if you're interested. As you learn more about CF, and get used to the idea that you (your child) have (has) it, and as you see that in most cases people can live quite a normal childhood, adolescence, and beyond, your emotions will become less raw, times will be less hard.

HOW CAN PEOPLE LEARN ABOUT CYSTIC FIBROSIS?

The purpose of this book is to help you learn about all aspects of CF, including how it is inherited, the problems it causes, how it is treated, and current research. Cystic fibrosis centers and the Cystic Fibrosis Foundation can provide information also. Some of you will want to plow through the book cover to cover now, while some others may not be able to face even the first chapter just yet. But the book will be here when you're ready for it, and can certainly be referred back to when a new question comes up, or if you find you've forgotten something. Encyclopedias and many general medical books are *not* a good source of information, since they are likely to be out of date. Newspapers, especially the tabloids we all see in the checkout line in the grocery store, are also not good sources, for they are likely to announce the discovery of a cure that bears little relation to medical truth. Even if you hear something that sounds encouraging on a national TV news show, be sure to check it out with your CF center, or someone who is knowledgeable and up to date on research developments.

There have been several instances of incorrect information—even dangerous information—being reported as medical truth on supposedly reputable news shows. In one of these instances, it was announced that CF was caused by a deficiency of *selenium* (a mineral we all need, and one which most of us—CF or no—get plenty of in the diet), and that a cure existed in taking huge doses of selenium; several babies died as a result of that report, after being given massive overdoses of selenium. Usually, information about CF that appears in the news is not harmful, and is even fairly accurate. But it is wise to be cautious about "dramatic breakthroughs" that are announced. Most often, medical progress is not made by dramatic breakthroughs, but rather by tiny steps, with one group of scientists building upon the work of previous researchers. Your CF center and the CF Foundation are informed of all the reputable work in the field worldwide, and will be happy to provide you with this information.

ORGANIZATION OF THE BOOK

The goal of this book is to cover all the important topics that concern people with CF and their families. The opening chapter (which follows this Introduction) discusses the basic defect in the cells of people with CF, going over some of the amazing discoveries that have been made just within the past few years. (My coauthor on this chapter, Dr. Ray Frizzell, is responsible for a lot of the exciting research that is unlocking the secrets of the cellular abnormalities in CF.) Next comes a short chapter (Chapter 2) summarizing how the diagnosis of CF is made. The respiratory system (lungs), how it normally works, the changes brought about by CF, and the treatment of the lung problems are the subject of Chapter 3. Chapter 4, on the digestive and gastrointestinal system, also reviews both normal functioning and that affected by cystic fibrosis. Chapter 5 briefly discusses the other body systems affected by cystic fibrosis. Then follows a chapter on nutrition (Chapter 6).

Chapter 7 discusses hospitalization and other types of elaborate treatments, and is followed by a very long chapter (Chapter 8) on everything you wanted to know (and then some) about organ transplantation for CF (mostly about lung transplantation, and a bit about liver transplantation), and then a short Chapter 9 dealing with various aspects of daily life including day care, school, sports, home responsibilities, and travel. Exercise is considered separately in Chapter 10. Chapter 11, on the genetics of CF, describes the manner in which it is inherited, and a lot of the very new information about molecular genetics, how researchers determine the abnormalities seen in CF, and even prospects for gene therapy. (My coauthor on this chapter, Dr. Francis Collins, is the codiscoverer of the CF gene.)

We then switch gears for Chapter 12, which deals with emotional and psychological issues (growing up with CF, effects on the family of a child with CF, etc.). Teenagers get their own chapter—Chapter 13. The special problems of the adult with cystic fibrosis are discussed in Chapter 14. Chapter 15 discusses the difficult issues surrounding dying with CF.

Research—past, present, and future—and some speculation about future treatments are the subjects of the next chapter. The national Cystic Fibrosis Foundation is discussed by its President and Chief Executive Officer, Dr. Robert Beall, in the final chapter.

The volume includes several appendixes: a glossary of technical terms; a listing of commonly used medications, giving brand names and generic names, uses, and side effects; diagrams illustrating the proper techniques for performing chest physical therapy, and discussions of other airway clearance techniques; a short but chubby group of high-calorie recipes; a brief appendix on major historic landmarks in CF; a list of CF centers in the United States; a list of CF centers worldwide; and a list of CF organizations worldwide. The final appendix is a brief bibliography of some outstanding readings (mostly technical) on CF.

A FINAL NOTE ON THE ORGANIZATION AND CONTENT OF THIS BOOK

Each of the chapters starts with a section labeled, *The Basics,* which includes just a few of the most important points of that chapter. Some of these chapters are very long, and have much more detail than you'll need or want at any one time. Some of the science presented—particularly in Chapter 1, *The Basic Defect,* and parts of Chapter 11, *Genetics*—is *very* difficult to understand, and can be daunting, especially the first time round. Try not to be intimidated by it, but keep in mind that it's been hard even for most physicians to keep up with the torrid pace of CF research, and it's taken some of us months or years to become comfortable with these concepts.

For each chapter, *The Basics* may give you an idea of what's there, and you can skim the chapter for what you want to get out of it. The details will be there when you want them.

Preface

I wrote this book (with a lot of help) for people interested in cystic fibrosis, whether they be patients, the friends and family of patients, or health professionals who work with patients and their families. It is designed to be of particular use to parents in the initial months that follow their child's diagnosis of cystic fibrosis. It is also written with the intention that it serves as a "refresher" course for people to review areas of treatment and physiology they may have forgotten. The relatives and friends of a patient may also benefit from this introduction to cystic fibrosis.

An important group for whom this book is written is teenagers who were diagnosed in infancy. While teenagers grow up knowing a lot about cystic fibrosis, they seldom receive the in-depth explanation that their parents received immediately upon diagnosis. A final goal of this volume is to provide a foundation for understanding cystic fibrosis that will enable patients and families to understand more fully the advances that are being made so rapidly in this field.

I have tried to stress throughout this book that cystic fibrosis is a serious disease, yet it is one that can be effectively controlled for long periods of time in most patients. It is a life-shortening disease, yet it is also one in which the outlook for patients' length and quality of life has improved dramatically in a relatively short time and continues to do so. There is currently no cure for cystic fibrosis, yet the treatment available is very effective. It is a disease that creates demands on patients and families for daily treatments; it is also one in which the efforts of patients and families can greatly influence the health and quality of life of the patient. Cystic fibrosis is commonly accepted as inhibiting normal life, yet the reality is that most patients go to school, play sports, and grow up accomplishing all the tasks, and experience all the joys and sorrows of childhood, adolescence, and young adulthood. It is my hope that patients and their families will find this volume to be of help in all these stages of life.

Many patients, families, and health professionals have responded generously to the First Edition of this book and have made suggestions that I have tried to incorporate in this edition to make it more useful. I have been extremely fortunate and honored to have been able to convince several of the leaders in the fields of cystic fibrosis research and clinical care to help with this edition. It is the hope of all of us that patients, families, and health-care workers will find this volume useful.

David M. Orenstein, M.D.

Acknowledgments

In addition to all those teachers, parents (of mine and of my patients), and colleagues who made the First Edition possible, quite a few generous and talented people helped with this edition.

The Arrington, Burns, Feldman, Gibson, Kennedy, Kinney, Michel, and Rubin families, George Attridge, Megan Petrick, and Angela Havyer have given generously of their time, and made helpful suggestions. Thank you to Nancy Smizik, Sinikka Davis, Drs. Joel Weinberg, Joe Pilewski, Gary Cutting, Stacey Fitzsimmons, Bob Beall, and Glenna Winnie for their assistance. Amanda Young gets special credit for her in-depth study and suggestions. Stefani Ledewitz provided the wonderful drawings that help clarify the difficult science. Ms. Michelle Roche of the ICF(M)A provided important information on international clinics and associations. The entire staff of our own CF Center provided a warm, nurturing place to work, and set the tone for much of the book.

Arthur and Anna Orenstein proved themselves unequaled in the T-D method of writing assistance. Thanks are due my wife, Susan Orenstein, M.D., for just about everything.

1

The Basic Defect

THE BASICS

1. The main problem with the cells that make up the lungs, pancreas, and sweat glands in people with CF is that chloride (part of what makes up common salt) cannot pass through the cells normally.
2. Another problem is that sodium (the other part of salt) may be pumped through the cells more than normal.
3. Both of these problems probably cause lung and pancreatic mucus and fluid to be drier than normal, and sweat to be saltier than normal.
4. The cells work abnormally in different ways in people with CF, depending on which CF gene they have.
5. Possibly, new treatments can be designed to get around these cell abnormalities.

INTRODUCTION

Until recently, it was not known what caused the various problems that people with cystic fibrosis (CF) have. One fact *almost* explained all of the problems: Examinations showed that extra thick and sticky mucus seemed to be in most of the organs of the body affected by CF: thick mucus clogged bronchial tubes in the lung, blocked ducts and tubes leading from the pancreas to the intestines, and sometimes blocked the intestines and liver. But one of the most noticeable abnormalities in CF patients is their salty sweat. The salty sweat is why the sweat test is still the best test to diagnose CF, even though it has been around for 40 years. [In the sweat test, as most people reading this book already know, sweat is collected from a patient and is then analyzed for its salt (sodium and chloride) concentration: a "positive" sweat test is one in which the saltiness of sweat is more than three times higher than normal.]

Mucus—thick or thin—has nothing to do with sweat glands, and so can't be blamed for this part of CF. When CF doctors used to try to explain CF, there was always that little stumbling block: "All the problems are caused by thick mucus: the lung problem, the pancreas and digestive problem, the intestine problems, and so on. . .Oh, and by the way [we'd say softly], there's the little matter of the sweat glands that seems different."

ELECTRICAL CHARGES IN THE NOSE!

In the 1980s, researchers in North Carolina made important discoveries that for the first time seemed to tie together *all* the abnormalities in CF. These researchers happened to be interested in measuring the electrical charge in people's noses. They measured what we now refer to as the nasal PD (for *p*otential *d*ifference), or simply the electrical charge across the mucous membrane in the nose. As it turns out, everyone has a negative electrical charge across these mucous membranes. In almost everyone, this is a small charge (–5 to –30 millivolts [mV]), but virtually everyone with CF has a much larger PD (–40 to –80 mV). The measurement of nasal PD is somewhat difficult to do correctly, but if experienced people perform the measurements, the PD result distinguishes people with CF from those who do not have CF at least as well as—and maybe even better than—the sweat test.

At the same time as the PD discovery in the nose, other researchers in California found the same elevated electrical charge across the cells lining the sweat glands of people with CF. Not long afterward, the cells making up the lining (the *epithelial surface*) of the intestines and pancreas were also found to have similar changes in their electrical properties. For the first time, all the organs that are affected by CF were found to have a single abnormality: the electrical charge across the cells making up their epithelial surfaces was much greater than the electrical charge seen in these glands in people without CF.

One of the things that made these discoveries, taken together, even more exciting than they might have been individually was that they appeared at about the same time as molecular biologists were discovering the CF gene (more about this in Chapter 11, *Genetics*). The scientists who discovered the CF gene predicted that the protein produced by this gene was like a number of previously discovered proteins that direct the traffic of various chemicals across cell membranes. The electrical charge across membranes has much to do with the speed of sodium (positive charge) and chloride (negative charge) movement across these membranes. Sodium and chloride make up salt, and we're back to the salty sweat. In the next section we give a few more details about what we've now learned about traffic across cell membranes in the organs affected by CF.

MOVEMENT OF SALT AND WATER ACROSS
CELL MEMBRANES

The protein whose production is directed by the CF gene has been called CFTR (for *c*ystic *f*ibrosis *t*ransmembrane conductance *r*egulator), and, as you might guess by its name, this protein is extremely important in regulating how much salt (sodium and chloride) gets across cell membranes.

Here's what seems to happen: For the proper functioning and cleansing of the lungs, there needs to be a certain amount of fluid and mucus lining the airways. This fluid comes from within the cells that line the smallest bronchi, far out in lungs, and the mucus comes from the specialized mucus-secreting cells that lie along the airways. The cells lining the smallest bronchi secrete fluid, that is, they push fluid out onto the airway surface. Although each of these airways is very small, and doesn't hold much fluid, the total amount of fluid in all the thousands of small airways is tremendous, and is as much as 4,000 times greater than the volume of the larger airways. (This is because there are fewer of the large airways.) Since the fluid is constantly moving upward toward the trachea, eventually reaching the back of the throat, this means that the cells in the larger bronchi are required to absorb the fluid in order to keep the fluid lining thin all along the airway.

The way healthy bronchial cells secrete fluid (Figure 1.1) is that they allow chloride to pass out through the luminal membrane of the cells (the part of the cell's membrane that lies on the airway surface, where the air flows). There are several different channels in the cell's luminal membrane through which the chloride can flow. One is opened by the presence of calcium in the cell, and is called the *calcium-dependent chloride channel;* another is called the *outwardly rectifying chloride channel,* usually abbreviated ORCC; but the main one for chloride flow onto the airway surface is CFTR itself. Remember its name ends with "*trans*-membrane conductance *regulator*," meaning that it is responsible for conducting chloride across the membrane. Every little chloride ion carries a negative charge, and since (as in many aspects of life) opposites attract, the negative charge of chloride pulls a positively charged ion with it, namely, sodium. There is a law here— the law of electrical neutrality—that says the number of positive charges in a solution should be the same as the number of negative charges. So, whenever a negative charge (chloride) leaves, a positive charge (sodium) is pulled along with

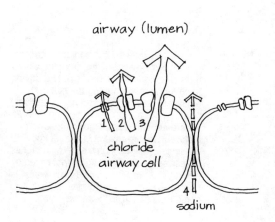

airway (lumen)

chloride
airway cell

sodium

Figure 1.1. Healthy cell chloride secretion. Chloride is secreted out of the cell into the airway lumen through several channels. The main chloride channel is *CFTR* (cystic fibrosis transmembrane conductance regulator) (labeled *3*). Two other channels shown are the *calcium-dependent channel* (*2*) and the ORCC (outwardly rectifying chloride channel) (*1*). When chloride leaves the cells, sodium passively follows, in this case probably between cells (*4*), in order to keep the positive and negative charges roughly equal, and (not pictured); where sodium and chloride go, water is pulled, so chloride secretion results in fluid being added to the airway.

it. Therefore, chloride **and** sodium are transported onto the airway surface. Actually, the easiest route for sodium is between cells, rather than through the cell's membrane. No matter; it gets to where it's supposed to go, and now, sodium and chloride (salt) are out on the luminal surface of the airways. Where salt goes, water follows, just as a dry sponge soaks up water. This is also how tree roots absorb water from the soil. So, getting back to the airways, fluid goes onto the airway surface following the sodium chloride. In summary, the secreting cells open channels to allow chloride into the lumen; the chloride **pulls** the oppositely charged sodium with it, and the combination of sodium and chloride pulls in water to form the airway lining fluid.

As the fluid moves up the tracheobronchial tree from the small bronchi (see Chapter 3, *The Respiratory System*), the thickness of the airway lining liquid is adjusted by chloride secretion (Figure 1.1) and sodium absorption (Figure 1.2). Since a lot of fluid is produced in the small airways, sodium absorption tends to be very important in controlling the volume of the airway lung fluid. As you can see in Figure 1.2, fluid absorption starts with sodium ions being pumped out of the airway fluid across the epithelial cells. As the positively charged sodium ion leaves, it pulls the negatively charged chloride ion, and also water, with it. Sodium absorption is a two-step process, where sodium enters the airway cell through a channel (a channel that can be blocked by the drug amiloride), and sodium is pushed out of the other side of the cell into the bloodstream by a protein that functions like a pump. In most circumstances, there is only a small force pulling on chloride to go with the sodium, and so the electrical charge difference across these membranes is normally small.

Changes in CF, and the CFTR Protein as a Chloride Channel and Regulator of Sodium Transport

This system does not work well in people with CF. As you can see in Figure 1.3, there are problems in both secretion and absorption of salt and water. Both

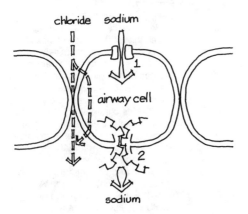

Figure 1.2. Healthy cell sodium reabsorption. Sodium enters the cell from the airway through a sodium channel (*1*). The driving force for sodium entering the cell from the airway lumen is that sodium is actively pumped out the other side of the cell (*2*). Where sodium goes, chloride follows (not pictured). In this case, it is not yet known if chloride passes *through* the cell membranes or *between* cells. Once again (not pictured), where sodium and chloride go, water is pulled, so sodium absorption results in fluid being removed from the airway.

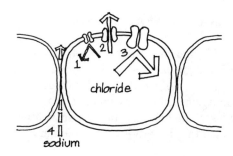

chloride

4 sodium

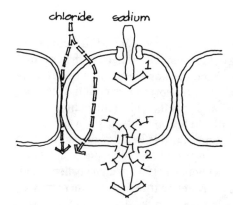

chloride   sodium

Figure 1.3. CF cell secretion and absorption. (**A**) Chloride secretion abnormality. With CF cells, the CFTR channel (*3*) is blocked or nonexistent, so chloride cannot exit. A small amount of chloride probably can exit through the calcium-dependent chloride channel (*2*), while probably none goes through the ORCC (*1*). With limited chloride secretion, there is also limited sodium (*4*) and fluid (not pictured) entering the airway lumen from the cell. (**B**) Sodium absorption abnormality. With CF cells, the sodium pump (*2*) is overactive, leading to excessive sodium being absorbed through the sodium channel in the luminal membrane (*1*), which also leads to excessive fluid absorption (not shown).

problems lead to less fluid in the airway lumen and drier, stickier contents of the airways, which are harder to move and perhaps more hospitable to bacteria:

1. The secretion problem is that the main channel to let chloride out of the cell is the CFTR protein. *In someone with an altered or missing CFTR protein* (because of having two abnormal CFTR genes, as everyone with CF has), *this channel is blocked or absent: chloride cannot easily exit from the cell.*

2. Then, the absorption problem is that the sodium channel, which is open to allow sodium to get into the cell and out of the lumen, is *over*active, so more sodium (and more positive charge) than normal enters the cells and gets absorbed. This makes the electrical charge (PD) across the airway larger in CF, and is the basis of the nasal PD test (see the preceding section). The hyperactivity of the sodium absorption system is determined—at least in part—by the changes in the CFTR protein that cause CF.

Together, these problems mean more salt and water have been removed from the airway lumen and gone into the cells and surrounding tissues, probably explaining the dry, thick mucus that we've long observed in people with CF.

WHAT ABOUT THE PANCREAS AND SWEAT GLANDS?

The lungs are not the only organs affected by the abnormal CFTR protein. The pancreatic ducts are affected in a very similar manner. The CFTR chloride channel is blocked or absent, and this leads to plugging of the ducts and eventual destruction of the pancreas. In the sweat glands, since chloride cannot be absorbed out of the gland fluid (see Chapter 5, *Other Systems*), that fluid retains a high concentration of chloride (and sodium), resulting in salty sweat, a hallmark of the disease.

WHAT CAUSES CYSTIC FIBROSIS AIRWAYS TO BECOME INFECTED?

We have long thought that people with CF got frequent bronchial infections because their airway secretions were drier, stickier, and harder to clear than normal secretions. This is still a likely explanation, and our knowledge about salt movement across the bronchial epithelial cells lends support to this notion. However, from what we know now, we cannot say that this is the only explanation for the ease with which the airways of patients with CF become infected. For one thing, although we are fairly certain about the abnormalities in chloride and sodium transport, we do not have proof that the airway secretions in people with CF actually have less water content than in those without CF. If we exclude patients with bronchial infection and inflammation, this may not be true. Further, there may be factors related to abnormal CFTR protein—other than the dryness of the airway fluid—that makes the airways easily infected. For instance, there is evidence that some bacteria (including *Pseudomonas*) can stick more tightly to airway cells when the electrical charge of proteins on the cells' surface is altered. In CF, there appears to be a different type of sugar coat on the proteins (with a different electrical charge) that is attached to the surface membrane, and this could make it easier for *Pseudomonas* organisms to stick to airway cells. If bacteria stick tightly to airway cells, they are harder to clear from the bronchi, and it's easier for them to set up housekeeping.

Another theory is that normal healthy lung cells respond in a very localized way to inhaled particles, including bacteria: perhaps the cell can detect when a foreign invader has landed, and it quickly opens its chloride channel to let chloride out of the cell; sodium and water quickly follow, in tiny amounts, but enough in this very small area to wash away the bacteria or dust particle. If the chloride channel can't open, the bacteria stay there long enough for the next line of defense, namely, white blood cells, to be called in to fight them off. Unfortunately, as you'll see in Chapter 3, *The Respiratory System,* these white blood cells can damage lung tissue along with the bacteria they attack. Under this theory, the airways don't have to start out as overall drier than normal, but because they can't wash away bacteria at thousands of individual sites, they eventually become damaged and filled with thick mucus and debris from dead bacteria, exhausted white blood cells, and damaged airway cells.

Whatever the exact details, it seems clear at this point that the lung problems must be somehow related to the abnormal CFTR and the abnormal movement of salt and water across bronchial cells.

ARE THERE DIFFERENCES AMONG THE DIFFERENT CYSTIC FIBROSIS MUTATIONS?

Chapter 11, *Genetics,* discusses the different ways in which the CFTR gene (and the protein it makes) can be abnormal. You'll see in that chapter that geneticists think that there are over 500 different ways that this one gene can be abnormal! You'll also see that there is a lot of interest in trying to find out how (or if) these different changes (mutations) make for different problems for patients. In this section, we'll discuss briefly what little is known about whether different mutations in the CFTR gene and protein make for differences in the basic defect, that is, in how the cells work.

The way the CFTR protein seems to work in healthy cells is shown in Figure 1.4. There are four steps involved: (1) The protein is made within the cell *(production),* then (2) it has to fold in a particular way so that its shape allows it to be transported to the cell membrane *(folding),* where (3) it responds to certain chemical signals that activate it *(regulation),* and it does its job, (4) including opening for brief periods to let chloride out *(conduction).*

Different mutations in the CFTR gene can cause it to get "hung up" on its way to the cell membrane or not work correctly, and usually a mutation interferes with one of these four steps. For example,

1. There are quite a few CF gene abnormalities that are known (or suspected) to prevent the CFTR protein from being made at all (defective *production*).

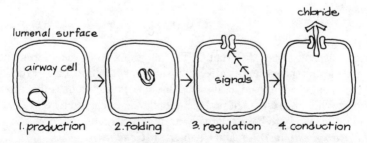

Figure 1.4. The four steps needed for functioning of the CFTR protein in healthy cells. (*1*) The protein is made within the cell *(production)*, then (*2*) it has to fold in a particular way so that its shape allows it to be transported to the cell membrane (*folding*), where (*3*) it responds to certain chemical signals that activate it (*regulation*), and it does its job, (*4*) including opening for brief periods to let chloride out (*conduction*).

These include mutations called G542X, 3905 insT, and R553X. With another abnormal form of the CFTR gene, one with the unwieldy name 3849+10kb C→T, CFTR protein is made, but much less of it than normal.

2. The most common CF mutation (ΔF508) results in the second kind of problem (abnormal *folding*): CFTR protein is made, but it folds into an abnormal shape, and therefore is not transported to the cell membrane to do its work. In the laboratory, when researchers have moved the abnormal ΔF508 CFTR protein into the cell membrane, it has worked fairly well (but not as well as the normal CFTR). Several other mutations seem to have a similar problem of not being delivered to the cell membrane, including ΔI507, N1303K, and S549R.

3. There have been several CFTR mutations that have abnormal *regulation:* the CFTR protein is delivered to the membrane, but is not able to respond normally to the usual chemical signals that should tell it to be active as a chloride channel (this means it doesn't open normally to let chloride pass out through the membrane). These mutations include G551D and several others that are very rare.

4. Finally, there are a few mutations with abnormal chloride *conduction:* these altered CFTR proteins seem to be made and transported to the cell membrane correctly; and under experimental conditions they respond normally to the chemical activating signals. Yet, under usual circumstances, they let a less-than-normal amount of chloride pass through the cell membrane (they open, but either not wide enough or not for a long enough time). The three most common of these mutations are R117H, R334W, and R347P. For the R117H CFTR protein, there is an explanation of its subnormal chloride current: although this protein-channel opens normally in response to the appropriate signals, it remains open for a much shorter time than normal.

There have not yet been ways identified in which the different CFTR mutations may affect the overactive sodium-reabsorbing channel. It is possible that the changes in sodium transport will be different for each different kind of CFTR mutation.

SO WHAT?

In most cases, the very different CFTR mutations do not seem to make much difference in how the patient is affected: patients with almost all of these different mutations have identical CF disease. One set of exceptions is that most of the CF patients with the last type of problem (conduction), caused by R117H, R334W, and R347P, are likely to have relatively normal pancreatic function (see Chapter 4, *The Gastrointestinal Tract,* and Chapter 11, *Genetics*).

What may be even more important one day is that if we know exactly how someone's abnormal CF gene affects his or her cells, there may be very specific ways to correct the problem. One example that may be useful in helping us to understand the situation (but not yet helpful to patients) is with the most common abnormal CF protein, produced by the gene ΔF508. Remember from a few paragraphs ago that this CFTR protein does not escape from the inner portion of the cell to be delivered to the cell membrane, but that if a scientist puts it into the membrane, it can function about half as well as the normal CFTR. What if there were a way to free the F508 CFTR from the cell interior so it could get to the membrane? Again, in the laboratory, there **are** a couple of ways:

1. In cells growing at normal body temperature (37°C, 98.6°F), the ΔF508 CFTR protein is trapped inside the cell; **but,** if the cells are grown at a cooler temperature (23–30°C; 73–86°F), some of the protein escapes and makes it to the cell membrane, where it functions. Now, it is not possible to lower everyone's body temperature 12–25°F, but it is helpful and encouraging to know that there is **something** that can make the protein act closer to normal.
2. There is also evidence that the chemical *glycerol* can do the same thing that the lower temperature does: ΔF508 cells grown in the laboratory in the presence of lots of glycerol have some CFTR protein that makes it to the cell membrane. Perhaps one day we'll have a safe drug patients can take to make this happen in their lungs.

Similarly, perhaps drugs could be discovered or developed that make CFTR protein more responsive to the usual chemical signals that tell it to open to let chloride pass, or to keep a quickly closing channel open a bit longer.

Even before treatments are designed that target the specific CFTR mutations, it might be possible to bypass the cellular problems that virtually all CF cells have: It might be possible to slow down the overactive sodium pump or to "rev up" the non-CFTR chloride channels. In fact, as this book is going to press, there are studies under way looking at drugs to do just that (see Chapter 16, *Research and Future Treatments*). Amiloride is a drug that's been around for a long time, and has been used as a diuretic (which makes you lose fluid by increasing the amount of urine made by the kidneys). Amiloride works by blocking the sodium channel. So far, there are conflicting studies as to whether inhaled amiloride is helpful over a several-month period. Another drug, UTP (uridine triphosphate), is being studied for its apparent role in increasing chloride flow through the calcium-dependent chloride channel in the cell membrane (not the CFTR channel).

DOES THE BASIC DEFECT EXPLAIN WHY THE CYSTIC FIBROSIS GENE HAS SURVIVED FOR SO LONG?

You'll see in Chapter 11, *Genetics,* that scientists always wonder how an abnormal gene sticks around, over centuries, instead of dying out. That question is especially puzzling for an abnormal gene that ends up with people dying before they're old enough to reproduce (as was true of CF until just the past decade or so, compared to the thousands of years that CF has been around). In a number of different genetic diseases, there has been something good found out about the mutation in the gene to offset its bad effects. That "good" is usually something that gives an advantage to the people who carry **one** copy of the abnormal gene. A well-known example is the case of sickle cell disease, a terrible problem afflicting some 10% of African-Americans. Like CF, sickle cell disease is a recessive disorder (more about this in Chapter 11, *Genetics*), meaning that to have the disease, someone has to have two copies of an abnormal gene, inheriting one from each parent. The parents almost always have one abnormal gene and one normal gene (as do many other people as well). Having one normal and one abnormal gene for sickle cell disease is called having the "sickle trait," and people with sickle trait are quite healthy. As it turns out, not only are they healthy, but having sickle trait *protects* them from the ravages of malaria. So, if whole villages were being wiped out by malaria, someone with sickle trait had a survival advantage, and would be more likely to live through the malaria epidemics, and *continue to pass on the abnormal gene.*

For CF, any number of different advantages for carriers (parents of CF patients, and others who carry only one abnormal CFTR gene) have been guessed at over the years. Within the last year or so, researchers working with CF mice (see Chapter 11, *Genetics*) found that carrier mice (those with one normal and one abnormal CFTR gene) were protected from having the terrible diarrhea that comes with being infected with cholera. Cholera causes severe illness and death in many places around the world. Its damage is done by a chemical made by the cholera bacteria ("cholera toxin"), which makes the intestines secrete chloride in huge amounts. As we've seen above, when cells secrete a large amount of chloride, sodium and water will follow. We said that airway cells secrete into the lumen of the lungs' airways; intestinal cell do the same thing into the lumen of the intestine. A large amount of chloride, sodium, and water pouring into the intestinal lumen creates a watery diarrhea. So people with cholera become dangerously—often fatally— dehydrated. It now appears that the intestinal cells of CF carrier mice do not secrete so much salt and water after they've been exposed to cholera toxin. We know that having two abnormal CFTR genes makes chloride secretion very much below normal. It looks like having one normal and one abnormal CFTR gene may allow for normal, healthy levels of chloride secretion under usual conditions. But under unusual conditions (for example, infection with cholera), perhaps the cells cannot increase their chloride secretion much above the usual level; that is, they can't increase their chloride secretion to the point where they become dangerously dehydrated because of too much fluid lost in diarrhea. Since this is different from the noncarriers (who increase chloride and water secretion dangerously), it is not "normal," but since it protects against fatal dehydration, it certainly is an advantage for the CF carrier. This is an attractive hypothesis: if carriers of the abnormal CFTR gene have been protected from cholera or other similar intestinal infections over the centuries, while people with no "CF trait" were being wiped out, that would explain the persistence of the abnormal CFTR gene that causes so much trouble. (It is not a *perfect* explanation, though, since the worldwide distribution of cholera is not the same as the distribution of CF. However, perhaps the intestinal protection extends to other infectious diarrheas, with a geographical distribution more similar to that of CF.)

In summary, the basic defect in CF is becoming better understood. It involves abnormal traffic of salt and water across and through cells that line the airways, pancreas, intestinal tract, and sweat glands. The ways in which the salt and water transport are abnormal may lead to effective new treatments.

2

Making the Diagnosis

THE BASICS

1. The sweat test is the best test for CF, *if* it is done in a laboratory that has a lot of sweat testing experience.
2. Genetic testing can help to tell if a patient has CF.
3. With genetic testing, "a positive" test means the person probably has CF, but a "negative" test does not completely rule out CF.
4. If there is any question about the possibility of a person's having CF, that person needs to be tested.

INTRODUCTION

Making the diagnosis of cystic fibrosis (CF) is one of the most important things that can be done for the health of people with CF. It can clear the way for starting extremely effective treatment that will have a tremendous influence on how healthy they will be and how long they will live. The earlier the diagnosis is made, the sooner treatment can begin, and the better the outlook for the patient. Making the diagnosis will also have a big impact on the patient's family, in several ways. It will have a big emotional impact, perhaps overwhelming at first. For some families, it will actually be a relief or a vindication, since they might have known for a long time that *something* was wrong, yet they had not been able to discover what. (In Chapter 12, *The Family*, there is more discussion of the emotional impact of CF on patients and families.) It will certainly influence the family's time, finances, insurance, perhaps even employment (since having good insurance will become a very important part of job considerations).

For these and many other reasons, making the correct diagnosis, and making it early, are extremely important. Yet many patients are seen in CF centers who have received an incorrect diagnosis of CF. Some have had negative test results, and their families were told they did not have CF (or CF was never mentioned), when they really *did* have CF; while others had positive test results, and they were told they had CF, when they really *did not* have it.

In this chapter, I'll discuss the various ways of making the diagnosis of CF, including sweat tests, newborn screening, and DNA analysis (sometimes called genetic testing). I won't discuss prenatal testing and carrier testing, since these are covered in Chapter 11, *Genetics.*

Before a CF test can be done, someone has to think about ordering one, so I'll begin with a brief consideration of who should be tested.

WHO SHOULD BE TESTED?

Not everyone needs to be tested for CF. Anyone with any of the signs or symptoms that are part of CF should be tested for it. The most important of these signs and symptoms are listed in Table 2.1, and are discussed throughout the book.

One other situation where testing is done is in hospitals (and some entire states) that have included CF in their newborn screening programs.

TABLE 2.1. *Reasons to Test for CF*

Family History of CF
(*Every* sibling of a CF patient should be tested; cousins should be tested if there are signs, symptoms, or worry of CF)

Respiratory System
Upper Respiratory System
Nasal polyps
Sinus disease with x-rays showing "pansinusitis" (all the sinuses abnormal)

Lower Respiratory System
Recurrent or severe bronchiolitis
Severe or nontypical "asthma"
Frequent productive cough
Persistent cough, especially with hard coughing spells
Coughing up blood
Recurrent pneumonia
Throat or sputum culture positive for *Pseudomonas*
Collapsed lung or partially collapsed lung

Gastrointestinal System
Meconium ileus (bowel obstruction in the newborn)
Frequent bulky, loose, oily, foul-smelling stools that float in the toilet
Failure to gain weight, especially with a big appetite
Rectal prolapse (see Figure 4.2)
Liver disease
Pancreatitis (inflammation of pancreas)

Miscellaneous
Tastes salty when kissed
Finger clubbing (see Figure 3.10)
Male infertility

WHAT CONFIRMS A DIAGNOSIS OF CYSTIC FIBROSIS?

To make the diagnosis of CF, most experts require a positive sweat test (discussed below) from a reliable, experienced laboratory, PLUS one or more of the following: (1) pulmonary symptoms, (2) gastrointestinal symptoms, (3) family history of CF.

In some cases, genetic testing that shows two abnormal CF genes can substitute for any of the items on the list. In most cases, CF experts will be willing to say that someone has CF if the person has two abnormal CF genes.

In the case of newborn screening, most experts will make the diagnosis on the basis of a "positive" newborn screen and a "positive" sweat test, or a "positive" newborn screen and genetic testing positive for two abnormal CF genes.

Let's now consider the different tests.

Sweat Tests

The sweat test has been the "gold standard" for diagnosing CF for over 40 years, and *when it is done in an experienced, reliable laboratory, the sweat test is still the best test for CF.* It is a superb test. It is painless, relatively inexpensive, and gives definitive answers within a few hours. There are almost no false positives (people who test positive for CF, but don't really have it) or false negatives (people whose tests say they don't have CF, but really do have it). Furthermore, in almost every case, the result of the test is positive or negative: there are almost no people who have test results in an "in-between" range (or "gray zone" or "intermediate range"). The test can be performed—with accurate results—on patients of any age. Many physicians mistakenly believe that sweat tests are not reliable in young infants. Some young babies may not make enough sweat for the laboratory to analyze, but most will produce enough. If a baby doesn't produce enough sweat on a sweat test, it should be repeated, either the same day or, at most, a week later.

Details of how the sweat test is performed and interpreted can be found in Chapter 5, *Other Systems*. Sweat is collected from the arm or leg and then is analyzed for its salt (sodium chloride) content. To do this the laboratory measures the concentration of chloride (and/or sodium). A positive test is one where the concentration of chloride (or sodium) is 60 milliequivalents per liter (mEq/l) or higher. Almost everyone with CF has values between 60 and 110 mEq/l. A negative test is one where the concentration of chloride (or sodium) is 40 mEq/l or lower. Very few people have values between 40 and 60 mEq/l. (Later in the chapter, we'll talk about what to do with these few difficult cases.) There are very few cases of positive sweat tests caused by rare diseases other than CF. These diseases are readily distinguished from CF. Lists of these diseases can be found in any pediatric textbook.

Once a test result is positive, it is always positive. Sweat test values do not change from positive to negative or negative to positive as a patient grows older. And sweat test values do not vary when the patients have colds or other temporary illnesses. There is no point in saying, "it was positive now, but the baby was sick; let's repeat it when she feels better."

I need to stress again the importance of the experience of the laboratory doing the tests. Most CF centers find that CF has been misdiagnosed in about half of all the patients they see who have been tested by inexperienced laboratory personnel. The mistakes happen in both directions: people who don't have CF are told they do, and vice versa. Sweat test laboratories associated with an approved CF center have passed accreditation by the national CF Foundation, and can be trusted. Many other laboratories are also good, but it's harder to know about those that are not in CF centers.

Newborn Screening

Since early diagnosis is so helpful to the long-term health of patients with CF, some states have mandated newborn screening. In states where this screening is not required by state law, some hospitals have taken it upon themselves to offer newborn CF screening as a service to their obstetric patients.

The test used for newborn screening is called the *IRT*. Those initials stand for *immunoreactive trypsinogen*, and the test is discussed in Chapter 4, *The Gastrointestinal Tract*. For our purposes here, it will suffice to say that the test is done on a spot of blood that is taken from the baby's heel within the first days of life. Almost every baby with CF has a high level of IRT. In a couple of weeks, when the laboratory discovers an elevated IRT, they notify the baby's doctor, who calls the family to bring the baby for a repeat test. The repeat test is needed, because many, many babies (not just those with CF) have high IRT levels on the first test. By the time the test is repeated, the IRT levels for most babies *without CF* will have fallen to normal, while most babies *with CF* will still have high IRT levels. If the level is still high on the second test, then sweat testing is needed. In some cases genetic testing is done on the blood spot, and that can help confirm the diagnosis (more about this in the next section).

This newborn screen has its good and its bad features: *good* is that very few babies with CF are missed by this test; *bad* is that *lots* of babies who don't have CF have to come back for the second test, and some who don't have CF have to get a sweat test. This means that lots of families have days or weeks of worrying that their little ones have CF, when it will turn out that they don't. Most families and CF experts now think that the *good* of getting babies diagnosed and started on treatment early outweighs the *bad* of some temporary worry for the families whose babies end up getting a clean bill of health.

Gene Testing

Gene testing is discussed further in Chapter 11, *Genetics*.

We all have two CF genes, one from our mother and one from our father, that determine whether or not we have CF. Both of these genes must be abnormal (have *mutations*) for us to end up with CF. If one is abnormal, we are said to be a "carrier," meaning we don't have the disease, but we *carry* the gene, and can pass it along to our children. (Then, if we do pass the abnormal CF gene on to our children, whether our children get CF depends on whether they also get an abnormal CF gene from our spouse.)

There are more than 500 different types of abnormal CF genes that can cause CF! A few of these are fairly common, and are found in different combinations in most CF patients; many of the CF gene mutations are very uncommon. There are even some that occur in only one family. There are patients with CF whose abnormal gene has not yet been discovered. This means that we can analyze blood or other tissue and see if people have abnormal CF genes of a type that has already been described. Most CF patients have two fairly common abnormal CF genes that would be identifiable on genetic testing. But some patients have abnormal CF genes that the genetic testing won't find, because they are rare, and have not yet been identified.

If we wonder about the diagnosis of CF, and we do genetic testing, finding two known abnormal CF genes pretty much tells us the person has CF. But finding *one* or *no* known abnormal CF gene does not give a definite answer. It may say the chances are *a little better* that the person doesn't have CF, since *most* people with CF have two of the abnormal genes we've been looking for, but it doesn't tell us for sure.

Some newborn screening programs automatically test all blood spots for the most common abnormal CF gene (called ΔF508, pronounced delta-F 508). Finding two of this particular abnormal CF gene (as happens in about 50% of people with CF in North America) pretty much confirms the diagnosis.

There are some unusual situations where genetic testing might be done instead of sweat testing. These situations might include a patient who does not make enough sweat for analysis, or who lives far removed from a reliable sweat testing laboratory. In these cases, it would probably make sense to send a blood sample (or a simple painless Q-tip rubbed on your inner cheek) for genetic analysis. If the test comes back with two abnormal CF genes identified, the diagnosis is almost certain. If the test comes back with one or no abnormal CF genes found, you won't know whether there's CF or not, and you'll have to go to a good sweat testing laboratory after all, but nothing's been lost.

Other Testing: "Nasal PD"

A very few specialized laboratories can perform a test called a "nasal PD." This test is discussed a little more in Chapter 1, *The Basic Defect*. The test measures the electrical charge (also called the *potential d*ifference) inside someone's nose. People with CF have a large electric charge, while people without CF have much lower values. This test is probably even better than the sweat test in separating those with CF from those without. The problem with it is that it is very difficult to do correctly, and *very* few centers are set up to do this testing.

What About the Unusual Cases?

In some cases, it might be difficult or impossible to make the diagnosis in the usual way. Examples might be a patient who doesn't make enough sweat to analyze or someone whose sweat test results are in the "gray zone"—neither clearly positive nor clearly negative—and genetic testing has been inconclusive. We'll assume that nasal PD testing is not available. In these cases, the physician has to consider the whole picture: what are the patient's lungs like? What germs grow on throat cultures? Does he or she have abnormal sinuses on x-rays? Are the stools abnormal? Is there finger clubbing? (All these signs and symptoms are discussed in Chapter 3, *The Respiratory System,* and Chapter 4, *The Gastrointestinal Tract.)* Occasionally, the physician and family will decide that the wisest course of action is (1) to accept the fact that for the time being a definite diagnosis cannot be made, and (2) to decide to treat the child *as if he or she has CF*. This makes sense because the treatments are not harmful for someone who *does not have CF,* but *not* getting the treatments could be very harmful for someone who *does have CF.*

3

The Respiratory System

THE BASICS

1. The lungs are the most important part of the body in people with CF, and they cause most of the sickness, and more than 95% of the deaths from CF.
2. Thick mucus blocks the bronchial tubes in people with CF, causing infection and inflammation.
3. The lung problem is progressive, meaning it keeps getting worse as time goes by.
4. With very good treatment, the progression of the lung disease can be slowed dramatically, and the lungs can be kept relatively healthy for long periods of time.
5. Regular treatment to keep the airways clear of mucus and infection is extremely important.
6. New or increased cough is usually the first sign of worsened infection and inflammation. If cough increases, you should call your CF doctor for treatment.

The respiratory system is the most important organ system for patients with cystic fibrosis (CF). Problems with this system account for over 95% of the sickness from CF, and also for more than 95% of the deaths from this disease. In the 60 years since CF was first recognized, treatment of lung disease has improved considerably, resulting in the tremendous improvement in longevity and quality of life that CF patients can now expect.

The three sections of this chapter are devoted to (1) a discussion of the normal anatomy and functioning of the respiratory system, (2) an explanation of how CF changes the functioning of this system, and (3) a review of the treatments that are aimed at preventing, correcting, or minimizing the changes that CF brings about in the respiratory system.

ANATOMY AND FUNCTION OF THE RESPIRATORY SYSTEM

All tissues in the body, especially the brain and exercising muscles, need oxygen to function. It is the task of the respiratory system to bring in oxygen from the air that surrounds us and transfer it to the bloodstream. Once oxygen is in the bloodstream, the cardiovascular system (heart and blood vessels) delivers it to all the parts of the body that need it. It is a further responsibility of the lungs to dispose of excess carbon dioxide, which builds up in the process of normal metabolism. These tasks are essential to life, since all body tissues need oxygen to survive, and if too much carbon dioxide builds up in the bloodstream and brain, it can put someone so deeply to sleep that he or she will not breathe.

The Airways

The actual transfer of oxygen from the air we breathe to the bloodstream (and carbon dioxide from the blood to the air we exhale) takes place deep in the lungs, in the **alveoli** (air sacs), which are located at the end of a long series of tubes. (One air sac is an *alveolus*, two or more are *alveoli*.) At the beginning of these air-carrying tubes, or "airways," are the nose and mouth, followed by the throat, then the larynx (or "voice box," another name given to this area, which includes the vocal cords), and the trachea (also called the "windpipe"). As the trachea enters the chest, it divides into two branches, and each branch leads into a lung. These branches are referred to as the **bronchial tubes**, or simply, **bronchi** (Figure 3.1). Each bronchus reaches into its lung where it divides again, and yet again, forming a network of bronchi that extend into the various **lobes**, or sections, of the lung, and the *segments* of each lobe, the **subsegments** of each segment, etc. Each time the bronchi branch, they become smaller, and are thus able to distribute air to the smallest and farthest reaches of the lungs. [The word "branch" is frequently used to describe the bronchial system, for it does look very treelike. Pulmonary physicians (lung specialists) and anatomists often adapt words used in forestry to describe this bronchial "tree."]

The bronchi divide, or branch, approximately 20 times before they reach the alveoli. It is in these air sacs that oxygen finally leaves the inhaled air and enters the bloodstream. Throughout most of this branching network, the bronchial tubes are referred to as "bronchi," or, for the smaller ones, "small bronchi." Toward the end of this network, however, the bronchi become quite small and are referred to as **bronchioles**. Bronchioles are the last segment of tubes through which air passes before it reaches the alveoli.

The difference between bronchi and bronchioles, aside from their size, is that bronchi have **cartilage** in their walls and bronchioles don't. Both bronchi and bronchioles need something to stiffen their walls so that they maintain their shape and, particularly, so that they stay open. In healthy lungs, there is a tendency for the bronchi and bronchioles to enlarge slightly as the chest expands with each

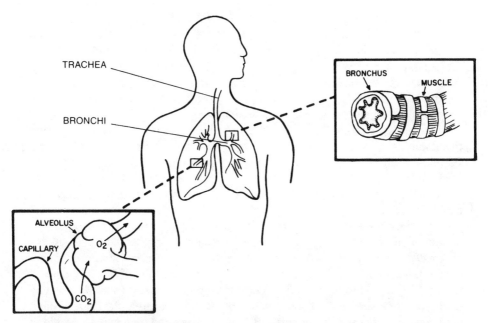

Figure 3.1. The lungs, including bronchi and alveoli. Note the muscles in the bronchial wall. Oxygen enters the bloodstream by passing from the inhaled air through the wall of the alveoli and into the blood cells in the capillaries.

breath *inhaled,* and to narrow with each breath *exhaled.* If breathing is particularly strenuous, or if the support of the bronchial walls is not very strong, the bronchi and bronchioles can collapse during exhalation, making it difficult for the proper amount of air to leave the lungs.

In addition to cartilage, other tissues help support the bronchi. One of the most important is **muscle:** the bronchi and bronchioles have bands of muscle running around their walls. If a dangerous substance threatens to enter the lungs (such as a chemical with toxic fumes), these muscles can contract, squeezing down and making the bronchial opening much smaller than normal. With the bronchial passage blocked in this way, it is difficult for anything to get deeply into the bronchial tree. This action protects the lungs only if it happens briefly, and only if it happens when there is a true danger. However, this "protective" mechanism can actually be harmful if the bronchial muscles squeeze down at inappropriate times.

Gas Transfer and Delivery

The transfer of oxygen from the inhaled air to the bloodstream takes place at the alveoli. Running past each alveolus is a tiny blood vessel called a **pulmonary capillary**. The walls of the alveoli and the capillaries are membranes, so thin that oxygen and carbon dioxide can pass directly through them. It is through these walls that oxygen passes from the alveoli to the bloodstream, and that carbon dioxide passes from the bloodstream to the alveoli. There are 20 million of these tiny air sacs in a newborn infant's lungs, and 300 million in an adult. The enormous extent of these figures can be better grasped by imagining that, if you were to lay out the working surfaces between the alveoli and capillaries side by side, they would span an area the size of a tennis court.

After the oxygen has been supplied to the blood, the task remains of getting the blood to the tissues that need the oxygen (the brain, exercising muscles, etc.). Fortunately, there is an excellent system that accomplishes the task of pumping the blood to where it is needed. The pump, of course, is the heart.

Actually, the heart is a muscular double pump. The right side of the heart pumps blood through the lungs, where the blood becomes oxygenated through the process just described (and where the carbon dioxide is dumped out of the blood). After the **hemoglobin** molecules, which are the oxygen-carrying elements in the blood, are loaded with as much oxygen as possible (that is, they are fully *saturated* with oxygen), the blood flows back to the heart. It then enters the left side of the heart, where it is pumped to the rest of the body. Oxygen is removed from the blood by the tissues that need it. The deoxygenated blood then returns to the heart through the veins, and enters the right side of the heart. The heart then pumps the blood back to the lungs, where it is loaded with oxygen once again. At rest, an adult's heart will pump 4 to 5 liters of blood per minute (1 liter is approximately equal to a quart). During heavy exercise, that amount can increase to 25 or even to 30 liters per minute.

The condition can arise in which the oxygen levels are too low and the carbon dioxide levels are too high. This is called **respiratory failure,** and can result from several circumstances. If someone with normal lungs is paralyzed in a car accident, for example, the breathing muscles (see the section *The Respiratory Muscles* below) could also become paralyzed and thus be unable to accomplish the work of breathing. Brain injury or brain disease, or drug overdoses, may also result in respiratory failure by damaging the brain's ability to direct the muscles to move the chest, in which case breathing will not occur. Serious lung disease can also cause respiratory failure if oxygen cannot be brought into, or carbon dioxide removed from, the bloodstream.

Control of Breathing

Among the many amazing things our body can do without our awareness is regulating how much we breathe. The main job of the lungs is to bring in the right amount of oxygen and eliminate the right amount of carbon dioxide that has been produced. This is a balancing act that is controlled with astounding precision.

In general, the more we breathe, the more oxygen we bring into the body, and the more carbon dioxide we breathe out. When we exercise, our muscles use as much as 10 to 20 times as much oxygen as when we're resting, and even more carbon dioxide is formed, which needs to be eliminated. During strenuous exercise, we breathe 5 to 10 times as much air as when we're resting, and our heart pumps 5 or 6 times as much blood each minute, yet all the while the levels of oxygen and carbon dioxide in the bloodstream remain almost exactly the same! You'd think that a little extra oxygen would come in, or not quite enough, or that a bit too much carbon dioxide would be breathed out, or not quite enough, but this doesn't happen. In healthy people as well as in most people with lung disease (including those with CF), the blood levels of oxygen and carbon dioxide remain steady, regardless of what the person is doing.

This tight control is achieved by the brain's response to the two gases that the lungs manage—oxygen and carbon dioxide. Carbon dioxide is usually the more important regulator. If the breathing slows down (as it does in all of us now and then), less carbon dioxide will be breathed out and it will begin to build up in the body. As soon as this happens, the brain senses the buildup and sends the signal to the breathing muscles to breathe more, until the carbon dioxide level is back down to normal. The opposite occurs also: if the carbon dioxide level gets too low, the brain sends out the signal to slow down the breathing. Most of the time this is very fine tuning, requiring such small changes in breathing effort that we are unaware of the adjustments that are being made.

If the lungs are severely affected by disease and are not able to eliminate carbon dioxide effectively, the carbon dioxide level will build up and the brain will "instruct" the body to increase the rate and depth of breathing. After a while, however, the brain acts as though it has "gotten tired" of the message that the carbon dioxide level is too high, and it ignores the message. In its place, the brain will respond to another signal that regulates breathing—the oxygen level. It notices that the oxygen level is too low, and continues sending the message to the breathing muscles to increase breathing more. It is in this way that severe lung disease (from whatever cause) may alter the way the brain controls breathing patterns. Various drugs may also affect breathing patterns, either by making us breathe more, or by making us less sensitive to breathing commands, and therefore breathe less.

The Respiratory Muscles

Once the message to breathe is sent, it must be carried out. The work of breathing is done by the **respiratory** (or **ventilatory**) **muscles**. The most important ventilatory muscle is the **diaphragm,** which separates the inside of the chest from the abdomen. Since the chest wall (ribs, chest muscles, skin, etc.) is relatively firm, when the diaphragm contracts and moves downward, it leaves more space inside the chest for the lungs to expand. This action creates a vacuum inside the chest, and air rushes into the trachea and bronchi (through the nose and/or mouth) and fills that extra space. When it is time to breathe out, most of the force comes as the lungs and chest wall just naturally spring back into their usual resting size. With hard breathing, exhalation gets a boost from the expiratory muscles, which include the abdominal muscles, the muscles between the ribs, and some muscles in the neck. During very hard breathing, inhalation gets extra help, too (even the tiny muscles that widen the nostrils contribute to inhalation). All of these muscles are called the **accessory muscles** of respiration, since they are helpful, but are not absolutely necessary, for normal quiet breathing. It is possible to see these muscles at work during hard breathing: when the muscles between the ribs (the **intercostal muscles**) are used, the skin seems to sink in between the ribs (this is called *retracting*), and when the neck or abdominal muscles are used, they stick out prominently. If the nose muscles are pitching in, you can see the nostrils widening, a sign called "nasal flaring," or simply "flaring."

Lung Defenses

The air we breathe has an abundance of potentially harmful elements in it (in addition to the good), such as cigarette smoke, pollution, dust, and bacteria and viruses and other germs. And yet, in most people, the lungs stay fairly clean, remaining unclogged by these substances and free from infection. This is the result of a very efficient lung protection system at work.

The Nose and Mouth

The defense of the lungs begins in the nose and mouth. Many of the largest particles breathed in get trapped here, especially in the hairs of the nose.

However, some of the smaller particles do make it past the air conditioning and filtering system of the nose and mouth, and reach the trachea or bronchi. When they reach the bronchi, they get stuck in the mucus that lines the airways. Fortunately, the lung defenses are very active in these lower airways, and can remove small particles through coughing, and the action of the **mucociliary escalator**.

Cough

A cough is an explosive release of air from the lungs. It is something we can do voluntarily, but it can also happen without our conscious control. The steps to producing a cough begin with the stimulation of nerves in the nose, throat, trachea, bronchi, or diaphragm. Some of these nerves can be triggered by pressure, others by noxious chemicals, and others by being touched by inhaled particles. Once the cough signal is sent out, there is a deep breath in, followed by a sudden forcible attempt to breathe out at a time when the upper portion of the airway (around the vocal cords) is tightly shut. Since air cannot get out through this closed door, pressure builds up within the lung. Then, after about one-fifth second, the upper airway suddenly opens and the air bursts out, at a speed reaching 600 miles per hour! This burst of air is very effective in carrying mucus (with its trapped particles of dirt or bacteria) to at least as far as the back of the throat, where it can be spit out or swallowed into the stomach. This tremendous air force is only effective in the largest bronchi and trachea, for the air moves much more slowly in the smaller bronchi farther out in the lungs. Coughing is therefore not an effective method for mucus clearance in the smaller bronchi, and another action is used, which involves the mucociliary escalator.

The Mucociliary Escalator

Many of the cells lining the trachea and bronchi have tiny hairlike projections, called **cilia**. A thin layer of fluid bathes these cilia, and reaches partway up their length, but not to their tips (Figure 3.2). Resting atop the cilia—and atop the fluid layer—is a blanket of mucus, which has been produced by special glands within the bronchi and bronchioles. This layer of mucus protects the airways by trapping substances that might be harmful to the lungs, and removing them through the action of the cilia. The cilia beat approximately 1,200 times per minute in a coordinated action that sweeps the mucus (and everything trapped in the mucus) toward the largest bronchi. When the mucus reaches the large central bronchi, it is carried up the trachea in a movement that is similar to that of an escalator. Hence this system is sometimes referred to as the mucociliary escalator. When the mucus reaches the top of the trachea (the back of the throat) it is swallowed, usually without our being aware of it. This amazing escalator clears about 2 teaspoons of mucus each day. Cigarette smokers and others with extra mucus are often aware of the mucus that has been carried to the back of the throat. If there is an espe-

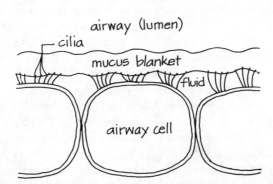

Figure 3.2. Cilia project into the airway from atop airway cells. The cilia are bathed in airway fluid almost—but not quite—to their tips. Above the fluid, and just at the tips of the cilia, is a blanket of mucus and trapped inhaled particles.

cially large amount, or if it is particularly thick, it may be coughed up once it gets to the large central bronchi. Once it is coughed up, it can be spit out, or it can be swallowed down into the stomach, sending it on its way through the digestive tract, where it will do no harm. The functioning of this wonderful airway-cleaning escalator depends in part on the composition of the mucus, in part on the composition of the fluid layer, and in part on other factors. If the mucus is too thick and sticky, it may be hard for the delicate cilia to move. If the fluid layer is too deep, the tips of the cilia may not reach the mucus, which is now floating above them. If the cilia don't reach the mucus, they can't grip the mucus blanket to move it. On the other hand, if the fluid layer is too shallow, the cilia may not have enough support to be effective. As you've seen in Chapter 1, *The Basic Defect*, the composition of the fluid lining the airway is controlled in part by the protein (CFTR) made under the direction of the CF gene. This protein helps regulate both *secretion* of fluid and salt from the airway cells into the airway, and *absorption* of fluid and salt from the airway back into the cells. Abnormal CF genes—as everyone with CF has—make for defects in this CFTR protein, which in turn makes for abnormal secretion and absorption of salt and water by these cells, almost certainly leading to abnormal fluid, and very likely interfering with the functioning of the mucociliary escalator.

Other Protection Against Lung Infection

It is thought, but not yet proven, that airway cells may be able to sense when they are touched by inhaled particles (including bacteria). The theory goes that when they sense an "invader," they suddenly secrete a burst of fluid that washes it away. If this doesn't happen (for example, if there is a defect in the ability of the cells to secrete fluid—as seems to be true of CF airway cells), then bacteria may not be removed immediately, or not completely, by the mucociliary route. When this happens, further steps are taken to protect the lungs. One such step is the delivery of **white blood cells** to the area where there are foreign substances and bacteria. These blood cells work in two ways: they can completely surround the bacteria and other particles, capturing them within the blood cells. Then, when the blood cell is removed from the lung, the bacteria or other particles are removed also. They can also release chemicals that attack and destroy the bacteria. These are potent chemicals, some of which degrade structural proteins of the bacteria, and are called *proteases* (the *-ase* ending means *breaks down. . .*). A particular one of these proteases is called *elastase,* and its main target is *elastin,* an important structural protein. It is unfortunate but true that these proteases can also attack proteins that make up airway cells—not just bacterial protein. The lungs have a finely tuned system that produces antiproteases to keep the proteases in check and to prevent degradation of proteins that are important for the structure of the airways.

There are certain proteins in the blood that also protect the lungs against infection. These are the **immunoglobulins** (gamma-globulin is one such protein). Immunoglobulins are part of a system that recognizes materials that are foreign invaders in all parts of the body, and produces antibodies that attack the foreign substances.

Another factor that influences infection in the airways is how tightly bacteria stick to airway cells. The stickiness of these cells seems to be related in part to the electrical charge on the surface of the cells.

THE RESPIRATORY TRACT IN CYSTIC FIBROSIS

The Upper Respiratory Tract

There are two major differences between the normal upper respiratory tract and that in people with CF. The first difference is in the condition of the **sinuses**, and has relatively little to do with the person's health or day-to-day comfort. The second difference is the presence of **nasal polyps**, which affects only about 20% of people with CF.

The Sinuses

The sinuses of people with CF almost always look abnormal on x-rays. In the x-rays, the sinuses appear as though they are badly diseased, indicating a condition called **pansinusitis** (*-itis* meaning "inflamed," *pan-* meaning "all"; thus, "all the sinuses are inflamed"). It is useful to understand the meaning of the appearance of pansinusitis on sinus x-rays for several reasons. First, because it is very unusual to find in children, except in children with CF, the appearance of pansinusitis on the sinus x-rays may help make the diagnosis of CF. Second, the appearance of the x-ray will suggest that problems exist such as sinus headaches. However, in children with CF, this is rarely the case. There may be some sinus infection, but this, too, is relatively uncommon. (Sinus infections are discussed in more detail below: *Infections of the Upper Respiratory Tract.*)

At some point a child may have skull x-rays taken, and if the child has CF, the x-rays will most likely show abnormal sinuses. It is important for parents to know that the appearance of sinus abnormality is primarily a problem with the x-ray, that (in the absence of symptoms) it is not something that bothers the child, and that nothing needs to be done about it.

Typically, treatment is not needed for the sinuses in people with CF. Some patients—particularly adults—with CF may have sinus infections that actually cause discomfort. In these cases, antibiotics might be helpful, but this is relatively uncommon. In rare cases, CF patients with repeated or persistent sinus problems may benefit from surgery to help the sinuses drain better. However, there is little evidence that sinus surgery is of any use to the majority of patients with CF. If a specialist who is not very experienced with CF suggests surgery for the sinuses, a second opinion should be sought.

The Nose

About 20% of CF patients at one time or another will have **nasal polyps**. Polyps are growths of extra tissue that form in various parts of the body. The formation of polyps in the nose occurs much more commonly in CF patients than in people who don't have CF. In fact, this can be another diagnostic clue: if a child has a nasal polyp, this is a strong indication that she or he has CF. Nasal polyps are also found in people who don't have CF, especially in those who have many allergies. In children, however, it is very uncommon to find nasal polyps, except in those with CF.

Generally, having a nasal polyp is not a major problem. It is *never* life-threatening, and it *never* becomes cancerous the way other polyps can in people without CF. What it may do is block up one side of the nose. When there is one polyp, there are often others, and both sides of the nose may become blocked. Rarely, they can become so large that they can protrude from the nostril. In either of these cases (when the polyp blocks the nose or sticks out of the nostril), it is a nuisance but not a threat to the person's health. Since it is usually a significant nuisance at this point, it is advisable to have the polyps removed. One other instance in which it is wise to remove polyps is when, after some time, the bridge of the nose grows wider in response to the increasing size of the polyps inside the nose.

It is not yet known why 20% of CF patients do get polyps, why most people without CF don't get polyps, or why some CF patients get a polyp once, while others get them often.

Treatment of Nasal Polyps

Polyps are strange growths that have a mysterious course of development. They frequently get larger or smaller without treatment, making it difficult to tell if medications are effective. If a polyp gets smaller after medication, one can't be sure that it wouldn't have gotten smaller on its own. Nonetheless, some medications *may* help shrink polyps. These medications are steroid sprays, such as beclomethasone (see Appendix B: *Medications*).

If the medicines don't work, and if the polyp is completely blocking one or both nostrils, or protruding from the nostril, or is widening the outside of the nasal bridge, then surgery to remove the polyp or polyps (*polypectomy*) is advisable. This surgery is best done by an ear, nose, and throat surgeon, in the hospital, and under general anesthesia. Simple polypectomy (just removing the polyps the surgeon sees in the nose) or a more extensive procedure called *FESS* (*functional endoscopic sinus surgery*) can be done. With the FESS, the surgeon uses an *endoscope* [a tube for looking (*-scope*) into (*endo*) things] to enable her to see further into the sinuses, to get at the roots of some of the polyps. It is not clear yet if the more extensive procedure actually gives better results. In most cases, a very short (overnight) hospital stay is all that is needed for either procedure. After the surgery, the nose is packed with gauze for several hours to make sure the bleeding has stopped, and once the gauze is removed, the patient can go home. In older patients, the simple polypectomy procedure may even be done in the surgeon's office, with local anesthetic. Most often, CF physicians, surgeons, patients, and families feel more comfortable if the surgery is done in the hospital, while the patient is asleep under a general anesthetic.

Surgery is very effective in removing the polyps, and once they are gone, they may never reappear. In some people, though, they may come back, once, twice, or many times.

The Lower Respiratory Tract (The Lungs)

More than any other factor, the lungs determine the health and life span of the large majority of patients with CF. In little more than one generation, the greatly improved treatment of the lungs has transformed the outlook for CF infants from one consisting of a few difficult months to one entailing many bright years. Infants with CF are born with lungs that appear normal, but, at varying times after birth, they begin to develop problems. In some, these problems may become noticeable within the first weeks, whereas in others, it may take years or even decades before any problems become apparent. Without treatment, lung problems will eventually appear in everyone with CF and the problems will progress. With treatment, this progression can be slowed, in some, almost to a halt.

The problems in the lungs can almost certainly be blamed on the abnormal movement of salt and fluid through the airway cell membranes. This abnormal traffic of salt and fluid, and the abnormal electric charge associated with it (see Chapter 1, *The Basic Defect*) are caused by the abnormal CFTR protein whose production was dictated by the 2 abnormal CF genes that everyone with CF has. The salt and fluid and electrical abnormalities lead to inflammation and infection and mucus clogging the smallest airways (the bronchioles). Infection and inflammation of those bronchioles is called *bronchiolitis*. The inflammation then readily spreads to the larger airways, the bronchi (*bronchitis*). If the mucus is too thick to be cleared by the normal mechanisms, such as the mucociliary escalator, it is very easy for germs (viruses and bacteria) to take hold, making it hard for the lungs and body defenses to combat them.

The more inflammation there is within the bronchi and bronchioles, the more swelling there is (Figure 3.3), and the narrower the opening becomes to these airways; or, said another way, the greater the bronchial (and bronchiolar) obstruction. With increasing obstruction it becomes more difficult for air to move in and out, which forces the respiratory muscles to work harder. Also, when the airways become obstructed, it is difficult to clear them of mucus. Other mucus-clearing mechanisms, especially cough, are then used more frequently to force the mucus up and out of the bronchioles and bronchi. *Increased cough is often the first sign that the bronchial infection and inflammation are getting out of control.*

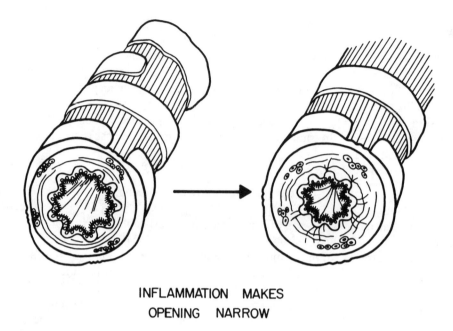

INFLAMMATION   MAKES
OPENING   NARROW

Figure 3.3. Inflammation within the bronchi makes the bronchial opening ("lumen") smaller.

If the bronchial and bronchiolar infection and inflammation remain out of control for too long, they can damage the bronchioles and bronchi. Bacteria can cause direct damage to the bronchial walls; and the body's response to the bacteria can cause even more damage: you've seen above (*Other Protection Against Lung Infection*) that white blood cells are sent to kill bacteria. These white blood cells release different chemicals that cause inflammation to attack and destroy the bacteria. Unfortunately, these chemicals (sometimes called *mediators of inflammation*, including proteases like elastase—see above) cannot distinguish between bacteria and airway tissue, and they can also damage the cells lining the airways. In recent years, we've come to understand that this damage from inflammation from our own white blood cells is just as harmful as—or even more harmful than—the harm from the bacteria (which also release chemicals that cause inflammation). If the damage to the airways continues, it can weaken their walls so that they become floppy, and the airways enlarge (**dilate**). The word-ending for abnormal dilatation or distention is *-ectasis*, and these changes in the airways are referred to as *bronchiolectasis* and *bronchiectasis*. If the lung damage progresses, it can lead to permanent changes such as infected cysts and scar tissue (*fibrosis*), which are indicated by the name of this disease.

The progression of lung damage is most often very slow and subtle, but it can be relentless. This is why the lung disease of CF is often referred to as "progressive"—if left to its own (and even in the majority of cases with treatment), it gets worse and worse. If this progression of infection, inflammation, and lung destruction continues uninterrupted for too long, it will eventually reach a point where there is no longer enough healthy lung to bring oxygen into the body or to eliminate carbon dioxide.

As a particular episode of increased infection and inflammation develops, or as the lung disease increases over the years, the following progression occurs: first, there is more cough. Someone who usually doesn't cough at all may develop a mild cough for a few minutes in the morning, or someone who coughed only in the morning may now cough during the day or through the night. Morning is a common time for people with CF to cough, since they have been in one position for many hours, making it easier for the lung mucus to stay down in the lungs. During the day, when people are active and breathing harder, mucus is more easily shaken loose and sent on its way out of the lungs.

Along with increased cough (and part of its cause) there is often an increase in lung mucus production and an increase in *sputum* (mucus that is coughed up and spit out of the lungs): the patient is more likely to feel "crud" in the lungs that feels like it needs to come up. The airways now contain mucus made by the bronchial glands and increasingly large amounts of other material. This other material includes DNA (genetic material contained in all cells) that has been released from white blood cells (*neutrophils*) that have died fighting the bronchial infection. There is also a stringy substance called *actin*. The neutrophil DNA and the actin account for a lot of the thickness of CF sputum. There are also numerous dead bacteria and old airway cells that contribute to the thickness and stickiness of CF airway secretions.

With the progression of the lung disease patients often have decreased exercise tolerance, with quicker tiring and even some shortness of breath (difficulty breathing).

As the particular episode of infection and inflammation subsides—on its own or with treatment—the symptoms also subside, either fully or partly, depending on whether any new lung damage has been caused. The goal of treatment is to get back to the *baseline* (the condition prior to the onset of the problem) after each episode of worsening (*exacerbation*) of lung infection. This is often, but not always, possible.

Asthma

Asthma affects people with or without CF, and is a condition in which the muscles that surround the bronchi squeeze down readily. This ability of the muscles to tighten and make the opening of the bronchi smaller is basically a protective mechanism (see above, *The Airways*), since it can prevent dangerous substances that have been breathed in (*aspirated*) from getting deep into the lungs. But if bronchial wall muscles go into spasm (*bronchospasm*) when there isn't a real threat to the lungs, the end result is that this "protective" mechanism does more harm than good. The bronchi become partly squeezed shut, making it difficult to move mucus out and to breathe air in and out. The airways also become inflamed in people with asthma. When the bronchi are narrowed from bronchospasm and inflammation, there is often a characteristic whistling sound to the breathing. This sound is called *wheezing*, and is heard especially when someone breathes out.

Asthma episodes can be related to allergies, infections, exercise, cold air or to breathing irritating substances such as cigarette smoke or air pollution. In some babies, a condition known as *gastroesophageal reflux* ("GE reflux," simply "reflux," or "GER") can also cause bronchospasm (see Chapter 4, *The Gastrointestinal Tract*). Between 10% and 40% of patients with CF also have asthma.

Infections of the Respiratory Tract

This subject can be confusing since there are many different kinds of respiratory infections (which may or may not present serious problems for people with CF), and it is not always clear which are the potentially dangerous ones and which are merely a nuisance.

Infections of the Upper Respiratory Tract

Sinusitis

Sinusitis is an inflammation of the sinuses, usually caused by infection. This is not often a problem for children with CF, even though sinus x-rays always look as though there is an active sinus infection. Many people attribute their cough (or their child's cough) to sinus problems ("mucus drips down my throat and makes me cough"), and this may be, but much more of the cough in people with CF is caused by lung (bronchial) infection. Some patients—mostly adults—do have bothersome sinus problems, and these can usually be controlled with antibiotics. In a very few patients, sinus surgery may be able to allow the sinuses to drain better and prevent recurrent sinus infections.

Colds

Colds are often referred to as "URI's," for *upper respiratory infections.* Everyone gets colds and has experienced first hand what they are: They are infections of the nose and throat that may produce mucus in the nose, sneezing, and a sore throat. The person with a cold feels generally bad. There may or may not be a fever. Fairly often there is some cough, and scientists don't agree about the cause of the cough. Some say the cough means that there is inflammation in the trachea and bronchi, as well as in the nose and throat, while others say that it results from nose (or sinus) mucus dripping down the back of the throat and tickling the nerves that activate the cough.

Colds are caused by viruses. The main source of cold viruses is other people. People catch colds from other people, who have the cold viruses in their noses and throats. The closer the contact with the infected secretions, the easier it is to catch cold. Sneezing on someone is probably one way to give that person your cold, but the most common way the cold virus is passed around is from one person's respiratory secretions to his or her hand, to the next person's hand, and to that person's mucous membranes in the nose or eyes. Despite what everyone's grandmother has said, *you do not get colds from going out without your galoshes* (or from playing in the snow, or from being outside in cold weather)! In fact, it's probably safer to be outside during cold weather than inside, where there is less ventilation and closer contact with people who might have cold viruses in their noses and on their hands. During the fall and winter seasons, children in day care or school are almost constantly in contact with cold viruses, and are likely to carry those viruses home with them to share with the whole family.

Avoiding Colds. Unfortunately, there is little that can be done to avoid catching colds. It is possible to try to avoid colds by staying away from all public places, such as shopping malls, church or synagogue, and school. However, even this will not be effective in avoiding all contact with the cold viruses. While it is probably sensible to avoid snuggling with someone who has a terrible cold, this also won't do the trick completely, since people can have the cold viruses—and pass them on—*before* they feel sick with a cold themselves.

Most colds for people with CF are no worse than colds for other people: You feel miserable, but they do not damage the lungs and they have no long-lasting consequences. Some colds definitely can lead to bronchial infection and can be serious, especially in infants, whose bronchi are tiny and therefore harder to clear of infection. Bronchial infections can be more serious than an infection that stays in the nose and throat, but most often bronchial infections can be successfully treated. In some cases, it may actually be helpful to get a cold. When we are exposed to viruses, our body's immune system produces antibodies that will prevent infections with these same viruses when we are exposed to them at another time. Many infections are more severe later in life, so it's good to get them early and get them over with (mumps and chickenpox are viral infections that are more severe in adults than in children). This doesn't mean that people with CF should try to get as many colds as possible. It just means that it's not worth losing sleep worrying about colds, and no one should disrupt the patient's or family's life in attempting to avoid all colds.

Infections of the Lower Respiratory Tract

Colonization and Infection

Most patients with CF have some bacteria in their lungs most of the time (people without CF do not). Whether the bacteria are merely colonizing the lungs (that is, the bacteria are there and have set up colonies, but aren't causing any inflammation or destruction) or whether there is actual infection (that is, bacteria are present and the body has set up an inflammatory reaction to those bacteria, possibly with tissue damage) may be hard to say at any one time. This question has become even harder to answer now, because recent studies have shown that some CF patients may have bronchial inflammation even *without* any bacteria or viruses present.

Bronchiolitis

Bronchiolitis (infection and inflammation of the bronchioles) is most commonly seen during the winter months in babies, with or without CF, and is most often caused by viruses. As many as four babies in 100 without CF will get bronchiolitis in the first 2 years of life. Babies with bronchiolitis may cough and wheeze, become very sick, and need extra oxygen. They may tire to the point of being unable to breathe independently, and require *assisted ventilation,* also called *mechanical ventilation.* Both of these terms mean that a machine is used to do the work of breathing for the baby by blowing air and oxygen into the baby's lungs. Of course, like most other infections, bronchiolitis can also be a mild disease, and can cause just a little cough and wheezing. Many infants with CF have bronchiolitis as the first sign of a lung problem.

Bronchitis

Bronchitis (infection and inflammation of the bronchi) is a term that is often used incorrectly, referring to a cough that has no obvious cause. Many children and adults with CF have true bronchitis, which is caused by bacteria. As was mentioned above, bronchiolitis and bronchitis are the main types of infection that affect the lungs of people with CF. It is these infections that, if not controlled, can lead to lung damage and scarring (*fibrosis*). Therefore, controlling the episodes of increased infection and inflammation in the bronchi is the most important part of the treatment of someone with CF. The more lung damage can be prevented or delayed in someone with CF, the better and longer that person's life is likely to be.

Pneumonia

Pneumonia occurs when bacteria, or the blood cells sent to fight bacteria, get into the air sacs (alveoli) or in the lung tissue between the sets of airways. Bacteria and white blood cells are frequently found in these areas in people with CF, but since the infection starts and is mostly confined to the airways, CF lung infections are most accurately thought of as bronchiolitis and bronchitis, and not as pneumonia. Even if someone with CF is diagnosed as having "pneumonia," it is almost never the dreaded kind of pneumonia that kills elderly nursing home patients.

Causes of Lung Infection in Cystic Fbrosis

Often it is not clear why a particular lung infection occurs, or why it gets out of control when it does. In some instances it is clear, as, for example, when someone has a cold, and a slight cough that develops into a worse cough remains long after the runny nose has disappeared. In a case such as this, the virus infection that caused this cold has thrown off the balance of the lung defenses enough for some of the hardier bacteria in the lung to multiply and cause problems. In someone who has asthma, the asthma may become worse because of pollution, allergies, cigarette smoke, etc., and lead to a serious infection (it may be difficult in this case to tell how much of the problem is asthma and how much is infection, and which came first). In some cases, there is no explanation of why a lung infection has gotten worse.

Bacteria, Viruses, and Fungi

Bacteria and viruses are the most important types of germs that cause infection in people with CF; fungi can occasionally cause problems as well.

Bacteria. Bacteria are probably the major cause of bronchial infection (and lung damage) in people with CF. Bacteria are larger than viruses, and can usually be killed by antibiotics. Normally, the number of bacteria in the lungs of someone with CF is relatively small, and the body's defenses (immune system) are able to keep these bacteria under control. But when something happens to offset this balance, the bacteria can multiply and cause inflammation. In this situation, there is bronchial infection and not just colonization.

There are several different bacteria (which seem to change their names as often as some people change their socks) that most often colonize and infect the lungs of people with CF: *Haemophilus influenzae,* sometimes called H. flu (not to be confused with the influenza virus); *Staphylococcus,* or "staph"; and *Pseudomonas aeruginosa.* Other bacteria that can be found include *Klebsiella, E. coli, Serratia, Stenotrophomonas maltophilia* (formerly called *Xanthomonas maltophilia* and before that *Pseudomonas maltophilia*—!), and *Burkholderia cepacia* (formerly called *Pseudomonas cepacia). Streptococcus,* which causes strep throat, and *Pneumococcus,* sometimes called the "pneumonia germ" because it is the most common cause of pneumonia in people with normal lungs, are not especially common in people with CF.

The most prevalent bacteria affecting people with CF are staph and the various types of *Pseudomonas.* The *Pseudomonas* family has a reputation, which is only partially deserved, of being particularly dangerous bacteria. Though most *Pseudomonas* are harder to kill than other bacteria—especially with antibiotics that are taken by mouth—it is *not* true that *Pseudomonas* (or any other particular bacteria) are the kiss of death. The important factor is not *what bacteria* are in the lung, but rather *what harm* they are causing. Many people with CF have *Pseudomonas* colonization of the bronchi for many years and experience little or no trouble. If someone has no cough, no problems exercising, and no trouble breathing, it doesn't much matter if a throat or mucus culture has shown *Pseudomonas.* On the other hand, if someone does have all those problems, and the culture grows only staph, the person is still sick.

Recently, it appeared that *Burkholderia cepacia* was an especially dangerous form of bacteria, causing death shortly after colonization, and some forms of these bacteria *are* very bad. It is now clear, however, that this is not always the case, and that some types of *Burkholderia cepacia* are no worse than other CF bronchial bacteria, like *Pseudomonas.* The major issue is how much damage they cause, and how readily they are killed by antibiotics.

Viruses. Viruses are smaller than bacteria, and generally cannot be killed by medicines. Antibiotics have no effect on viruses. Viruses are the most common cause of upper respiratory infections (colds), and may affect the bronchi as well. Not only can viruses cause infection, but infection with viruses makes it easier for bacteria to take hold in the bronchial tree, perhaps because the viruses interfere with mucociliary clearance. Some 20% of episodes of increased bronchial infection in patients with CF are associated with virus infections (either viruses alone or together with bacteria). Some of the common respiratory viruses are *respiratory syncytial virus* (RSV), parainfluenza virus, rhinovirus, and influenza virus. This last virus, influenza ("flu"), causes epidemics in the winter, afflicting many people with miserable coldlike symptoms. Influenza can cause a very serious pneumonia, which can even be fatal.

Some of the common childhood illnesses, such as chickenpox, measles, mumps, and rubella (German measles), are caused by viruses. On rare occasions, measles can cause a very serious pneumonia. This is true of chickenpox (varicella) as well, although chickenpox pneumonia is extremely rare in people with CF.

Fungi. Fungi, especially the fungus *Aspergillus fumigatus,* are sometimes found in the bronchi of CF patients. They can cause trouble, but not usually in the same way as viruses or bacteria. The problem with *Aspergillus* is not infection with tissue damage, but rather an allergic reaction (*allergic bronchopulmonary aspergillosis,* or *ABPA*), which induces swelling within the bronchi. In many patients with CF, *Aspergillus* may be present and cause no problems at all. As many as 80–90% of CF patients have *Aspergillus* in their airways at one time or another.

Treatment of the Lungs in Cystic Fibrosis

Since the main problems in the lungs are obstruction of bronchioles and bronchi and the resulting infection and inflammation, treatment is aimed at relieving bronchial blockage and fighting infection and inflammation. There are also some general principles to be observed.

General

CF is unusual in how very much of the outcome (how healthy someone is, indeed, how long people live) can be influenced by what the patient and family do for care of the patient's lungs. Being careful not to miss treatments (or to miss as few as possible), getting adequate rest and exercise, paying attention to good nutrition, avoiding cigarette smoke, and getting regular CF clinic visits all have been associated with better outcomes.

Cigarette Smoke

Everyone knows that smoking is not good for the smoker. More and more people are beginning to realize that it's also harmful for "innocent bystanders," who breathe the smoke coming from the end of the cigarette (*sidestream smoke*) or the smoker's exhaled smoke (*second-hand smoke*). This has been shown very clearly for CF patients: those who are exposed to smoke in the home have worse lungs than those who aren't. Period. So, parents who smoke should not, or—at a minimum—should not smoke in the house (even from another room the smoke can get to where it can do harm) or in the car. Parents who have thought about quitting for their own health but haven't been able to *are* often able to stop for their children's health and life. (In many cases, the drive to protect our children is even stronger than the drive to protect ourselves.) Certainly, teenagers and adults with CF who feel peer pressure to take up smoking should resist that pressure.

Medical Care

Regular check-ups with your CF physician are extremely important to be able to detect small signs of lung infection and inflammation, before these problems have caused irreversible damage. When someone appears to be doing well it is very tempting to put off a time-consuming (and perhaps expensive and anxiety-producing) visit to the CF center, but these visits are important. One study showed a clear difference in actual patient *survival* between centers that saw their patients frequently (best survival) and those that saw their patients less frequently (worst survival). Visits to your regular pediatrician or family doctor are also important for good health maintenance.

Relieving and Preventing Obstruction: Airway Clearance Techniques

Chest Physical Therapy

A major portion of most treatment programs is aimed at keeping the airways as free of mucus as possible. The methods seem crude, but are quite effective. The most common method is based on a principle taken from everyday life, namely, the "Ketchup Bottle Principle": If you want to get a thick substance out of a container with a narrow opening, you turn the container upside down so that its opening is pointing downward, and then you clap it, shake it, and vibrate it. If the thick substance is mucus, and the container is the various segments of the lungs, the procedure is the same, and may be equally effective: you turn the child (or yourself) in various positions, with each position allowing one of the major portions of the lungs to have its opening pointing downward, and then you clap firmly on the back or chest over that part of the lung, and actually shake the mucus loose (for details on positioning for these treatments, see Appendix C: *Airway Clearance Techniques*). Once it's shaken loose, the mucus can fall into the large central airways, and then be coughed out. This form of treatment goes by many different names, a few of which are *postural drainage* (PDs), *chest physical therapy* (chest PT, or just CPT), and *percussion and drainage*. Often, children and families invent their own pet names: "exercises," "clapping," "boom-booms."

PD treatments are not painful; in fact, they can be very soothing and relaxing in the way that a massage is. Babies who may be crying at the beginning of their PDs are often asleep halfway through the procedure. The treatment can be time-consuming, however (from 1 to 2 minutes for each of 10 or 12 positions), and can be a bother to children, adolescents, and adults alike, since it interferes with the day's agenda. It may also keep an older child or adult tied to home, since it is awkward to perform on oneself and may require accommodating to someone else's (usually a parent's) schedule.

There are several pieces of equipment that make these treatments easier to perform at home. The first is the mechanical percussor/vibrator. This tool comes in a variety of models, the simplest of which is like an electric jigsaw that instead of a blade has a rod with a firm cushion on it. The cushion is held on the chest and bounces firmly and repeatedly where it is aimed. Most models have variable force and speed; some models are driven by electricity and others by compressed air. The action of some models is a pounding motion, whereas others vibrate; some models can do both, depending on the setting selected. Treatments with the good mechanical percussors are probably just as effective as those done by hand, if conscientiously performed. Some children (and adults, too) have a strong preference for the hand, whereas others prefer the machines. Clearly, a treatment by either method is considerably more effective than no treatment at all. Another mechanical device that some patients have found effective is the percussor vest. This looks a bit like a life-vest, and it is hooked to high-pressure air hosing that rapidly inflates and deflates the vest, causing a vibrating that seems to help shake loose airway mucus. In the category of devices-you-wear is a percussor pack, which you slip on like a backpack. This device works like the mechanical percussor, with pistons inside the pack pounding on the back. Some patients have found these packs useful.

The mechanical devices have two advantages over the manual method. Most of the mechanical percussors or vibrators come with extension handles or straps, which enable teenagers or adults to reach areas of the back that they could not reach by hand. This makes it possible for them to give themselves a full treatment independently. This of course is also true of the vests and packs. Another advantage of the mechanical percussors, vests, and packs is that they are gentler on the elbow and shoulder joints of the person who performs the treatments—a particularly great advantage for a parent who has more than one child requiring treatment each day.

Another device that simplifies treatment is a PD table. Treatments for infants and small children are done most comfortably with the child on a parent's lap, but when the patient is an adolescent or an adult the table becomes very useful. The person receiving the treatment can sit or lie on the table, which can be set at different angles, thereby making proper positioning easier to achieve. Tables and percussors can be bought from commercial suppliers, and are relatively expensive. However, since some CF centers have tables available for no charge (supplied by charitable organizations), it is worth checking with your center before you purchase one.

There are several airway clearance techniques that do not involve hitting the chest, but seem to be very effective for adults, adolescents, and children old enough to cooperate: The first of these uses the *Flutter* valve. This is a hand-held device, small enough to carry around in your pocket, that looks a little like a kazoo. It has a stainless steel ball in it that vibrates up and down (flutters, you might say) as you blow into the tube. The vibrations are transmitted backwards down through the patient's mouth into the trachea and bronchi, where they shake mucus free from the bronchial walls. Many teenagers and adults who had done traditional PDs for years have become "Flutter converts," saying that the Flutter is more effective in helping them bring up mucus, letting them feel when there's excess mucus there, and to know when they've cleared their airways. Like some of the mechanical devices, the Flutter has the advantage of enabling patients to work on airway clearance without help (except perhaps the reminder from a parent that so many children seem to need to do *any* job).

Other techniques have had more use in Europe than North America. These techniques include one called a *PEP mask* (positive expiratory pressure). The patient breathes through a special mask that has an exhale-valve that requires some air pressure to open. It is thought that this expiratory pressure is transmitted back down the airways and helps to prop them open during the exhalation, allowing mucus to be pushed out along with the air (remember that usually during exhalation, the airways tend to narrow a little bit, so this keeps them wider open than they'd normally be). Another method is called the *active cycle of breathing tech-*

nique. This technique has three phases, *breathing control* (quiet breathing), *thoracic expansion* (deep breaths in), and *forced expiration* or *huffs* (quick, strong—but never violent—breaths out, with the mouth and throat open). *Autogenic drainage* involves a series of breaths controlled so that some are done with very little air in the lungs, some with a medium amount, and some done with the lungs filled almost to capacity. This technique requires instruction by someone very skilled in its use before it can be effective in mobilizing mucus.

Exercise

Many people believe that vigorous exercise may be helpful to loosen mucus and to keep bronchi clear. Certainly, hard exercise, or laughing or crying, often result in a coughing spell that brings up mucus, even in people who do not raise mucus during the traditional PD treatments. Since there is not yet any scientific evidence that exercise can successfully replace the time-honored PD treatments, it is best to encourage patients to be very active *and* to do their treatments. (Exercise is discussed at greater length in Chapter 10, *Exercise.*)

An Important Note on Airway Clearance Treatments

One important point to keep in mind is that a method may be helpful even if it does not result in the immediate expectoration of large amounts of mucus. Mucus might be shaken loose from the smallest bronchioles and started on its way to the central bronchi, but it will not cause a cough until it actually reaches the large, central bronchi. There is good evidence that regular airway clearance treatments are helpful, even though a single treatment makes little or no apparent difference. In one study, a number of children stopped their PDs for 3 weeks, and had a significant deterioration in their lung function (even though they didn't *feel* any different); when they resumed their treatments after the 3-week experimental period, their lung function returned to its previous level. This can be a problem for patients with CF and their families: the treatments are time-consuming, and it is not uncommon to see or feel no obvious results right after the treatments. That means it's easy to convince yourself that skipping the treatments won't hurt. But it will! All too often, people have realized too late that they have harmed their lungs by not keeping up with their treatments. Of course, for many CF patients, the benefit of the treatments is very obvious even during the individual treatment sessions.

Breaking up Mucus

For decades, the idea of somehow breaking up, thinning, or watering down the thick CF airway secretions has been appealing, and numerous attempts have been made to accomplish this end, most of them not very successful. For many years, CF patients slept all night in *mist tents,* which surrounded them with a dense fog of water. It turned out that this didn't really help. The next approach—still used by a very few patients—was a medication called acetylcysteine (Mucomyst®), which is inhaled as an aerosol. When Mucomyst® is mixed with CF mucus in a test tube, it does make the mucus thinner and easier to move. However, human bronchi and tracheas are different from glass test tubes, and may react with inflammation when Mucomyst® is inhaled. Some people have developed increasing bronchial obstruction because of inflammation, or even bronchospasm, after inhaling Mucomyst®. While some people do improve with this treatment, most are neither helped nor hurt by it.

There is now a new era in thinning bronchial mucus, based on our better understanding of what makes CF mucus thick. Remember that DNA that's been released from white blood cells is an important component of CF mucus; it happens to account for some 40% of the stickiness of CF mucus. There is now a genetically engineered medication that breaks down this DNA: DNase (the ending *-ase* refers to enzymes that break down other substances). DNase (*Pulmozyme®*) is extremely effective in liquefying CF mucus in the test tube (as was true of Mucomyst®). Taken by aerosol, it also seems to be very safe for most CF patients (with the possible exception of those with very severe lung disease and huge amounts of mucus in their airways—these patients do better if all that mucus is not mobilized all at once). So, it works in the test tube, and is *safe.* Does it work in people with CF? Is it *effective* in helping people get mucus out of their lungs? The answer is yes, *for some patients.* Studies in large numbers of patients have suggested that breathing in DNase once a day does seem to bring about a small (5%) improvement in lung function, as compared to the gradual deterioration that might be expected. However, not everyone does benefit, and the drug is extraordinarily expensive: about $12,000 a year in 1996. The approach many CF doctors have taken is to have patients try DNase for a month or so, comparing pulmonary function before and after. If the patient *feels* better, and/or the pulmonary function tests have shown an improvement, then it makes sense to use it. There are some patients who do feel better, without any *measurable* improvement, and we don't know how to explain this.

It is possible that even better mucus-thinning medications—or combinations of medications—will be developed.

Treating Asthma

When asthma is present in addition to CF, there is increased bronchial obstruction with which to contend. Bronchospasm makes the opening of the bronchi smaller than normal, making it much more difficult to get the mucus out. Several very effective bronchodilator medications that dilate (open) the bronchi are available. These medications can be inhaled as an aerosol, or taken by mouth or injection. The aerosols are delivered by an aerosol machine, which is composed of an air compressor, a length of tubing, and a *nebulizer* (Figure 3.4). The compressor sends air through the tube to the nebulizer, which holds the liquid medicine. As the air rushes by, it lifts the medicine, breaks it into a mist, and blows it out through the mouthpiece or mask to be inhaled. Some medications are available in hand-held metered-dose inhalers (Figure 3.5). These devices deliver a measured amount of medicated mist with each puff. Since the puff of medicine is only available for breathing in for a fraction of a second, the timing of the puffing and breathing in is crucial, and may be quite difficult to coordinate, especially for small children. Extension devices are available that attach to the opening of the inhaler, and temporarily trap the medication until the next breath, making the timing less crucial. Some aerosol bronchodilator medications are albuterol (Ventolin®, Proventil®) metaproterenol (Alupent®, Metaprel®), and salmeterol (Serevent®) (see Appendix B: *Medications*).

Oral bronchodilators include some of the same medications that are inhaled. These are all in the family of *beta-adrenergic* drugs (albuterol, metaproterenol). Another family of bronchodilators that can be taken by mouth are the theophyllines. Theophylline is related to caffeine, which is actually a weak bronchodilator. Theo-

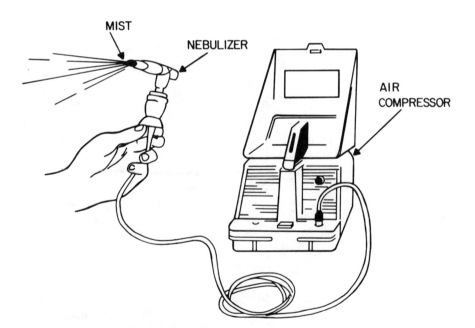

Figure 3.4. Aerosol machine. The machine blows compressed air through the tubing, over the liquid medication that is held in the cup of the nebulizer, creating a mist from the liquid medication. The patient then breathes the medicine.

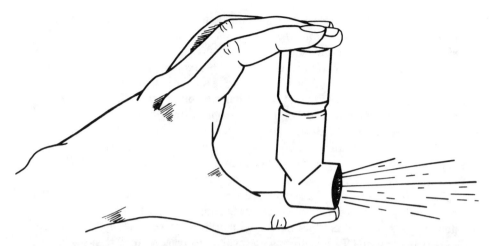

Figure 3.5. Hand-held nebulizer (also called metered-dose inhaler or MDI). Pushing down the top of the inhaler causes a puff of medicated mist to shoot out into the air, for the patient to breathe.

phylline comes in the form of a liquid, tablet, or capsule (fast-acting or sustained-release) (see Appendix B: *Medications*).

Reducing Airway Inflammation

Airway inflammation often accompanies infection and/or asthma (see above, *The Lower Respiratory Tract*), making the airway opening that much smaller, and possibly damaging the cells that line the airway. Although inflammation is a normal part of fighting infection (see above, *Other Protection Against Lung Infection*), if it gets out of control it can do more harm than good. Excessive inflammation appears to be a very important cause of the progressive damage to CF airways, and therefore prevention and treatment of airway inflammation has become an important focus of CF research. Some medications, most notably a group of drugs called *steroids*, can reduce inflammation wherever it occurs, including in the bronchial tree. Within the past few years, prednisone (one of the steroids) has been studied in a number of people with CF, and has appeared to be effective in improving their lung function.

Prednisone, however, is a very potent drug that has many possible side effects (see Appendix B: *Medications)*. One of the most serious of these side effects is *oversuppression* of the immune response, which makes the body unable to fight infection. Prednisone can also bring out a tendency to develop diabetes, and can interfere with growth. Although the chances of dangerous side effects are much lower if prednisone is given on alternate days (Monday-Wednesday-Friday, etc.), instead of every day, there are still some risks. In fact, in the largest study done to date in CF patients, prednisone was given on alternate days, and improved pulmonary function, but did cause side effects in some patients, so if prednisone is to be used, patients need to be checked fairly frequently.

Steroids have been developed in a form for inhalation, and these drugs have been very helpful in preventing airway inflammation in people with asthma. It is not yet known if they will be helpful for people with CF. Similarly, an inhaled drug called *cromolyn* (Intal®) has been known for years to be useful in preventing airways inflammation in people with asthma. Cromolyn has not yet been shown to be helpful for people with CF, but it has barely been studied. (Unlike most drugs, cromolyn has close to zero side effects.)

There are other drugs that reduce inflammation without interfering with the body's ability to fight infection. These drugs include aspirin, ibuprofen, and related drugs, which are used for people with arthritis. A small study with ibuprofen in patients with CF gave promising results: the drug seemed to slow the rate of decline of pulmonary function over a four-year period. However, ibuprofen has its own problems, as well. Many patients taking the high doses of ibuprofen needed for the beneficial effects have had bleeding ulcers, while others have had kidney failure. Studies are currently under way to see if other medications might have anti-inflammatory effects without side effects.

Reducing Bronchial Infection

Antibacterial Drugs (Antibiotics)

Antibiotics are probably the most important single factor responsible for the tremendous improvement in the outlook for people with CF, both in terms of length of life and quality of life. Antibiotics are very effective in reducing airways infection, and therefore in preserving lung health. (See Appendix B: *Medications*, for a more complete discussion of antibiotics.) Most CF physicians agree that antibiotics should be used when there is evidence of increased airways infection (such as increased cough and mucus production and decreased exercise tolerance). There is no agreement, however, on whether it is helpful to give antibiotics on a regular basis to *prevent* infection. One large multicenter study suggested that the *preventive* ("prophylactic") use of continuous antibiotics was *not* helpful for young patients with CF.

Oral antibiotics are usually taken when the infection is caused by staph or *Haemophilus*. (See Appendix B for a review of these antibiotics.) Oral antibiotics may also be helpful for *Pseudomonas* infections, but most often throat and sputum culture results will say that they will not work, and in fact, in many cases they will *not* bring these infections under control. If this is the case, someone may need treatment with aerosol or intravenous antibiotics. Compared to oral antibiotics, the aerosol and IV antibiotics are more powerful, more likely to get to the site of infection within the bronchial tubes, or both. Intravenous antibiotics most often require a hospital stay (see Chapter 7, *Hospitalization and Other Special Treatments*).

Preventing Bacterial Infection

There is no very effective method for preventing bronchial infections caused by bacteria. There is, however, a vaccine available that is moderately good at preventing infection with the *Pneumococcus* bacteria. Since this is the most common cause of pneumonia in the general population, the vaccine is often called "the pneumonia vaccine." People who are at risk from pneumonia, such as the elderly and people with sickle cell disease, are encouraged to get this vaccine. Since people with CF are not very likely to get pneumococcal pneumonia, or if they get it they do not usually have trouble getting rid of it, there is no particular need for them to get the "pneumonia vaccine."

Contact with Other Cystic Fibrosis Patients and Their Bacteria

The sources of bronchial infection in CF patients are not completely understood. Some of the bacteria and viruses that cause these infections are all around us, in the air, in soil, and so on. But we have found out that some of the bacteria can be passed directly from one CF patient to another. A prime example of this "person-to-person transmission" of CF airway bacteria is *Burkholderia cepacia*. And it these particular bacteria that have in some cases (see above) been associated with an especially bad sickness. Because of dangers from *cepacia* for some people (and possible dangers from other bacteria as well), and because of the possibility of person-to-person spread of these bacteria, most experts are now recommending that CF patients limit their contact with other CF patients. These recommendations have been carried out in different ways by different individuals; and different CF centers and organizations have all set up different guidelines (or none at all).

Some typical recommendations include:

- No direct or very close contact (like kissing, or perhaps even hand-shaking) between CF patients

- No prolonged close contact between CF patients (no rooming together in the hospital or elsewhere, no being in the same room during aerosols or chest PT, no long car rides together, etc.)

- Careful hand-washing for CF patients and their caretakers

- Careful hygiene: cover your mouth and nose during coughing spells, carefully dispose of tissue that has sputum in it, etc.

Other recommendations have been made by some—but not all—experts, including no playing together for young children with CF, no holiday parties, or CF group picnics.

This is a very difficult issue to deal with. CF patients and families have always received information, friendship, and a sense of shared experiences from contact with each other. It would be a shame to lose that. It would also be a shame for someone who is relatively well to get dreadfully ill if that could have been avoided. Discuss this problem with your own CF physician. It should be possible to find a safe and humane approach that's right for you and your family.

Fighting Viral Infections

There are very few safe drugs that kill viruses, and, therefore, no safe, effective drug treatment for viral bronchiolitis or bronchitis. One possible exception is ribavirin, which seems to be effective for some very sick babies with bronchiolitis caused by the respiratory syncytial virus (RSV). This drug is delivered by an aerosol, and must be breathed in for as long as 12 hours at a time. Ribavirin is not effective for infections caused by most other viruses, and specifically, it provides little benefit to people with colds.

One other exception is amantadine, which appears to be helpful in fighting the influenza virus. It is taken by mouth, and is used primarily by people who become infected with influenza during an epidemic. People who are at risk for influenza infection, such as CF patients who have not had the flu vaccine, may also take the drug as a preventive measure, during a community outbreak of influenza.

Preventing Viral Infections

See also *Avoiding Colds,* above.

The most common type of viral infection, namely, the common cold, cannot be effectively prevented (see above, *Infections of the Upper Respiratory Tract*). There are other viral infections that *can* be prevented, though, including measles and influenza ("flu"). All children should be immunized against measles, and all children with CF (or other abnormal lung conditions) should receive a flu shot each year. These vaccines are effective and are safe except in people with very severe egg allergy.

There is a new varicella (chickenpox) vaccine available, and the American Academy of Pediatrics recommends it for all children. It is safe for children with CF. Another chickenpox-related medication is *zoster immune globulin,* or ZIG. It is not a vaccine, but rather a gamma-globulin-like shot that is given to prevent chickenpox. Most CF physicians feel, however, that this is unnecessary for people with CF, since the chances that someone with CF would have lung complications from chickenpox are very small. In addition, a major drawback to ZIG is that once it is given, it has to be repeated every time there is an exposure to chickenpox. Nonetheless, some CF physicians recommend ZIG for nonimmunized patients who have been exposed to chickenpox. Others recommend "chickenpox parties" for children who have not yet had chickenpox. In this way, they will come in contact with a "poxy" child and contract chickenpox in childhood when it's likely to be mild, instead of in adulthood when it often follows a much more severe course.

Steps in Treating Worsened Lungs

In CF, the lungs get worse from time to time. These periods of worsening, called *pulmonary exacerbations,* are most often caused by increased airways infection, and can usually be brought under control if proper steps are taken.

Recognition

In order for pulmonary exacerbations to be treated, they must first be recognized, which is not always easy. The signs that the lungs are worse may be very subtle, and may at first escape attention. These signs include more cough than usual, more mucus, decreased energy, poor appetite, difficulty exercising, and shortness of breath. In most people, the amount of cough is the single most important clue. Many people will *not* have lessened activity or shortness of breath, nor will they have fever, so the absence of these clues should not be taken as a reassuring sign. It is important to recognize when there are more signs of infection than are usual for *you,* since everyone is different. For example, if your usual pattern is to cough only a little bit in the morning, but you begin to cough after laughing or crying and find that the cough lasts just a bit longer, then you will know that your condition is not quite as good as it usually is. On occasion, someone else, such as your doctor or a relative who doesn't see you every day, may point a difference out to you that you haven't noticed. Sometimes, however, it may take an x-ray or pulmonary function test to show that a change has occurred. For this reason, it is quite important to make fairly frequent clinic visits. It's very tempting to say, "I [or my child] am doing so well that there's no need to go for a checkup." There are far too many CF patients (usually teenagers) and parents of patients who have used this reasoning, only to return to regular care after irreversible lung damage has been done. Regular visits, which would include physical examinations, throat or sputum cultures, and periodic chest x-rays and pulmonary function tests, can often spot a problem while it is still reversible. Since the progression of lung disease in CF is usually very gradual and subtle—and is *not* characterized by sudden dramatic deterioration—it is easy for patients and families to miss signs of deterioration. Your physician may be able to recognize these signs, because a change in the weeks or months since your last visit is easier to detect than small day-to-day changes, and because sensitive laboratory tests (pulmonary function tests and x-rays) help clarify your condition.

Once you have recognized that there is a problem, it is important not to wait until you're terribly ill to do something about it. That wait can give the infection and inflammation an opportunity to destroy a small portion of lung, leaving a little scar tissue behind. A little scar tissue with each inadequately treated infection adds up over the years. Scar tissue can never become normal lung tissue, so it's important to prevent its formation. It is impossible to tell at any one time whether bronchial obstruction is because these tubes are filled with mucus and bacteria and white blood cells—that could be gotten rid of, or because of permanent irreversible scarring.

Oral Antibiotics

During a period of worsening, your physician will probably prescribe an oral antibiotic, or change the antibiotic if you are already taking one. The choice of antibiotics is based on several factors, including how the individual patient has responded in the past, how sick the person is at the time, and what recent throat or sputum cultures have shown (what bacteria are there and which antibiotics kill those bacteria in the laboratory). The physician may also increase the number of airway clearance treatments you're doing, in order to clear out the extra mucus that builds up with infections.

If an infection does not improve quickly, and certainly if it becomes worse, it is advisable to take the next step of changing antibiotics. This change will be to a more powerful antibiotic, or to one that is better at killing the particular bacteria a culture has shown to be in your system. If a more powerful or appropriate oral antibiotic is not available, or if the physician feels that an oral antibiotic would work too slowly, then he or she may recommend an aerosol antibiotic, or even intravenous antibiotics. Most often, symptoms will improve nicely with oral antibiotic treatment. In fact, patients are often back to their *baseline* (usual state of health) even before the antibiotic prescription has run out. In these cases, it's tempting to stop the medicines as soon as you feel better, but this is usually not a good idea. Infectious disease experts tell us that one of the surest ways to make bacteria become resistant to an antibiotic (not be killed by it) is to give antibiotics for too short a time. So if your doctor has prescribed 2 weeks of antibiotics, and your cough is gone (or back to your usual) in 1 week, you should take the second week of antibiotics anyway.

Aerosol Antibiotics

Several different kind of antibiotics can be breathed directly into the lungs as aerosols, using the same kind of machine that we use for bronchodilator aerosols

(Figure 3.4). The most commonly used aerosol antibiotics are gentamicin and to-bramycin. There are widely varying doses of these medications, and you should be sure you know how much your doctor wants you to take.

Intravenous Antibiotics

If these steps do not work, or do not work fast enough, it may be time for intravenous (IV) antibiotics. In almost every case, putting antibiotics into a vein is the most effective way of treating infection, especially if the infection is caused by *Pseudomonas*. Typically, the administration of IV antibiotics requires a hospital stay. In some cases, it is possible to get IVs at home. (For more information about IVs and hospitalization, see Chapter 7.)

The length of time to give IV antibiotics should be determined by how the patient is responding to treatment. Patients seldom improve (and may perhaps even worsen) in the first 4 or 5 days on IVs. Thereafter, most people improve for several weeks, then return to their usual condition or even to an improved condition. On occasion, someone may stop improving without having returned to his or her previous baseline. Studies have shown that the level of lung function achieved after in-hospital IV treatment of a pulmonary exacerbation can be maintained for at least several weeks, but will not continue to improve after discharge from the hospital. Therefore, it makes sense to get the most mileage possible from the IV and hospital treatment, and not to stop after a predetermined number of days have gone by. Some people will have gotten the maximum benefit from the intensive treatment in as short a time as 10 days, but most people take about 2 weeks, and quite a few people take even longer. Keep in mind that this investment of time can pay off in the long run if it keeps even a small portion of lung from becoming scarred. Figure 3.6 shows a time curve for when someone should enter the hospital, and when he or she should leave.

Other Treatments

In some cases, other treatments may be used with IV antibiotics or tried before them. One example is trying medications to decrease bronchial inflammation, like prednisone. Another example is altering anti-asthma medications by increasing their dosage, or by adding different ones. The best steps to take will differ under different conditions.

General Questions About Using Antibiotics

How Do We Know Whether to Give Antibiotics or Not? For individual episodes of increased cough, we will often have the question, is this a cold that does not involve the lungs, and therefore shouldn't need antibiotics, or is it a bronchial in-

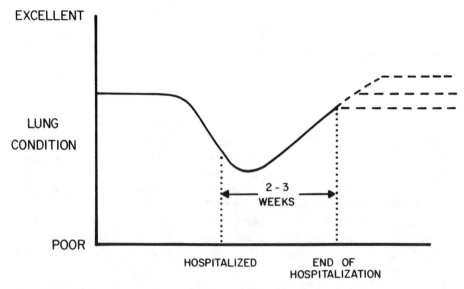

Figure 3.6. Timing of hospitalization. When it is recognized that the patient is not doing well out of the hospital, she or he is admitted to the hospital for treatment. Improvement begins within four or five days. Hospital treatment then continues until the patient has returned to her or his usual state of health.

fection, which definitely should be treated with antibiotics? And we can't always tell. Given that we can't tell for sure, we have to base treatment decisions on an educated *guess*, and keep in mind the possible consequences of a *wrong* guess. If we guess this is bronchial infection and it's really only a cold, we would have given unneeded antibiotics. The consequences of that mistaken decision would be: (1) financial (had to pay for antibiotics that weren't needed), (2) small risk of allergic or other reaction to the antibiotic, and (3) small theoretical risk of encouraging the bacteria to become resistant to the antibiotic. If, on the other hand, we guess this a simple cold with no bronchial infection, and we don't give antibiotics, and we've guessed wrong (there really was infection), then the consequences are much worse: possible lung damage, some of which could be irreversible. Given those choices, we'll almost always take the chance of giving antibiotics when they might not have been needed rather than not give them when they might have been needed.

What's Too Much Antibiotics? Will I Become "Immune" to the Effects of the Antibiotic? People often worry that they or their bacteria will "become immune" to the antibiotics (or as physicians say, the bacteria become *resistant* to the antibiotics). This *can* happen over time, but not nearly as easily as many people fear. Further, if the choice is between treating an infection that we *know* can cause lung damage—even irreversible damage—or not treating it because of the *remotely possible* development of resistance to a single antibiotic, most experts would go with the treatment every time. In fact, the history of CF has shown this to be the correct approach: we use a lot more antibiotics now than a few decades ago, and there are more resistant bacteria now, but patients live well into adulthood instead of dying before school age. One important study showed that the survival of patients was much better in centers that use a lot of antibiotics than in those that are stingy with their antibiotics.

What If We "Run Out" of Antibiotics That Are Effective? On occasion, a patient's cultures (see the end of this chapter) may show that one or more of the bacteria in the lungs have become *"resistant"* to some, many, or even all of the available antibiotics. When this happens, it can be frightening to a patient or parent, for it may signal to them the end of effective treatment for lung infections. While it is undeniably better if the bacteria are all *sensitive* to readily available antibiotics, the problem of *resistance* is not completely straightforward, and therefore not always as bad as a culture report may make it seem. We have known for decades that patients often respond well to antibiotics that *"shouldn't"* work. Chloromycetin® is an example of an antibiotic that has been used frequently and very successfully for CF lung infection, even when cultures showed only *Pseudomonas* that were resistant to it. Why should this be so? There are several possible explanations: One (as you'll see at the end of this chapter) is that "resistant" is not an absolute term; that is, although it may sound as though it means that the antibiotic in question has *no* effect on the particular bacteria, this is not the case. Often it means that the antibiotic doesn't kill *all* the bacteria, or that you need a lot of the antibiotic to kill the bacteria. So, some killing may be possible. Another important part of the explanation is that the testing for bacterial *sensitivity* or resistance takes place in a test tube or culture plate—*not* in the body. The body has its own defenses, including white blood cells, antibodies, and so on, that help to kill invading bacteria, and these aren't measured in the bacteriology laboratory. Finally, it has come to light in recent years that antibiotics have important effects other than their ability to kill bacteria. Erythromycin, for example, has usually been shown in the laboratory to be good for killing *staph*, but not *Pseudomonas*, yet has seemed to be effective in improving the lungs of CF patients whose only cultured bacteria are *Pseudomonas*. Why? Well, we now know that erythromycin has powerful anti-inflammatory effects separate from its ability to kill bacteria. Since *Pseudomonas* causes damage largely through inflammation—from the chemicals it itself releases or those released by white blood cells that have come to fight it—lessening the inflammatory response to *Pseudomonas* may do just as much good as killing it.

What if the culture reports are right, and the antibiotics really don't work any more? This happens occasionally, and is very serious. In these cases, when the antibiotics really seem unable to make any dent in a patient's symptoms of lung infection, the physician may try other means to fight inflammation (for example, steroids). In some unusual situations, physicians have been able to stop antibiotics for a while, and let the bacteria become sensitive to the antibiotics again, so that when the antibiotics are resumed, they are effective once again.

This is a risky business, and you should definitely not try it without your doctor's direction, for there is a strong chance that it won't work, and stopping the antibiotics will allow the infection to worsen, without changing the sensitivity pattern of the bacteria.

Finally, there is the helpful fact that the pharmaceutical industry is well aware of the problem of emerging resistance, and is continually at work developing new antibiotics. As with so many other aspects of CF care, there is almost always hope even when things might appear bleak. If you're worried about your (or your child's) culture results and their implications for the future, be sure to let your doctor know.

Complications

There are several problems that can be an indirect result of CF. These problems are often referred to as *complications* of CF. The most important complications related to the lung disease of CF are hemoptysis, atelectasis, pneumothorax, respiratory failure, heart failure, and chest pain. Other complications which relate to the lung disease of CF affect the bones and/or the joints.

Hemoptysis

The literal translation of this term is to "cough up blood" (*heme* is the Greek word for "blood," and *ptyein* translates as "to spit"). Hemoptysis is very uncommon in young children with CF, but as many as 50% of adults with CF will on occasion have some streaks of blood in the mucus they cough up and spit out. A relatively small proportion of patients (3–5% of those older than 15 years) will cough out large (more than 10 ounces) amounts of blood at a time. This problem, called *massive hemoptysis,* can be fatal, although it rarely is, even in people who bring up very large amounts of blood. In most cases, the significance of hemoptysis is the same as that of an increased cough, namely, both are signs of increased infection. A major difference, however, between having a bit more cough than usual and bringing up bright red blood is that it is very frightening to see the blood, especially the first time it happens. One's first reaction is to panic and to assume that all of one's lungs must be bleeding. This is not the case: It's extremely important to know that *hemoptysis is a fairly common problem that is almost always simple to treat.*

What is happening is that the increased infection in one small area has irritated a capillary or small artery and made a small hole in its wall, causing blood to leak out into the airway. Remember that the size of the working surface of the lungs is about the same as a tennis court; the problem area in someone with hemoptysis is about the size of a little pebble on that tennis court. It helps to keep this in mind if you should see some blood mixed in with mucus sometime. If you see *pure* blood, you should notify your doctor, because you do need treatment, but there's no need to panic.

In unusual cases, hemoptysis can mean something other than just increased infection. It can indicate a more general bleeding problem. Bleeding problems can be caused by inadequate vitamin K (this would be uncommon in someone with CF who is getting a good diet and taking the prescribed enzymes), by advanced liver disease, or rarely by a drug side effect. In some unusual situations it may be difficult to tell where spit-up blood has come from. Bleeding in the stomach or esophagus can be confused with bleeding in the lungs. Fortunately, bleeding in the stomach or esophagus is not common in people with CF.

Treating Hemoptysis

The treatment required for someone who coughs up bloody mucus, or pure blood, depends on the cause of the bleeding. In most cases, the cause is an increase in bronchial infection which has irritated a blood vessel, and the treatment therefore is the same as the treatment for any increased infection, namely, antibiotics and airway clearance treatments, like PDs. There is little or no controversy about the need for antibiotics (or for stronger antibiotics in someone who is already taking antibiotics). Not all CF specialists agree on the usefulness of PD, and, in fact, some experts recommend stopping PD treatments in someone who has brought up a large amount of blood. However, in most cases, the clapping and vibrating are very unlikely to cause any bleeding and should be continued.

In some people who bring up blood, a gurgling sensation is felt in the chest (they can sometimes even tell which part of the lung it's coming from) just before the blood comes up. If someone feels a gurgling every time he or she goes into a particular position, the head-down position, for example, then that position should be avoided. In general, though, the treatments should be continued as much as possible, for three reasons: (1) the blood is not good for cilia and should therefore be removed; (2) the blood can make an infection worse by providing a hospitable environment for bacteria; and (3) even if the blood itself is not a problem, one of the underlying principles of treating bronchial infection in someone with CF is to lessen bronchial mucous obstruction as much as possible.

In most cases where a person has brought up a large amount (more than a cup) of pure blood, hospitalization is recommended. In the hospital, IV antibiotics can be given easily, and patients can be watched carefully to make sure the bleeding is under control. If the bleeding is very severe and much blood has been lost, blood transfusions may be necessary, just as they would be if the bleeding were caused by a car accident, for example. It is quite uncommon, however, for a transfusion to be required.

Extra vitamin K is usually given to someone with CF who has hemoptysis, since a lack of that vitamin can cause bleeding problems. If the bleeding is not controlled fairly quickly it may be necessary to do various tests. These tests would check for a generalized bleeding problem (as might occur in someone with severe liver disease) or examine the possibility that the bleeding is a side effect of a drug or drug combination.

In a few cases of massive hemoptysis that can't be controlled by the above means, more difficult methods may be needed. One such method is *bronchoscopy,* which allows the physician to look into the lungs with a flexible tube that goes through the nose and down the back of the throat, or with a rigid tube that is passed directly down the throat. Most physicians, however, doubt that bronchoscopy is very helpful, and a relatively new procedure is more likely to be recommended. This procedure is called *bronchial artery embolization,* and has been helpful in people with massive hemoptysis. An *embolus* is a clot or other plug in a blood vessel that blocks the circulation in that vessel (*embolos* is the Greek word for "plug"). Emboli are usually harmful, but they can also be helpful when a bronchial artery is leaking. In this case, a radiologist may be able to thread a catheter (a thin, flexible tube) into the artery and inject a plug (typically made of a synthetic substance called *Gelfoam®*) through the catheter that will then seal the leak and stop the bleeding.

There are several problems that make this procedure less than perfect. The first is that it is not always possible to find the artery that is leaking, even with the sophisticated radiologic technology that is available. The second problem is that, in some people, arteries to the spinal cord may come from the bronchial arteries. If the *Gelfoam®* plug blocks off the blood supply to a portion of the spinal cord, serious problems could result. Fortunately, with modern techniques, the radiologist can nearly always tell beforehand if the patient has such a spinal artery, and can plan the plugging accordingly. Lastly, a fair proportion of people whose bleeding has been stopped with bronchial artery embolization will bleed again from that spot in the future.

In a very few cases—when there is massive bleeding and bronchial artery embolization cannot be performed or is not successful—surgery may be necessary to remove the lobe of the lung that is the source of the bleeding. There are numerous problems with this approach, a major one being that, although the person will obviously not bleed again from the removed lobe, he or she will also not have the use of that lobe for breathing. In addition, general anesthesia and chest surgery carry their own risks, especially in someone with severe lung disease. Finally, even with the chest open, it may not be possible to identify the lobe that is the source of bleeding with absolute certainty. There are too many cases of CF patients who have had a lobe removed in a hospital inexperienced in CF care, only to be transferred to a CF center because the bleeding didn't stop. Nonetheless, there *are* some cases in which surgery is necessary and very successful.

Because of the problems and uncertainties with the invasive means of dealing with hemoptysis, many CF experts prefer to treat patients—even those with massive hemoptysis—as conservatively as possible, with antibiotics, PD, vitamin K, transfusions if necessary, and careful observation.

Pneumothorax

This complication is also called *"collapsed lung."* The term actually means *"air inside the chest,"* which doesn't sound all that abnormal, since that's where air is supposed to be. But it actually refers to air that's within the chest, but *outside the lung* (Figure 3.7). That is very abnormal, and can be dangerous, since once air gets outside the lung, it can press in on it and cause it to collapse. If

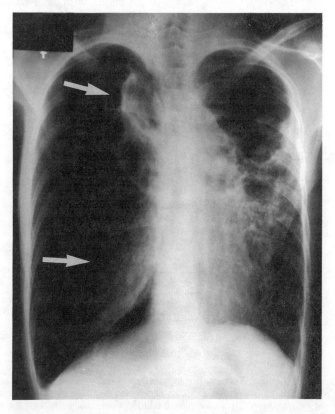

Figure 3.7. X-ray appearance of pneumothorax. The air outside the lungs appears black, while the lungs are lighter in color. Arrows show edge of collapsed lung.

there is enough air under enough pressure or tension, it can even squeeze the blood vessels (*venae cavae*) that bring the blood back to the heart. This will mean that there won't be enough blood to pump out to the body to keep it functioning normally. This does not usually happen with a pneumothorax in someone with CF. It is unusual for pneumothorax to occur in someone under the age of 10, and after age 10, between 10% and 25% of CF patients will develop a pneumothorax. Pneumothorax is much more likely to happen in someone with CF if there is relatively severe lung involvement than if the lungs are in very good shape.

Pneumothorax develops when mucus partially blocks a bronchus or bronchiole, and functions as a one-way valve or "ball-valve" (Figure 3.8). This kind of blockage allows air to go in only one direction past the blockage. Bronchi enlarge with inhaling, and get smaller with exhaling (see *The Airways*). When mucus fills up a portion of a bronchiole, the bronchiole will enlarge enough with each breath that some air can get beyond the mucous plug. But during exhaling, the bronchus may collapse to the same size as the plug, so no air will escape. When this happens, the alveoli beyond the blockage will get bigger with each breath in, until, like an overfilled balloon, they finally burst. If these overfilled alveoli are at the edge of the lung (especially at the *apex*, or top, of the lung), when they burst, the air leaks out of the lung.

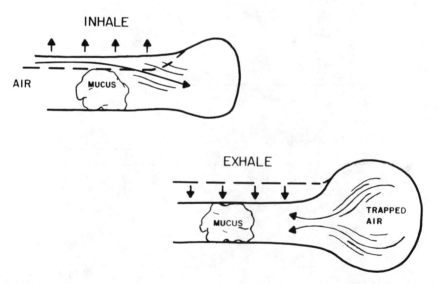

Figure 3.8. Partial obstruction of bronchi may cause progressive overinflation of a portion of lung, leading to pneumothorax. The bronchi enlarge slightly when one inhales, allowing air to get into the lungs past the mucus. When one exhales, the bronchi get smaller, trapping the air behind the blockage. With each breath, more and more air can become trapped, leading to progressive overinflation, and eventual tearing of the tissue, allowing air to escape from the lung.

A pneumothorax almost always causes sudden sharp pain in the chest, side, or back, and difficulty breathing (shortness of breath). The only way to tell for certain if someone has a pneumothorax is with a chest x-ray (Figure 3.7). The x-ray will show an area inside the chest that is completely black, rather than the usual combination of white and gray; there will also be a clear outline to the edge of the collapsed lung. Some people "score" pneumothoraces on the basis of how much of the lung is collapsed on the x-ray. A "25% pneumothorax" means that air outside the lung takes up 25% of the space that the lung normally occupies, and that the lung itself has collapsed to 75% of its normal size. If someone with relatively healthy lungs develops a pneumothorax, this can be a useful description. But when a pneumothorax occurs in someone with CF, it's less helpful, since the lungs tend to be stiff in people with CF, and therefore may not collapse readily, even with quite a bit of air outside, under quite a bit of tension. So, what looks like a small amount of air may actually be a lot.

Since pneumothoraces need to be treated, you should let your doctor know if you ever develop sudden chest pain and shortness of breath.

Treatment of Pneumothorax

The treatment for pneumothorax usually requires hospitalization, and is directed toward accomplishing three goals: (1) relieving the pressure on the lung by evacuating the air from around the lung, (2) sealing over the hole through which the air has escaped, and (3) ideally, preventing recurrence. There are rare instances in which there is a tiny pneumothorax—just the smallest bit of air outside the lung, with the leak already sealed off by itself—and no treatment is needed. Much more commonly, if there is a pneumothorax, all three treatment goals should be met.

The pressure is usually relieved by a *chest tube*. This is a tube that goes through the skin, between the ribs, and into the *pleural space*, which is the space between the chest wall and the outside of the lung. This is the space where air accumulates if it leaks out of the lung. The tube is hooked up to a vacuum that sucks the air out continuously and allows the lung to expand to its normal size. The system of tubing used to evacuate the air from the pleural space must have a good valving system (most often provided by having the tubes pass through a series of vacuum jars or a water seal) so that air can pass only out of the chest, and not back into it. The physician makes a small skin incision to place the chest tube, then pushes the tube into place and hooks up the vacuum. Placement of the tube can be painful, and having a tube in place is also uncomfortable. If the treatment chosen is only chest tube placement, the treatment is often successful in the short run, but very unsuccessful in the long run. Since most air leaks will seal themselves eventually, a chest tube can evacuate the air, and sooner or later the air will stop accumulating, and the tube can be pulled out. Unfortunately, it may take many days for this self-sealing to occur, and during this time, the painful chest tube will interfere with the deep breathing and coughing needed to keep the lungs clear. Even when the leak does seal itself, between 50% and 100% of these pneumothoraces will recur within months or years unless further steps are taken to prevent this from happening.

There are two main approaches to sealing the leak and preventing recurrences of pneumothorax. Both approaches purposely cause inflammation of the pleural surface (the covering of the lung), almost like a burn, so that when the irritated, inflamed surfaces heal, the healing scar tissue will cover over any weak, leaky area. The first approach is called *chemical sclerosing* or *chemical pleurodesis*. For this method, it is necessary to have a chest tube in the pleural space (the space between the lung and the chest wall). An irritating chemical (such as tetracycline, talc, or quinicrine) is sent through the tube once a day for three days in a row. When the chemical is pushed through the tube, the patient rotates through different positions, holding each one for several minutes in order to distribute the chemical to all surfaces of the lungs. The head-down position is particularly important, since the weakest spots are usually at the apex (top) of the lung. If the treatment is successful, it causes intense inflammation, and therefore is often very painful. Pain medication prior to the daily procedure is essential.

Another method of causing inflammation of the surface of the lung is with a surgical operation, during which the patient is asleep under general anesthesia. The surgeon makes an incision between the ribs, spreads the ribs, and examines the lung for weak spots (*blebs*). These areas are then cut out, and the remaining hole is sewn closed. The next step is to strip the pleura off the upper part of the lung, which leaves the lung surface raw and irritated. The side and lower portions of the lung are more difficult to strip of their pleural covering, so the surgeon will take a piece of gauze and rub the surface roughly to set up the same kind of irritation and inflammation. (This whole procedure is referred to as *open thoracotomy, apical pleurectomy, and pleurabrasion,* which means "cutting the chest open, stripping the membrane off the uppermost portion of the lung, and rubbing the rest of the lung surface.")

When the chest is closed, a chest tube must be left in to drain the extra air outside the lung. Usually that tube can come out when the air has been fully evacuated, and when it is clear that the leaks have been sealed. Although this procedure sounds brutal, the patient is asleep and feels no pain. After the surgery, the main discomfort is from the chest tube, which is usually removed within a few days. It is surprising, but true, that most people have less discomfort with the surgical treatment than with the chemical sclerosing. This treatment by an experienced surgeon is nearly 100% successful in preventing recurrences of pneumothorax in the involved lung. This time-honored procedure can in some cases be accomplished without actually opening the chest. Some specially trained and skilled surgeons can accomplish the pleural stripping and bleb-sewing through a *thoracoscope,* a tube that can be inserted into the chest, through a small incision in the chest wall. (This is similar to an *arthroscope,* which has allowed sports medicine orthopedic surgeons to operate on football players' knees without large incisions.) The surgeon looks through the thoracoscope while he or she manipulates special surgical *forceps* through another small hole in the chest wall. These forceps can grasp the pleura, and a similar tube can insert a device to staple over blebs. The surgeon can also inject a chemical (talc, for instance) through the thoracoscope to cause the necessary inflammation. Doing the procedure this way avoids a large chest incision, and greatly speeds recovery.

Treatment of pneumothorax has changed with the advent of lung transplantation (see Chapter 8, *Transplantation*), since the best treatment for preventing pneumothorax (surgery) may make future transplant much more difficult. The scar tissue that is purposely promoted to seal leaking blebs and prevent future leaks will make it very difficult for a transplant surgeon to remove the lungs in order to put new ones in. Therefore, some physicians recommend a stepwise approach to pneumothorax in a patient who may one day consider transplant, starting with no special treatment, and getting progressively more aggressive, ending with surgery, if steps short of the definitive surgery do not seal the leak.

Atelectasis

This term is derived from two Greek words (*ateles* + *ektasis*), meaning "incomplete" and "expansion," and refers to different kinds of incomplete expansion of the lung or part of the lung. Like pneumothorax, atelectasis is a kind of *collapsed lung*, but is very different from a pneumothorax. In someone with CF, atelectasis is almost always caused by mucus which completely blocks a bronchus leading to one of the lobes or segments of a lung (much more often in the right lung than the left, and more often in the upper lobe than in other lobes). If the opening to a lobe or segment is blocked, air cannot get into that portion of the lung. Eventually all the air that was in that lobe or segment gets absorbed, leaving the lobe or segment airless. On an x-ray it will appear white (solid) instead of the usual combination of white and gray (Figure 3.9). About 1 of every 20 people with CF will develop atelectasis at some point. This problem is more common in infants than older people, probably because their bronchi are smaller and therefore more readily blocked. Usually, atelectasis does not cause any specific signs or symptoms, but is likely to occur during a period of worsened lung infection.

Treating Atelectasis

Since atelectasis occurs when mucus totally blocks the opening of the bronchi in a segment or lobe of a lung, the treatment is similar to the maintenance care

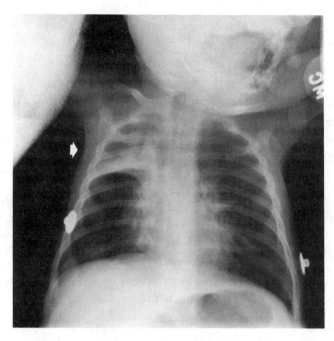

Figure 3.9. X-ray appearance of atelectasis of right upper lobe (x-ray taken as though we are looking at the front of the child, so his right side is on our left). The portion of the lung with more mucus and less air (the atelectatic portion) appears white, while the rest of the lung is darker.

designed to keep the bronchi clear on a regular basis. The mainstay of the treatment is airway clearance techniques, especially PD and percussion. Once atelectasis is identified, the physician will recommend increasing the frequency of PD treatments, perhaps to as often as four times a day. Most physicians will also recommend antibiotics, since infection may have caused the bronchial obstruction (by generating more mucus), and may also result from the obstruction. Physicians who don't usually advise their patients to inhale mucus-cutting drugs such as DNase (see Appendix B: *Medications*) may make an exception in treating atelectasis. There is little or no information to support its use in this particular circumstance, however.

Bronchoscopy (see above, *Hemoptysis*) with *lavage* (washing out mucus from the bronchi) is often employed in treating atelectasis. This is an appealing kind of treatment based on the logic that if mucus is blocking the bronchi, why not just go in and wash it out? Though it is logical, this treatment, unfortunately, is rarely successful.

The most inclusive study to examine the results of treating atelectasis with many different methods has shown that the traditional methods of PD and antibiotics are just as successful as invasive methods such as bronchoscopy. Successful treatment of atelectasis, regardless of the method chosen, may be slow, and it may take weeks or even months before the condition resolves.

Low Oxygen Level

Most people with CF who have any more than the mildest amount of lung disease will have a lower-than-normal blood oxygen level. In most cases, this causes no problems. If someone lives at sea level, extra oxygen is needed only when the lung disease is very severe. At higher altitudes, the air pressure is so low that it's harder to move oxygen from the air in the alveoli into the bloodstream. At the top of Mount Everest, the air pressure is less than half of what it is at sea level; up there, *everyone* needs to breathe extra oxygen. In Denver (and in the passenger cabins of commercial airliners), the pressure is about four-fifths of the sea level pressure. For people with normal lungs, this presents no problems; however, for someone with lung disease, it is likely to mean that extra oxygen will be needed.

With the appropriate treatment, which is simply getting extra oxygen to breathe, it's remarkable how much better a person can feel. The various ways to obtain oxygen are outlined in Appendix B: *Medications*.

Respiratory Failure

As its name implies, respiratory failure is the condition where the job of the respiratory system is not being accomplished, which is usually defined by the blood oxygen level being too low, and the blood carbon dioxide level being too high. This problem can occur in different people for different reasons (see *Gas Transfer and Delivery*). Most often, respiratory failure occurs at least partly because of lung disease. If the lungs are very severely affected by CF, it may be difficult for oxygen to be absorbed into the bloodstream at the alveoli; there will also be airway obstruction which can be so great that the work of breathing becomes too difficult for the ventilatory muscles. Except in very rare cases, this does not happen suddenly in CF. When respiratory failure *does* occur in someone with CF, it is in someone who has had severe lung disease for a long time.

Treatment of Respiratory Failure

Respiratory failure is another complication of CF where the best treatment is simply a continuation and intensification of the usual treatments aimed at reducing bronchial obstruction, infection, and inflammation. In many cases, however, respiratory failure occurs only after the usual treatments have failed, and there is so little healthy lung tissue remaining that it cannot sustain the functions of bringing adequate amounts of oxygen into the body and eliminating enough carbon dioxide. If the oxygen level is low enough and/or the carbon dioxide level high enough, this is clearly a life-threatening situation. (You may want to refer back to *Anatomy and Function of the Respiratory System* to review why this is so serious.)

In desperation, physicians and families may consider using a mechanical ventilator to do the extra breathing for the patient. In some special circumstances, this may be effective, and may support the sick patient long enough for the lungs to improve, so that independent life is once again possible. These very unusual instances include respiratory failure that occurs suddenly and in a previously well patient, for example, as a result of an automobile accident or, rarely, as a result of a sudden serious viral infection like influenza. Respiratory failure in infants under the age of one year is also a special circumstance in which temporary support with a mechanical ventilator may be helpful.

However, in most cases where respiratory failure occurs, it is at the end of a long process, and the use of a mechanical ventilator does not reverse that process. The majority of patients with CF who are put on mechanical ventilators either die while still on the ventilator or are never able to come off it, despite weeks or even months of very intensive care. In order for a ventilator to work, a patient needs to have a tube in the trachea (either through the nose or mouth, or as a tracheotomy tube, through an incision in the neck). These tubes are uncomfortable, and make it impossible to talk. Ventilator support almost always means living in an intensive care unit, where there is usually little or no privacy, little differentiation between day and night, and constant monitoring by machines and people.

Lung transplantation is a fairly new procedure in which a patient's lungs are removed from the chest and a new set of lungs and heart put in their place. By 1996, this procedure had been performed in several thousand people with various kinds of lung problems, including a few hundred with CF. Some patients have done extremely well with this procedure, and have been able to go back to work and resume a reasonably active life, while others have had many complications, and some have died. As with any new procedure, results are poor at first and improve as more experience is gained with them. This topic is discussed in Chapter 8, *Transplantation*.

Clearly, *the best treatment for respiratory failure is* **prevention.**

Cor Pulmonale and Heart Failure

Cor pulmonale literally means "heart disease caused by lung disease or breathing problems." Whenever the lungs are very severely affected (from almost any disease, including CF), or when the blood oxygen level is very low (from any cause), the blood vessels in the lung narrow, and it becomes difficult for the heart to pump blood through these blood vessels. Since it is the right side of the heart that pumps blood through the lungs, the right side of the heart gets a lot more exercise than usual. As with any other muscle, heart muscle will get bigger after it's had a lot of strenuous exercise. People who have had fairly severe lung disease for a period of time will commonly have a thick right-sided heart muscle, a condition called *right ventricular hypertrophy*. Not only will the muscle become thicker, but the whole right side of the heart may also expand. This enlargement is the way the heart adapts to the excess work it's being asked to do. It is most often a *successful* adaptation. Since this is a successful adjustment by the heart to a difficult situation, it is not considered heart *disease*. Though there is an abnormal *shape* and *size* to the right ventricle of the heart, this is quite different from *disease*, which is, by definition, harmful. Right ventricular hypertrophy is the *healthy* adjustment to the abnormally great demands placed on the normal heart by the diseased lungs.

If the lung disease remains too severe for too long, the heart may no longer be able to meet all the demands placed on it. It may not be able to pump all the blood that's necessary, and some fluid may back up. This fluid can sometimes be noticed in the ankles and lower legs, and sometimes a feeling of fullness in the right side of the abdomen under the ribs signifies fluid buildup in the liver. When the heart muscle fails to pump its entire assigned load, we say there is "heart failure," which is a frightening and misleading name for the condition, because it makes one think of heart *stoppage*, which it is not. Heart failure is the failure of the heart to do its *full* job. It is a serious problem, but one that indicates a serious lung problem rather than a problem with the heart itself.

Treatment of Cor Pulmonale and Heart Failure

Once again, the most effective treatment for this complication of CF lung disease is the aggressive treatment of the lung disease itself. In some cases, where there is excess fluid, a diuretic medication may be helpful (see Appendix B: *Medications*).

Chest Pain

Chest pain is a fairly common complication of CF and has many different causes. The major cause is pneumothorax. This is usually a sharp pain, that occurs suddenly, is limited to one side, and is accompanied by shortness of breath. Other problems, while not as dangerous as pneumothorax, can be just as bothersome. The musculoskeletal system can be the source of chest pain in CF, especially when someone is coughing a lot: strained muscles, pulled tendons, bruised or even broken ribs can occur. Infection involving the pleura (the membrane surrounding the lung) can be very uncomfortable, especially with deep breaths or coughs. This problem is called *pleuritis,* or sometimes *pleurisy.* Although anatomy books state that bronchi do not have pain-sensing nerves, some CF physicians think that pain may arise from large mucous plugs caught in small bronchi: clearly, some patients experience pain that disappears after they have coughed up a large plug of mucus. In younger people, the chest tightness that may accompany an asthma attack or a pulmonary exacerbation may seem like pain. Finally, there are nonpulmonary causes for chest pain in CF (heart attack is *not* among these): inflammation of the esophagus from acid reflux (see Chapter 4, *The Gastrointestinal Tract*) can cause "heartburn," which may be accompanied by difficulty in swallowing; and psychologic stress can certainly cause chest pain.

Bone and Joint Problems

People with CF who have absolutely no lung problems will not have any skeletal problems that can be attributed to CF. However, almost everyone with CF who has even the slightest degree of lung involvement (and that means almost everyone with CF) will have a condition called *digital clubbing.* This is an unfortunate name for this condition, since it sounds rather grotesque, and while in its most extreme form it can be very noticeable, in most cases it affects only slightly the shape of the fingers and toes. As shown in Figure 3.10, two features distinguish clubbed fingers from nonclubbed fingers: the first is the angle at which the base of the nail meets the finger. This angle becomes progressively flatter as clubbing increases. The second characteristic of a clubbed finger is that the thickness of the tip of the finger, the part beyond the last joint, when measured from the base of the nail to the bottom of the finger pad, becomes thicker than the finger at the joint itself.

The cause of digital clubbing is not known. In general, as lung disease worsens, so does clubbing. However, many people with fairly mild lung disease may also have pronounced clubbing. Therefore, clubbing itself does not precisely reflect the degree of lung involvement.

There are other conditions aside from CF that are associated with clubbing, including some forms of liver disease, inflammatory bowel disease, and heart diseases in which the blood oxygen level is too low. Clubbing is a very helpful diagnostic clue when a child with lung problems is being evaluated, since clubbing is found in most CF patients over the age of 1 or 2 years, and is very rare in children who do not have CF. Any child with chronic or recurrent respiratory problems and digital clubbing should be tested for CF.

Another complication of CF which may affect the skeletal system is one that causes bone or joint pain in the legs, particularly the knees. This problem is called *hypertrophic pulmonary osteoarthropathy* (HPOA). The name indicates that it is

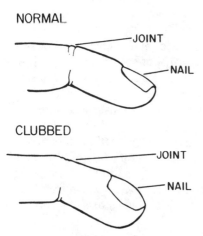

Figure 3.10. Digital (finger) clubbing. The clubbed finger is flattened at the angle where the nail meets the skin, and the tip of the finger is thicker than usual.

seen in people with pulmonary problems, and refers to "something wrong with" (*-opathy*) the bones (*osteo*) and/or joints (*arthro*). The term *hypertrophic* refers to x-ray findings in this condition, which include an elevation of the *periosteum* (the membrane covering the bone). This periosteal elevation makes it appear as though there is extra (*hyper*) *growth* (*-trophy*). The condition can be painful. It is not very common, and occurs mostly in people whose lung disease is severe. It usually improves as the lungs improve with treatment, but specific treatment for the bone/joint problem can also be helpful.

Finally, there is an uncommon and poorly understood arthritis—most commonly of the ankle or knee—that some people with CF get. The joint is tender, and may have a skin rash associated with it. It usually gets better with anti-inflammatory treatment, like aspirin or ibuprofen.

Treating Bone and Joint Problems

The degree of digital clubbing roughly corresponds with the degree of lung involvement, so treating the lungs may indirectly lessen the amount of clubbing. There is no treatment for clubbing aside from treatment of the lungs. Fortunately, a specific treatment is not required for clubbing, since it is not a painful condition. The only problem with clubbing is the embarrassment it can cause some people in adjusting to having fingers that look different from normal.

Osteoarthropathy may cause some physical discomfort, and people often will not mention it to their CF physicians, being unaware that leg or knee pain could be related to CF. As with clubbing, osteoarthropathy improves when the lungs improve. Regardless of the condition of the lungs, the discomfort of osteoarthropathy responds very well to aspirin, ibuprofen, and other similar anti-inflammatory drugs (see Appendix B: *Medications)*.

TESTS

Several kinds of tests can give important objective information about the lungs in someone with CF. These tests may be useful to confirm the physician's or patient's assessment of the patient's condition, to guide treatment, to measure the response to treatment, or in some cases to identify a problem before it has become evident to family or physician. Since most problems can be treated best if they are discovered early, many CF centers employ these tests on a regular basis, and not just when there is obvious trouble.

Pulmonary Function Tests

Pulmonary function tests (PFTs) are tests that measure various aspects of lung function. They can determine lung size, and presence and degree of bronchial obstruction. They can even give a good idea of which bronchi are blocked (the smallest bronchi or the larger central airways). They can identify asthma in children and adults, and they can measure the amount of oxygen circulating in the blood.

PFTs are a sensitive tool for following the condition of someone's lungs, showing subtle changes which might not have been detected otherwise. Since most PFTs require the understanding and cooperation of the patient, children under the age of 6 or 7 years may not be able to do these tests.

Spirometry

Spirometry ("measuring breathing") is the simplest PFT and is available in most hospitals and clinics. In this test, the patient breathes in and out through a tube while the machine records the amount of air breathed and the speed at which it is blown out.

Figure 3.11 shows two kinds of graphs that the spirometer can produce. The first (Figure 3.11A) records the amount (volume) of air blown out after the largest possible inhalation, and the time it takes to exhale it forcefully. Most of the air is exhaled in the first second, and all of it by 3 seconds. The most basic measurement from this curve is the *forced vital capacity* (FVC), the volume of air that is blown out in a single maximum exhaled breath. The next most commonly used measurement is the *forced expired volume in 1 second* (FEV$_1$), since this is a good indicator of whether there is blockage, and how much, particularly in the large central bronchi. The more obstruction there is, the more difficult it is to get air out of the lungs quickly, and the smaller the FEV$_1$. This is illustrated on the graph, where the solid line is from someone who has CF and normal lung function, and the dotted line is from someone who has CF and a moderate amount of obstruction.

The *maximum voluntary ventilation* (MVV) is similar to the spirometric tests just discussed. It calculates the maximum amount of air that someone can breathe in and out in 1 minute. The test doesn't last a whole minute, though. In most labs, the technician cheers and yells and vigorously encourages you to "Blow! Blow! Blow!" for either 12 or 15 seconds. The volume of air you've been able to breathe is then multiplied by 5 (for a 12-second test) or 4 (for a 15-second test) to give a value for 1 minute's worth of all-out effort.

These tests (FVC, FEV$_1$, MVV) are useful, but they have one important drawback, namely, they are very "effort-dependent," meaning that a half-hearted breath will give worthless information. Experienced technicians can very often tell from the shape of the curve whether the patient has given as good an effort as possible. Newer machines may print out numbers for the FVC and FEV$_1$, rather than a curve. With these machines it is extremely difficult to evaluate the information, since it is difficult to determine how reliable the effort was that went into the breath.

Another way of looking at the information from spirometry is the *flow-volume curve* (Figure 3.11B), which shows how quickly air flows out of the lungs at dif-

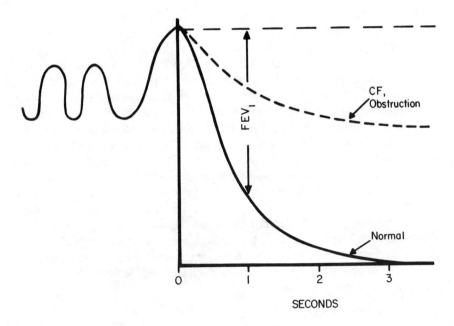

A

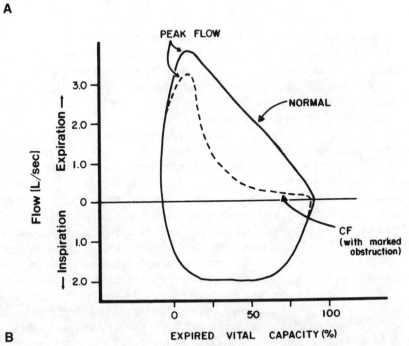

B

Figure 3.11. Pulmonary function tests. **A:** Spirometry. **B:** Flow-volume curve (see text for discussion).

ferent points during a maximum expiratory effort. This gives valuable information because air comes out much faster at the beginning of a breath, when the lungs are fully inflated, than it does later on in the breath, when the lungs are nearly empty. The flow-volume curve relates the flow rates to precise portions of the breath. For example, the MEF_{25} is the maximum expiratory flow rate at 25% of vital capacity, meaning it is the rate at which air flows out of the lungs during a maximum effort at the point when exactly 75% of the breath is gone (and 25% remains in the lungs). Another reason this information is so useful is that the flow rates during the second half of a breath out depend very little on how hard a breath is taken; that is, these flow rates are relatively effort-*in*dependent, and are therefore valuable even in someone whose cooperation is less than perfect. Finally, the flow rates at the end of a breath seem to be a good reflection of the amount of obstruction in the smallest bronchi: during the first part of the exhalation, the air quickly empties out of the larger bronchi, and during the last half or quarter of the breath the air empties out of the smallest bronchi. Therefore, a slower than normal second half of a breath can indicate some blockage in the smallest airways, even when the larger bronchi are unobstructed and the first half of the breath is perfectly normal.

Lung Volumes

Lung volumes are measured by two different methods and require complex machinery, which may not be available in every physician's office or hospital. Yet they can give valuable information that cannot be obtained with spirometry. Spirometry measures the air that moves in and out of the lungs, but indicates nothing about the actual size of the lungs or the amount of air left inside the lungs after a person has finished blowing out.

The *helium dilution method* for measuring lung volumes uses the "Iced Tea Principle." If you place a teaspoon of sugar into a full glass of iced tea, and mix it thoroughly, the sweetness of the tea will depend on the size of the glass. Clearly, an 8-ounce glass will be much sweeter with a teaspoon of sugar than a quart jar. Another way of saying this is—the smaller the glass, the greater the concentration of sugar. In fact, if you had tools precise enough to measure the exact sweetness or the exact concentration of sugar, and you knew the exact amount of sugar you put in (1 teaspoon, in this case) you could calculate the size of the glass.

For measuring lung volumes, the sugar-substitute is helium, a gas that is very safe to breathe in and which is not absorbed into the bloodstream. If you breathe in a known amount of helium for a few minutes, until it is thoroughly mixed with the air in your lungs, the concentration of helium in the air you breathe out can tell the size of your lungs. This method works fairly well for determining the size of your lungs at their largest (with the biggest breath in), and at their smallest (after you've breathed out all you can). These are the *total lung capacity* and *residual volume,* respectively. The method is not perfect because it requires that all of the bronchial tubes be open so that the helium can mix completely with all areas of the lung. If a portion of one lung is blocked off, the helium won't mix with the air in that part of the lung, and it will seem that the lungs are smaller than they actually are. What is measured by this method is the volume of lung which freely communicates with the mouth; that's the same as the total lung volume if the airways are healthy, but in obstructed lungs the volume will be underestimated.

The "body box" (*total body plethysmograph*) solves the problem of obstruction. It is an expensive piece of equipment that looks something like a space capsule. Not many hospitals are equipped with body boxes suitable for testing children. The person being tested sits inside the box and breathes through a tube. When the box is shut, it is completely airtight, which allows changes in pressure within the box to be measured very precisely while the person breathes. The changes in pressure reflect the changes in chest size. A mathematical formula is then applied that translates the pressure changes into accurate lung volume calculations, which include all of the lung volume, whether the bronchi are blocked or open. If someone does have bronchial obstruction, the total lung capacity will not be affected very much, but since obstruction (especially of small airways) makes it difficult to empty the lungs, the *residual volume* (the amount of air left in the lungs after a maximum exhalation) will be larger than normal. Normally, the residual volume is less than 25% of the total lung capacity, but in someone with severely blocked small airways, it can be as much as 70% of total lung capacity.

Asthma Testing

Asthma is a condition in which bronchi are blocked because of inflammation within bronchi and contraction of the muscles in the bronchial wall (this contraction of bronchial wall muscles is sometimes called *bronchospasm*). While the flow rates and lung volumes from the tests just described can tell if an obstruction is present, they can't tell what has caused it. However, if someone inhales a fast-acting bronchodilator, the bronchial muscle quickly relaxes, and the obstruction decreases. If the PFTs are repeated, the flow rates will show dramatic improvement within a few minutes. Since it's important to know how much obstruction is reversible, many laboratories will automatically schedule a bronchodilator inhalation and repeat spirometry as part of routine PFTs.

Some laboratories may go one step further, and try to identify people whose bronchi aren't yet blocked by bronchospasm but are *susceptible* to such blockage. These are people with *reactive airways*, which is another term for asthma. These people may have completely normal pulmonary function at a given time, but if they inhale certain chemicals, their bronchial muscles may contract much more readily than the bronchial muscles of someone with normal airways. To test for this, people may be asked to breathe in these chemicals (*methacholine* is the one most commonly used in this country; histamine is another), starting with a very dilute solution, and increasing step by step to a stronger solution, repeating the spirometry after each new challenge. The test is completed when the PFTs worsen. Someone has reactive airways disease if his or her PFTs get worse with a dilute (weak) solution of the chemical. These tests which measure airway reactivity are called *bronchial provocation* or *inhalation challenge tests*. Other bronchial challenge tests involve PFTs before and after exercise or before and after inhaling cold dry air.

Blood Gases

Since the major job of the lungs is to bring oxygen into the bloodstream and to eliminate carbon dioxide, it may be important to know the blood oxygen and carbon dioxide levels. To find this out, a blood gas test is performed by inserting a needle into an artery and drawing out blood. Since a needle inserted into an artery can be much more painful than one inserted into a vein, a small amount of xylocaine may be injected into the skin first, or the skin is prepared with EMLA® cream which numbs the skin and makes the test more tolerable.

Oximetry

Over the past few years, painless, noninvasive monitors have been developed which decrease the need for arterial blood gases. These monitors are called *oximeters* (either ear oximeters or pulseoximeters), and they work through a computerized method: a light is shined through the fingertip or earlobe to a sensor on the other side of the finger or ear; the amount of light that can pass through the tissues is determined partly by the amount of oxygen that is in the blood in those tissues. The oxygen saturation of the blood is calculated almost instantaneously by computer, and is indicated on a digital display.

Exercise Tests

Standard pulmonary function tests measure lung function while a person is resting. It may be useful in some situations to see how the lungs (and heart) function when they are put under some stress, as with exercise. Exercise tests can range from the very simple (listening to someone's lungs after he or she has been running in a hallway) to the very complex (measuring the precise amounts of oxygen consumed, carbon dioxide produced, oxygen exhaled, time it takes to inhale and exhale, rate of breathing, heart rate, etc.). Many physicians feel that the exercise test is more successful than regular PFTs in detecting mild problems. This is because a mild problem will not present itself unless the system is stressed, as when people exert themselves to the limit. For most exercise tests, the person being tested pedals on a stationary exercise cycle or walks/runs on a treadmill. The test begins with an easy pace, and gets increasingly difficult. While the test is going on, you may have to breathe through a mouthpiece like a scuba diver's, so that the air you breathe in and out can be analyzed. In other tests, you may have electrocardiogram (ECG) electrodes taped on your chest. In some tests, oximeters may be used, with a light taped to your finger or ear. In very special tests, there may even be a small plastic tube placed in the artery at your wrist. In other tests, none of those monitors may be used.

Exercise tests can show how physically fit a person is, and one study has shown that fitness level (as measured on an exercise test) was the test that correlated most closely with a CF patient's likelihood of surviving the next eight years or more.

Chest X-rays

X-rays are generated by a machine that functions similarly to a camera. The x-ray machine is directed at the object to be studied, and generates x-rays, which pass through that object, in varying amounts and intensity. The x-rays then strike and expose photographic paper which is situated behind the object. When there is no object in the way, and the x-rays hit the photographic paper directly, it becomes completely black. When an object such as lead is in the way, which totally blocks all the x-rays, the paper becomes completely white. The thicker or more dense a material, the more rays it absorbs, and the whiter the image of that material on the resulting x-ray film. When the object in question is a person's chest, there will be recognizable white/black/gray patterns determined by the bones, lungs, heart, etc. The bones are quite dense, and therefore will appear white on the final x-ray. The heart, because it consists of thick muscle and is filled with blood, also appears fairly white. The lungs are much less dense, since they are relatively delicate tissues largely filled with air, and therefore appear much blacker, or at least a darker shade of gray. The lungs do contain some dense tissue, including blood vessels, so they are not totally black. The diaphragms mark the lower edges of the lungs, and are white since they are fairly solid muscle.

Chest x-rays can give important information about the condition of the lungs. If, for example, a lobe of the lung is collapsed because it is filled with mucus, that lobe will appear much denser (whiter) than normal. If thick scar tissue has replaced healthy lung tissue, that too will be whiter than usual. Bronchial walls swollen by fluid or inflammation may have a similar appearance. In many cases it is possible to see "increased markings," meaning more white (dense) markings than normal, but it is not possible to tell if the increased density is caused by inflammation or mucus (which can get better), or by scar tissue (which cannot get better).

A pneumothorax, in which air has escaped through a leak in the lung but is still within the chest, will show up on the x-ray as a totally black area outside the lung, while the lung itself will be whiter than normal (see Figure 3.7). The totally black area is air, and the lung will appear denser (whiter) than normal since it is partly collapsed, with the solid parts of the lung closer together than normal.

Lungs that are obstructed and difficult to empty will be larger than normal, and will push the diaphragms downward (Figure 3.12). These over inflated

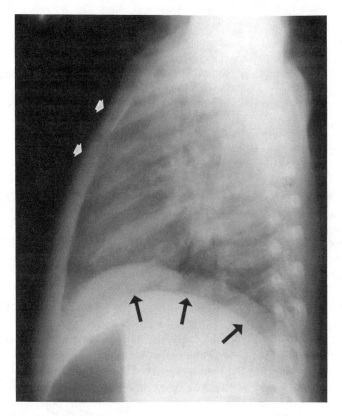

A

Figure 3.12. X-ray appearance of overinflation of lungs. These are lateral (side) views of the chest of two different children with CF. **A** shows normal lungs, with nicely domed diaphragms (*black arrows*), a normally straight breast bone (sternum—*white arrows*), and little air directly behind the sternum. In contrast, **B** shows severe overinflation of the lungs, with the diaphragms pushed downwards and flattened (*black arrows*), and the sternum "bowed" outward (*white arrows*), and excessive air (*blacker*) behind the sternum. Note, too, that the overall depth of the chest from the sternum to the spine is much greater in the overinflated chest. This is referred to as an *increased AP* (anterior-posterior) *diameter.*

(*hyperinflated*) lungs may not only push the diaphragms down into a flattened shape (compared with the normal dome shape), but may actually push the sternum (the front of the chest) forward. This is called *sternal bowing* (since the shape of the sternum comes to resemble an archery bow).

Cultures and Sensitivities

It is important to know what bacteria are in the bronchi of someone with CF, in case antibiotic treatment becomes necessary. To identify bacteria, small samples of mucus are sent to a bacteriology laboratory where they are placed in

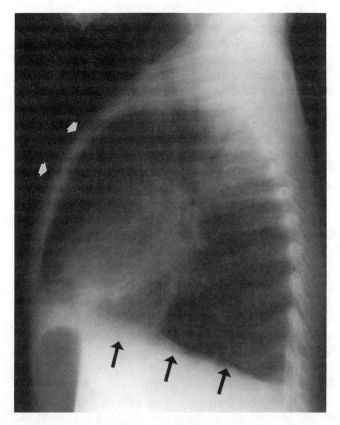

Figure 3.12. *(Continued.)*

different substances called *media*. Some media are good environments for all types of bacteria to grow in, and others will allow only certain bacteria to grow. After the bacteria have grown they are analyzed and identified, with the entire process taking several days.

Once the bacteria are grown and identified, the task remains of determining which antibiotics are the most effective in killing those bacteria. To find this out, various antibiotics are added to the cultures and their effects are observed. One method of introducing antibiotics is through the use of paper discs that have been soaked with the antibiotic. These discs are placed at intervals around the plate where the bacteria are grown (Figure 3.13). If the antibiotic kills the bacteria, there will be a clear area around the disc, where the bacteria have not been able to grow (this clear area is called the *zone of inhibition*). If the bacteria are not killed by the antibiotic, they continue to grow right up to the disc, leaving no clear

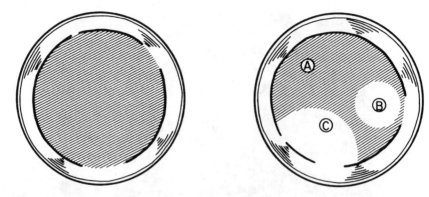

Figure 3.13. Culture and sensitivity testing, showing clear zones around the antibiotic discs. The larger the clear space around the disc, the more potent the antibiotic has been in preventing the bacteria from growing.

zone. Sometimes there will be a very small zone, sometimes a larger one. Most laboratories will define the response to the antibiotic based on the size of the clear zone. For example, when the antibiotic gentamicin is used in cultures of *Pseudomonas,* the bacteria are proclaimed *sensitive* to the antibiotic if the clear area is 15 mm or larger; if the clear area is 13–14 mm, it is considered *intermediate,* and if it is 12 mm or less, the bacteria are said to be *resistant* to the effects of the antibiotic. "Resistance" is thus a relative term, since the presence of even a very small clear space indicates that some bacteria have been killed. This also means that the laboratory might report a culture back as showing the bacteria to be "resistant" to a particular antibiotic, and your doctor might decide to use it anyway. Frequently in this kind of situation, the antibiotic has its desired effect despite the laboratory report.

SUMMARY

The respiratory system accounts for over 95% of the illness and deaths from CF, and therefore keeping it healthy is the most important thing that can be done for anyone with CF. Fortunately, there is much that can be done toward this end, and the tremendous improvement in life expectancy of CF patients can be attributed largely to better prevention and treatment of lung problems. Most of the problems that develop in the lung are the result of bronchial blockage caused by thick mucus, and of infection which follows the blockage. Physical means, such as postural drainage and percussion treatments, and medications, including bronchodilators, help prevent and reverse bronchial obstruction. Antibiotics, given by mouth, aerosol, or injection, are very successful in treating bronchial infection.

4

The Gastrointestinal Tract

THE BASICS

1. Most people with CF need to take pancreatic enzymes with their meals to help digest their food.
2. People who skip their enzymes (or whose enzymes are not working right) will have abdominal pain and frequent, large, smelly, loose bowel movements, and will have trouble gaining weight.
3. With help from the CF center, almost everyone can learn how much enzyme to use.
4. Some CF patients have intestinal blockage that needs to be treated promptly. The signs of this problem are "stomachaches" and fewer bowel movements than normal. If your child has no bowel movement for 24 hours, call the CF center immediately.
5. Some babies and children with CF have gastroesophageal reflux (acid moving backward from the stomach into the esophagus).
6. To minimize reflux, put your baby to sleep on its stomach.
7. A few CF patients have serious liver problems.

THE NORMAL GASTROINTESTINAL TRACT

The gastrointestinal tract is made up of the organs that digest food (Figure 4.1). One way to understand how the gastrointestinal tract normally works in people without cystic fibrosis (CF) is to think about what happens to the parts of a meal when they are eaten. For this purpose we can use a (not completely well-rounded) meal consisting of meat, potato with butter, a glass of whole milk, and a dessert

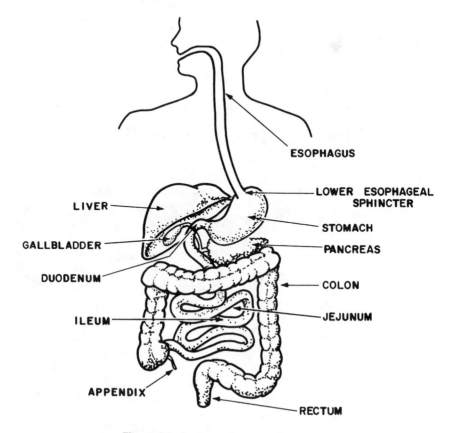

Figure 4.1. Anatomy of gastrointestinal tract.

of candy. Each of these foods has a mix of nutrients: *protein, fat,* and *carbohydrate.* For this discussion, however, the meat will represent its main component, protein; the potato, starch (a carbohydrate with complex branching chains of molecules); the butter, fat; and the candy, sucrose (a carbohydrate that is simpler than starch). The milk contains another simple carbohydrate, lactose, as well as fat and protein.

None of this food would stay in the body if it were not broken down into small particles that can be absorbed into the bloodstream. This breaking-down process is called *digestion.* When a person eats such a meal, digestion begins immediately in the **mouth**. Saliva contains digestive enzymes called *amylase* and *lipase,* and when these are mixed with the food during chewing, the amylase starts to break down the starch of the potato, and the lipase starts to break down the fat of the butter and milk. You will notice that most of the enzymes that break down food end in "-ase" or "-sin."

The **esophagus** is not actively involved in the process of digestion. It is a tube that moves the chewed food from the mouth to the stomach. It does have an important role, however, for it must move food down without air getting in, and it must let air or food come up when the need arises to belch or vomit. It is the esophagus that keeps food and liquid in the stomach, even when a person is upside down.

The chewed-up meat, potato, butter, milk, and candy have now passed through the esophagus into the **stomach**. Here, the protein in the meat and milk is acted upon by the enzyme *pepsin,* which is secreted by the stomach.

When the food has been ground up by the stomach into small particles, the partly digested food is released slowly into the **duodenum**, the first part of the **small intestine**. Several inches beyond the stomach, in the duodenum, is a tiny opening through which juices from the **liver** and **pancreas** flow into the duodenum. These juices contain large amounts of important digestive enzymes made by the pancreas, and bile salts (also called bile acids) made by the liver. Among the pancreatic enzymes are proteases, which digest proteins. *Trypsin* and *chymotrypsin* are two protein-digesting enzymes that continue the digestion of the protein from the meat and milk after it has passed from the stomach. Two other important pancreatic enzymes are *amylase,* which, like salivary amylase, continues to break down the potato's starch, and *lipase*, which digests nearly all the fat in the butter and milk. Lipase is a particularly important enzyme because it is the major fat-digesting enzyme in the digestive tract, and also because it is very fragile, and is destroyed when in the presence of too much acid. Lipase also has other requirements to function well: bile salts, made by the liver, and colipase, made by the pancreas, are both needed in the duodenum for lipase to work well.

The products of all of this digestion of protein and fat and starch are absorbed by the tiny cells of the wall of the small intestine as the muscles of the intestine squeeze the food slowly along toward the **large intestine** (also called the **colon**). There are enzymes attached to the cells of the wall of the small intestine that break down simple carbohydrates such as the sucrose of the candy and the lactose of the milk, just before they are absorbed by the intestinal cells. Other enzymes on these cells complete the digestion of starch and protein that was begun by the enzymes from the pancreas. Once the food has been broken down into these tiny particles and taken into the intestinal cells, it passes into the bloodstream and is carried to the various parts of the body where it is needed.

In a person whose gastrointestinal tract is working properly, nearly all of the nutritious food that is eaten is digested by the pancreatic enzymes and absorbed by the intestinal cells into the bloodstream. Very little of the food gets to the colon. That person's bowel movements contain indigestible fiber from the food, some water to keep the movement soft, and quite a lot of the bacteria that normally live in the large intestine. Very little of the carbohydrate and protein, and less than 7% of the fat, is wasted.

THE GASTROINTESTINAL TRACT IN CYSTIC FIBROSIS

The remainder of this chapter is devoted to the problems that occur in the gastrointestinal tract in patients with CF, with each problem being reviewed under the affected organ. Table 4.1 lists the problems and the frequency with which they occur.

TABLE 4.1. Incidence of Gastrointestinal Conditions in Cystic Fibrosis

Organ	Condition	CF Patients with Condition (%)
Pancreas	Pancreatic insufficiency	85–90[a]
	Pancreatitis	1
	Diabetes	1–5[b]
Liver and gallbladder	Cirrhosis	1–4
	Gallstones	10
Esophagus and stomach	Gastroesophageal reflux	10–20
	Ulcers	1–10
Intestines	Meconium ileus	10
	Meconium peritonitis	1
	DIOS[c]	10–30
	Rectal prolapse	10–20
	Intussusception	1

[a]At birth, only about 50% are pancreatic-insufficient.
[b]Diabetes is extremely uncommon before the age of 10 years; thereafter, it occurs in about 10% of patients until age 20 years, and in another 10–20% from 20 to 30 years.
[c]Distal intestinal obstruction syndrome.

Pancreas

Pancreatic Insufficiency

Abnormal mucus blocks the tiny tubes in the pancreas of people with CF, much as it does in the lungs. This means that the pancreatic digestive enzymes are not secreted into the intestine as they should be. (Remember that these enzymes are *lipase,* which digests fat; *amylase,* which digests starch; and the *proteases,* including trypsin and chymotrypsin and others, which digest proteins.) Pancreatic insufficiency refers to the inability of the pancreas to secrete *enough* digestive enzymes for normal digestion and absorption. This does not happen until nearly all (90%) of the normal enzyme activity is lost, so the pancreatic secretion must be quite low for pancreatic insufficiency to occur. In fact, most people with CF have extensive damage to their pancreas, so that it is largely replaced by scar tissue and fat, and they need to take enzymes by mouth with their meals. Until recently, it was thought that pancreatic insufficiency was present from birth. We now know that nearly 50% of infants with CF have pancreatic *sufficiency,* that is, they retain enough functioning pancreatic tissue for the digestion and absorption of their food, without needing enzyme supplements. In the first months and years of life, most of these *pancreatic-sufficient* infants lose pancreatic function, so that by age 8 or 9 years, fully 85%–90% of CF patients will have pancreatic insufficiency, and will need to take enzymes with meals to digest their food. Somewhere between 10% and 15% of patients with CF remain pancreatic-sufficient all their lives. This one characteristic—whether someone will be pancreatic-sufficient or pancreatic-insufficient—seems to be determined in large part by which particular abnormal CF genes he or she has received (see Chapter 11, *Genetics,* for more details).

Before effective treatment was available, most CF children died in infancy, in part from starvation (malnutrition) due to their pancreatic insufficiency.

The intestinal cells have a "backup" group of enzymes that do fairly well at digesting starch and protein when the pancreas is not working properly. In this case, however, the digestion and absorption of starch is not complete, and the remaining starch may cause gas when it gets to the large intestine (colon). The digestion of protein is also not complete, so that some patients, especially infants, may have low levels of protein in the blood. If protein levels are sufficiently low, fluid may leak out of the blood vessels and cause puffy skin (*edema*).

The intestinal cells do not have a backup means to digest fat, and the effectiveness of the lipase produced by the salivary glands is limited. Therefore, most CF patients do not digest and absorb fat well, and fat is passed out of the body in the bowel movements. Fat makes the bowel movements large, greasy, and more smelly than normal. Furthermore, all of the fat that comes out in the bowel movements is lost to the body. A given amount of fat has more calories than any other kind of food, so losing an ounce of fat means losing more than twice as many calories as would be lost in an ounce of carbohydrate or protein. Loss of fat in the bowel movements thus leads to malnutrition and poor growth, despite a huge appetite. The "textbook picture" of a youngster with undiagnosed CF is someone who is scrawny, has a huge appetite, and has frequent, large, smelly, greasy stools. This person is scrawny because most of the nutrients in the food consumed go directly into the toilet; the apparently huge appetite is really a way of compensating for losing half of what is eaten in the bowel movements—it's as if you've been fed a half portion, so you eat another portion to make up for that. Fat malabsorption may also lead to the lack of special kinds of fatty nutrients that are essential to health—"essential fatty acids," and fat-soluble vitamins (vitamins A, D, E, and K). (A detailed discussion of vitamins and fatty acids is in Chapter 6, *Nutrition*.)

Diagnosis

There are several ways in which a physician can determine if someone has pancreatic insufficiency. One method is simply a review of the history of bowel movements: frequent, greasy, smelly, large bowel movements usually indicate pancreatic insufficiency. Another method is a test that involves taking a small sample of stool (bowel movement), staining it with a dye that will make whatever fat there is in the stool an easily noticeable color, and then examining it under the microscope. A large amount of fat in the sample indicates that fat was not digested and absorbed, which suggests pancreatic insufficiency. A more accurate stool test is the *72-hour fecal fat test,* which—as you've probably guessed—involves collecting all bowel movements for three whole days and nights in a large, sealable container (usually the laboratory supplies a paint can). At the same time the stool collection is going on, the family keeps a careful food diary, listing every bite of every food the patient eats over the three days. The nutritionist can then calculate how many grams of fat were eaten, and the laboratory staff can see how many grams of fat came out in the stool. Most healthy people will absorb at least 93% of the fat they eat. Put another way, less than 7% of the dietary fat should appear in the stool. More than 7% fat excretion means there is *malabsorption* (not as much absorbed as normal), which suggests incomplete digestion, usually caused by insufficient pancreatic enzymes.

Pancreatic insufficiency can also be evaluated by analyzing the amount of trypsin and chymotrypsin in the stools. Absent enzymes, or very low levels of enzymes, suggest that the pancreas has not released the enzymes. However, this test can be misleading, since some of the bacteria that live in the intestines can produce trypsin, while others can destroy it.

A more reliable test for pancreatic insufficiency is the Chymex® (or *bentiromide*) test. In this test, the patient takes in a chemical by mouth. This chemical (bentiromide) is composed of two ingredients, *p*-aminobenzoic acid (PABA) and benzyl-L-tyrosine (BzTyr). This chemical is so large that it cannot be absorbed, so it passes through the body into the stools. But if PABA is separated from BzTyr, the PABA is small enough that it can be absorbed into the bloodstream, filtered by the kidneys, and then excreted in the urine. Pancreatic chymotrypsin is the only substance that can separate PABA from BzTyr. Therefore, if PABA appears in the urine, then chymotrypsin must have been available from the pancreas.

A final laboratory test for pancreatic insufficiency is more invasive than those just discussed. This test involves passing a tube through the nose, esophagus, and stomach into the duodenum, then collecting fluid directly from the point at which the pancreas empties its enzymes. The fluid can then be analyzed directly for enzyme content.

The test that is probably used more than any other is called a *therapeutic trial;* it is also called "trial and error," although physicians prefer the first term. In this test, enzymes are administered to the patient, and the physician observes what happens—particularly what happens to the patient's stools, appetite, and growth. Since enzymes in small doses are not harmful, and are not very expensive, this can be a good, sensible test. It may not always give the most accurate information in the fastest time, however.

There is a substance that French CF researchers have found, called PAP (for *p*ancreatitis *a*ssociated *p*rotein), which seems to be found in elevated levels in people with CF and pancreatic insufficiency. It is not yet clear whether this will become a widely used and reliable test for pancreatic insufficiency.

One further test that is being used primarily as a newborn screening test for CF also relates to pancreatic function. This is a blood test that is performed on the first or second day of life. A dried spot of blood is analyzed for *immunoreactive trypsin (IRT),* a substance that is found in higher quantities in the blood of newborns with CF than in those without CF. It is not known why this is so, but it may be that the trypsin, which can't get out of the pancreas into the duodenum, "backs up" into the bloodstream. One problem with this explanation is that even most CF babies with pancreatic sufficiency have an abnormal IRT. (Perhaps these pancreatic-sufficient babies have *some* pancreatic blockage—not total, and enough trypsin and other enzymes get into the duodenum to bring about normal digestion and absorption—but enough blockage that *some* trypsin backs up into the bloodstream and is detected by the IRT.) The test is not perfect for identifying CF, since there are many *false positives* (babies who don't have CF, but who test abnormal for IRT). Nevertheless, the test is being used in many hospitals (and even some statewide programs) in the United States and in several countries around the world. It is discussed a bit more in the *Introduction*, in the section *Diagnosis of CF*.

Treatment

Treatment of pancreatic insufficiency is fairly simple and the results are dramatic, now that pancreatic enzyme replacement is possible through the use of granules, powder, or capsules taken with meals. Although it may seem complicated when families are first introduced to enzymes, virtually everyone who has CF or who has a child with CF soon becomes an expert at using enzymes. These enzymes are often *enteric-coated,* meaning that they are protected from the stomach acid by a coating that dissolves only when it is in a nonacidic surrounding. These enzymes pass through the stomach and begin to dissolve in the duodenum, which is a nonacidic environment (see Chapter 6, *Nutrition,* and Appendix B: *Medications).* Since the raw enzymes (especially lipase) are easily inactivated by acid, the introduction of enteric-coated enzyme preparations was revolutionary, and made a huge difference in the effectiveness of this very important part of CF treatment. The quantity of enzymes to be taken is determined by evaluating such factors as bowel movements, appetite, and weight gain (and is discussed further in Chapter 6, *Nutrition,* and in Appendix B: *Medications*). On rare occasions, more formal tests, such as the 72-hour fecal fat test discussed above, may be needed.

The amount of enzyme taken must be adjusted properly, since too much enzyme can occasionally cause problems. Usually, taking too much enzyme has no medical consequences, and no change in bowel habits, appetite, or growth will result. The only consequences will be financial ones (paying for more enzymes than you need). On occasion, though, too much enzyme can cause one of two medical problems, one usually not serious, the other quite serious. A few patients who take too much enzyme will have a change in their bowel habits, most commonly with their stools becoming a bit looser than normal, and less commonly with patients becoming constipated. These problems are most often just a nuisance, and resolve quickly with lowering the enzyme dose. In recent years, with the availability of super-high-dose enzyme preparations, a new, serious, but rare, problem has been recognized: some patients taking very high doses of enzymes have had scarring of their large intestine, causing abdominal pain, often with bloody diarrhea, and many have needed surgery to correct the problem. This problem has never been seen except in those patients taking extremely high doses of enzymes. The usual enzyme doses, and those that have been associated with this problem, called *fibrosing colonopathy,* are discussed in Chapter 6, *Nutrition.* ("Fibrosing colonopathy" means something is wrong with the colon, which leads to the formation of scar tissue—*fibrosis*.)

Since the CF pancreas also does not produce the bicarbonate-rich acid-neutralizing juice found in the normal pancreas, stomach acid is not always neutralized when it passes into the duodenum. This means the duodenum may be more acidic than normal, and enteric-coated enzymes may not be properly activated (the coating may not dissolve). Therefore, some CF children need treatment with antacids (medicines that neutralize acid), or medicines that decrease the stomach's production of acid, like cimetidine, ranitidine, or omeprazole (see Appendix B: *Medications*) to make their enzymes work. Infants who are given the enzymes as non-enteric-coated granules or powder may develop an irritation around the mouth or buttocks, and mothers who are breast-feeding these infants may develop nipple irritation. For all these reasons, the enteric-coated enzymes are usually much better than the non-enteric-coated enzymes, especially in infants. (See Appendix B: *Medications,* for more details about taking enzymes.)

Pancreatitis

Pancreatitis is an inflammation of the pancreas that causes severe abdominal pain and usually vomiting. It occurs in people without CF, sometimes due to gallstones blocking secretion of the pancreas, sometimes due to drinking alcohol, sometimes as a side effect of medications, and sometimes for other, rarer, reasons. Pancreatitis is uncommon among CF patients, probably in part because most CF patients do not have enough intact pancreatic tissue to become inflamed. In fact, patients with CF and pancreatic insufficiency virtually **never** develop pancreatitis. Among the few CF patients with pancreatic sufficiency, very few will get pancreatitis. Pancreatitis is diagnosed with blood and urine tests and with x-rays. Eating calls on the pancreas to work, and this worsens inflammation, so the treatment of pancreatitis usually involves a stay in the hospital, during which time no food is given by mouth, and nutrition is given intravenously. Taking pancreatic enzymes may also help this problem to resolve. Although the problem is rare, it often recurs in those unfortunate enough to have it.

Diabetes

In addition to producing digestive enzymes and acid-neutralizing juices, the pancreas produces hormones, especially insulin. Insulin is needed by the body to move glucose, the body's main simple carbohydrate used for energy, from the blood into the body's cells. When insulin is not produced as it is needed, diabetes results, with elevated *blood glucose* (blood sugar) levels.

Diabetes involves many complicated processes in the body. The high level of blood glucose causes glucose to be lost in the urine, and this glucose takes water with it that is needed by the body. The loss of glucose and water from the body produces other changes that can make people with diabetes malnourished, dehydrated, and quite ill. Sugar in the urine pulls extra water with it, so people with diabetes lose water in addition to sugar and calories. They urinate a lot, and drink a lot, and may lose weight and feel "dragged out."

Nearly one-half of all people with CF have some limitation of the ability of their pancreas to produce insulin, which is detectable with special tests. However, only a very small proportion of CF patients have diabetes—that is, glucose lost in their urine. Almost no one under the age of 10 years has this problem, and between the ages of 10 and 20 years, approximately 10% of CF patients develop it. From the ages of 20–30 years, another 10%–20% develop it, and so forth, with an additional 10%–20% developing diabetes with every additional decade. Stresses like pregnancy, worsened lung infection, or medications—most notably, steroids, which are sometimes used to control CF lung disease—can bring on CF diabetes. Diabetes that appears during these stresses often goes away when the stress is removed. The diabetes in CF patients tends to be milder than the diabetes in other children, and is less apt to produce serious illness. The treatment for diabetes involves taking insulin by injection every day, in some cases several times a day, and cutting down on the amount of "simple sugars" (candy, soda pop, etc.) in the diet. There is conflicting information about the influence of diabetes on the overall health of people with CF, with some studies suggesting that CF patients with diabetes die earlier than those without diabetes. Other studies have shown no difference in survival between those CF patients with and without diabetes.

Intestines

Meconium Ileus

Meconium is a baby's first bowel movement, formed in the intestine while the baby is still in the mother's womb. Since the baby has had nothing to eat, this bowel movement is formed from bits of mucus and intestinal cells shed into the intestines before birth. It is usually darker and stickier than the infant's stools will be once he or she starts taking milk.

In infants with CF, the meconium is much thicker and stickier than usual, probably because of the abnormal sticky mucus that CF patients seem to make throughout the body, almost certainly related to the basic defect (see Chapter 1, *The Basic Defect*). In about 10% of babies with CF, this meconium is so thick that it clogs in the ileum [the third part of the small intestine, right near the appendix (see Figure 4.1)] and blocks up the intestines. This condition is called *meconium ileus*. This prevents the baby from having a bowel movement, and therefore causes the abdomen to swell—usually within the first 2 days after birth. In such babies, meconium ileus is usually the first clue that they have CF. Sometimes the intestines get so filled because of the blockage that a hole is broken in the intestinal wall, and meconium escapes into the abdomen. This is called *meconium peritonitis,* and can make the baby quite sick. It occurs in about 10% of infants with meconium ileus, meaning approximately 1% of all infants with CF.

Treatment for meconium ileus can be given with special x-rays and enemas, but sometimes surgery is required. The x-ray and enema, called a *Gastrografin®* *enema,* involves putting Gastrografin, or a similar product into the rectum, and letting it run back through the colon. Gastrografin is a liquid with three characteristics that make it ideal to use in this situation: (1) it is very slippery and can get by just about any obstruction; (2) it is very concentrated and acts like a dry sponge, pulling fluid into the intestines and watering down the thick meconium; and (3) it appears on an x-ray, so the progress of the whole procedure can be followed. When this procedure is carried out by radiologists experienced in its use in infants (ideally with the cooperation of surgeons and CF specialists), it is safe and very effective. However, in some infants, these enemas will not relieve the obstruction and surgery becomes necessary. All infants with meconium peritonitis require surgery. When the surgery is performed by surgeons with experience in infants, it is usually successful. Babies who have had surgery have a slightly higher likelihood of developing intestinal obstruction later in life because after abdominal surgery in *anyone* (infants or older people; CF or non-CF), scars (adhesions) may form and block the intestines.

Meconium ileus is a serious problem, but most infants who have it do very well after it is treated. If they make it through the difficult first few weeks, their outlook is similar to other CF babies who have not had meconium ileus. Meconium ileus occurs almost exclusively in infants with CF; therefore, a baby with meconium ileus should be diagnosed immediately, and general CF care should begin right away. A sweat test should be performed, despite a commonly held misconception that babies don't sweat enough for a valid sweat test. In fact, most babies do give plenty of sweat for analysis and diagnosis. In those few infants who do not produce enough sweat, the baby should be treated *as though he or she has CF* until a definite diagnosis can be made, perhaps with genetic testing, perhaps with a repeat sweat test (see the *Introduction* and Chapter 11, *Genetics,* for more discussion of tests used to diagnose CF).

DIOS (Distal Intestinal Obstruction Syndrome)

DIOS involves blockage of the intestines that is similar to meconium ileus, but occurs after infancy. Because of its similarity to meconium ileus, the problem used to be called "meconium ileus equivalent," even though intestinal contents are not referred to as "meconium" in anyone older than a newborn. The intestinal contents usually block the same area of the ileum (just before the colon) as in meconium ileus, but sometimes the blockage occurs farther along, in the colon.

DIOS may be brought on by too few enzymes (since that will make the stools very large and bulky), or by dietary changes, and it is somewhat more common in children who have had meconium ileus as newborns, especially if they had surgery. In rare cases, it may be caused by an excess of enzymes. In many cases, it is not known what caused the blockage, other than the thickening of the intestinal mucus.

Crampy stomachaches and constipation are the symptoms produced by DIOS, and often the blockage can be felt by the doctor, when he or she examines the patient's abdomen, or seen on x-rays. If a person with CF has severe abdominal pain and no bowel movements, it is most likely due to this problem. No bowel movements for 24 hours should prompt an urgent call to the CF center.

Treatment for this complication of CF may involve continuing to take enzymes, taking stool softeners or special laxative preparations, and having special x-ray examinations and enemas. Although it rarely requires surgery, it must be attended to promptly so that more serious problems, such as bursting or leaking of the bowels, do not occur.

Intussusception

Intussusception is a very rare problem that occurs when part of the intestine is pulled along inside another part of the intestine in much the same way that a telescope collapses in on itself (Figure 4.2). Intussusception can be a complication of DIOS, and the part of the intestine that is pulled along is usually the end of the ileum, which is pulled into the colon. What probably causes this action is that sticky stool and mucus, which adhere to the inside of the intestines, are pulled along by the powerful waves that pull the food along, drawing the intestine with

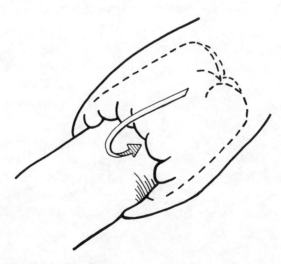

Figure 4.2. Intussusception. This condition occurs when the intestine slides within itself, like a telescope.

them. This "telescoping" may cause the blood vessels that normally nourish the intestines to be blocked off, which may damage the intestine, causing bleeding or even destruction of that part of the bowel. Intussusception, like DIOS, causes abdominal pain (which may be intermittent or constant), and may cause vomiting or a decreased number of bowel movements. Intussusception may be treated by barium enema x-ray, or may require surgery, but patients with this problem tend to do well if promptly treated.

Fibrosing Colonopathy

Fibrosing colonopathy is a relatively new problem, affecting only a very few patients, and only among the patients taking very large doses of pancreatic enzymes with each meal. People who develop the problem have abdominal pain and may have bloody diarrhea. It is a serious problem that may require surgery. It is discussed at greater length in Chapter 6, *Nutrition*.

Rectum

Rectal Prolapse

Rectal prolapse is similar to intussusception, involving the same "telescoping" action. In this case, the rectum is pulled along through, and right out of, the anus, to a point where it becomes visible (Figure 4.3). This usually happens during a bowel movement. Rectal prolapse may occur repeatedly in a young child, before the diagnosis of CF is made. It is fairly common, occurring in nearly 20% of patients with CF. Though it is frightening for a parent to see, it is seldom dangerous or painful.

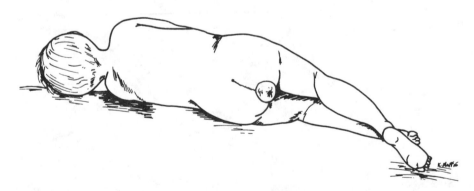

Figure 4.3. Rectal prolapse. This condition is similar to intussusception in that the bowel turns partly inside-out. In rectal prolapse, the last part of the bowel (the rectum) turns inside-out, and protrudes from the anus.

Rectal prolapse may be the first CF-related problem to appear before CF is diagnosed in a child. Several factors related to undiagnosed CF can cause rectal prolapse. Malnutrition affects the structures that usually support the rectum, and coughing and straining during sticky, bulky bowel movements increase the pressure on the rectum, pushing it out. Treatment of each episode of prolapse usually consists simply of pushing the rectum gently back into place by hand. If it is difficult to restore it to its normal position, then a doctor's help should be obtained immediately. The prolapse usually stops occurring when treatment of the CF (especially with enzymes) improves the bowel movements, reduces coughing, and increases overall nutrition. Rectal prolapse rarely requires surgery. Since rectal prolapse is very uncommon in developed countries except in youngsters with CF (and a very few with severe constipation or diarrhea), anyone with rectal prolapse should be tested for CF.

Esophagus

Gastroesophageal Reflux

Gastroesophageal reflux occurs when the stomach contents (consisting of acid made by the stomach and partially digested food) come back up into the esophagus ("gastro" refers to the stomach; and "reflux" indicates a fluid going backward from the way it's supposed to go). A certain amount of this is normal, and we are usually unaware that it is happening. However, when this occurs often, or when the acid from the stomach remains in the esophagus for very long, the mucous membranes of the esophagus become irritated and inflamed. *Esophagitis* (inflammation of the esophagus) then results, producing the feeling called "heartburn," which has nothing to do with the heart. In addition to the discomfort this causes, on rare occasions the damage can be severe enough to cause bleeding, or a narrowed area of scar tissue (*stricture*) within the esophagus, which can make swallowing very difficult.

Gastroesophageal reflux can lead to other problems in addition to the irritation of the esophagus itself. One problem occurs when the refluxed material comes up farther than the esophagus, and is actually vomited. Besides being messy, vomiting entails a loss of food and crucial nutrients and, if it occurs frequently, can lead to malnutrition. This is a particular problem in babies who have reflux, because a baby's esophagus is much shorter than that of older children. Although a certain amount of "spitting up" is quite normal in babies, too much may be harmful, such as when it interferes with normal weight gain.

In addition to the irritation of the esophagus and the loss of calories, gastroesophageal reflux can cause pulmonary (lung or breathing) problems. This may occur two different ways: (1) refluxed material may reach the back of the throat and actually be breathed (aspirated) into the lungs. There are normally quite good protections that keep refluxed material from getting into the lungs, so most breathing problems caused by reflux occur in the second way; (2) when nerves in the esophagus are irritated by stomach acid, they can send a signal to the bronchial tubes in the lungs to get narrower, making the bronchi squeeze down. [In certain instances, this reaction is actually a protective mechanism (see Chapter 3, *The Respiratory System*).] This reaction of the bronchi causes breathing difficulties that are similar to those of asthma, and may make the breathing problems of CF worse.

Several factors are responsible for the occurrence of reflux in people with CF. Some medications and treatments have a side effect of relaxing the muscle at the bottom of the esophagus (lower esophageal sphincter) (see Figure 4.1). If that sphincter relaxes too much, food is more likely to pass backward through it from the stomach into the esophagus. People with CF spend more time upside down (for treatments) than other people. If the muscle at the bottom of the esophagus relaxes when you are upright, gas escapes, and we call that a burp, but if it happens when you are upside down, the stomach contents escape into the esophagus. The esophagus enters the stomach from above, which is obvious from the diagram in Figure 4.1. What's not as obvious is that it goes into the *back* part of the top of the stomach. This means that lying on your belly is similar to standing up: what's in your stomach will fall to the front (away from the opening to the esophagus), and if the muscle at the bottom of the esophagus relaxes, it produces a burp; but if you lie on your back, the fluid in the stomach is right at the esophageal opening, just waiting for it to relax so it can go back into the esophagus. (It's not really *waiting* for this to happen, of course, but it might as well be. Studies have shown clearly that babies have much less reflux when they sleep on their bellies than when they sleep on their backs.) Coughing, which is helpful in clearing lung mucus, also tightens the abdominal muscles, and may put pressure on the stomach that forces material up into the esophagus. People with CF may produce more stomach acid than normal, and this may also make reflux worse.

Treatment for reflux is divided into three categories: simple measures, medications, and surgery. The simple measures include position and meal characteristics. Head-down positions and lying on the back or slouching while sitting make reflux worse. Infant seats, which put babies in a partly back-lying and partly slouching position, can cause infants to have more reflux than when they are lying face down. Sitting or standing straight up, or lying face down, make reflux less likely to occur. Babies with CF should be put to sleep on their stomachs, unless they are very unhappy that way, despite recent recommendations to put babies to sleep on their backs. In older children with CF, meals should be eaten at least two hours before they go to bed, and acid foods (tomatoes, soft drinks, juices) should be avoided. Thickening infants' formula with 1 tablespoon of dry rice cereal for each ounce of formula helps decrease spitting up, and also adds calories to the formula. Smoking (or being around smoke) and caffeine may make reflux worse, so children with CF and reflux should avoid exposure to these things. (Of course, the smoke has an even worse effect on the lungs themselves, so there are several reasons to avoid being around smoke.)

Medications used to treat reflux include bethanechol (Urecholine®), metoclopramide (Reglan®), and cisapride (Propulsid®) (see Appendix B: *Medications*), which strengthen the muscle at the bottom of the esophagus. Since bethanechol may add to lung problems, and since metoclopramide may be of more benefit by also causing the stomach to empty into the intestine faster, metoclopramide is probably better than bethanechol for CF patients. Its main side effect, when the dose is too high for a patient, is a restlessness, which may progress to back-arching and stiffening, with eyes rolling back. This rare side effect looks frightening, but is usually easily treated by stopping the medication and by receiving an injection of diphenhydramine (Benadryl®) from a physician. Cisapride is the newest of the three medicines and seems to provide at least as much benefit with fewer side effects. Other medications that may be used to treat reflux include cimetidine and ranitidine, which decrease the stomach's production of acid, and liquid antacids, which neutralize the acid that has been produced.

If the simple measures and medications do not produce enough relief from the reflux, a surgical procedure called a *fundoplication* (or a Nissen fundoplication) can be performed. This involves wrapping the upper part (the *fundus*) of the stomach around the bottom of the esophagus to strengthen the muscle at the bottom of the esophagus. When performed by a surgeon experienced in children's problems, this procedure is nearly always successful in treating reflux. It has also recently been done using a "scope," without as large an abdominal incision as previously required (a *laparoscopic fundoplication*), which helps make the procedure and recovery simpler for the patient.

Stomach

Increased Acid

There may be an increase in the amount of acid the stomach makes in CF. Though this does not seem to make ulcers common in people with CF, it may add to the problem of gastroesophageal reflux and cause pancreatic enzymes to be less effective. These possibilities have been discussed in other sections.

Liver

Fatty Liver

The livers of people with CF fairly often become enlarged because the liver cells get packed with fat. This also happens in malnourished people without CF and it may be due to the malnutrition itself. (It is not known why malnutrition, which makes the rest of the body lose fat, makes the liver gain fat.) Fatty liver may happen at any age, and may improve as nutrition improves. It does not by itself cause any problems.

Blocked Bile Ducts

In addition to blocking the small tubes in the lungs and in the pancreas, abnormally sticky mucus can block the bile ducts. The bile ducts are the small tubes in the liver that take the bile, including the bile salts needed for digestion, to the pancreatic duct and then to the duodenum. Thus, when the bile ducts are blocked, the digestion of fat may become more difficult, since fat digestion is more efficient if bile salts reach the intestine.

When the bile ducts become blocked in babies, the yellow bile cannot get out of the liver and backs up into the blood, where it is carried to the skin, causing a temporary yellow discoloration of the skin called *jaundice*. Jaundice in CF infants is much more common in those who have meconium ileus (blockage of the intestines, which was discussed in an earlier section). In older children, the blocked ducts are less likely to cause jaundice, but they may cause scarring in the liver (*biliary fibrosis*), which may often be present without producing any signs or problems. If this scarring becomes severe, it is called *biliary cirrhosis* and can cause serious problems. This problem is quite uncommon, occurring in only 1%–4% of people with CF.

The complex problems caused by cirrhosis of the liver include fluid (*ascites*) building up in the abdomen, and life-threatening bleeding from large veins (*varices*) that form in the esophagus. A third problem resulting from cirrhosis is called *hypersplenism:* The spleen, an organ in the left side of the abdomen, swells; as it enlarges it traps blood cells flowing through it. If it traps blood-clotting cells called platelets, it may cause bleeding problems; if it traps the red blood cells, anemia may result.

If cirrhosis becomes severe enough, the liver may fail to work at all. Since the liver is essential to life, this is a cause of death in a small percentage (1%–2%) of CF patients.

There is no definite way at present to interrupt the scarring caused by the duct blockage in the liver, any more than in the pancreas. However, there is a relatively new medicine, called ursodeoxycholic acid ("urso") or Actigal® that is showing some promise. Urso (which means "bear") is a bile salt found in bears. Whether urso or other newer medications prove to be helpful in reducing or delaying the liver scarring itself, there are effective treatments for some of the problems caused by the liver scarring. Bile salts are part of some enzyme preparations used for people with CF, such as Accelerase and Cotazym-B, although neither of these is enteric-coated (see Chapter 6, *Nutrition*) and the enteric coating seems to be more important to the function of the enzymes than are the bile salts. If hypersplenism causes dangerously low levels of a particular type of blood cells, they can be replenished by transfusion, but this is rarely needed. If varices form and bleed, they can be treated by *sclerotherapy*. In this procedure a flexible, lighted tube is passed down the throat, and a material is injected into these large vessels in order to close them by scarring. Sclerotherapy is usually repeated at intervals ranging from weeks to many months, and is quite effective in treating varices.

Another method used to treat varices is a surgical technique that directs the blood flow away from the varices; this is called a *shunt* or *portosystemic shunt*. These shunts are major surgical procedures, and make subsequent liver transplantation extremely difficult or impossible. A new procedure called *TIPS* (for *t*ransjugular *i*ntrahepatic *p*ortosystemic *s*hunting) can be performed by specially trained radiologists. This method can relieve some of the pressure that causes hypersplenism and esophageal varices, and it does not make it more difficult to do a liver transplant later.

Ascites, the collection of fluid in the abdomen, can be treated by changes in the amount of salt and water a person eats, and by drugs (diuretics) that increase urination. There are other treatments for the complexities of liver failure, which your doctor can discuss with you if they are ever needed.

Liver transplantation can be performed for someone whose liver function has failed, or whose problems from esophageal varices cannot be controlled. Dozens of liver transplants have been performed successfully in CF patients. Any transplant procedure is an extremely risky undertaking, often with unpredictable consequences, and should not be done if the risks are not fully understood by patient and family. Liver transplantation is discussed at greater length in Chapter 8, *Transplantation*.

Gallbladder

The gallbladder is a pouch attached to the bile ducts just outside the liver. It collects the bile made by the liver, and releases it into the intestine at the time of a meal, when it is needed. The gallbladder and the tube that connects it to the liver are abnormal in one-third of all people with CF, but this does not usually cause any problems. Approximately 10% of all CF patients may have gallstones. If they cause pain, which they sometimes do, they are treated by surgery to remove the gallbladder and the stones.

Abdominal Pain

"Stomachaches" are a common problem for people with CF, and there are many possible causes. Several of the complications listed in Table 2.1 cause abdominal pain. DIOS may be the most common cause of stomachaches, but gallstones, ulcers, pancreatitis (almost exclusively in those patients who do not need to take enzymes), and intussusception, all of which occur more often in CF patients than in other people, are also major causes of abdominal problems. For patients who take enzyme supplements, it is important to take them regularly, for skipping enzymes is almost guaranteed to result in discomfort. Other sources of abdominal pain include excessive coughing, which can cause the abdominal muscles to become sore, and medications, some of which cause abdominal pain as well. People with CF can have the same abdominal problems as everyone else, including constipation, gastroenteritis (this is an intestinal infection, often inaccurately called a "stomach flu," and is frequently accompanied by nausea, vomiting, and/or diarrhea), urinary tract infection, and appendicitis. Lactose intolerance (the inability to digest the main carbohydrate in milk) is a common cause for abdominal pain in children with or without CF. In young women, gynecologic problems can be responsible for abdominal pain, and a rare cause of apparent abdominal pain in boys is *testicular torsion* (a twisted testicle). Finally, psychological stress can be a cause of stomach problems in some people.

5

Other Systems

THE BASICS

1. Sweat glands make sweat that is very salty in people with CF. This gives us the sweat test, and occasionally babies lose excess salt in hot weather.
2. Thick mucus in the reproductive system means that most men with CF are sterile (although their sex life is completely normal), and women have a harder time getting pregnant than other women.
3. Both boys and girls may go through puberty later than their classmates, but most will develop normally, a year or two later.

SWEAT GLANDS

Normal Sweat Glands

Sweat begins in the coil of the sweat gland, below the surface of the skin (Figure 5.1) as a fluid that is chemically very similar to blood. As it makes its way toward the skin, sodium—with its positive electrical charge—is pumped out of the duct, and eventually back to the bloodstream. Whenever a positive charge leaves any tube or duct in the body, a negative charge accompanies it in order to maintain the same total electrical charge. In the case of the sweat, it is chloride and its negative charge that are carried out of the sweat fluid to follow the positive charge of sodium. By the time the fluid reaches the skin surface in the form of sweat, it still has some salt, but the sodium and chloride contents are very low compared with those in the blood. This helps the body conserve sodium and chloride, especially in hot weather or when someone is exercising heavily.

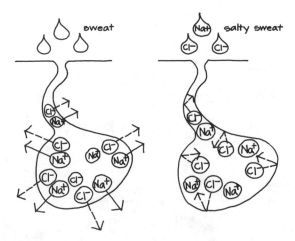

Figure 5.1. Sweat abnormality. In the normal (*left*) and CF (*right*) sweat gland, fluid begins in the base of the duct with a salt (sodium chloride) content close to that of blood. Then, in the normal sweat gland, as the fluid moves up the gland toward the skin, sodium (Na^+)—with its positive charge—leaves the gland, and chloride (Cl^-)—with its negative charge—follows, in order to keep electrical neutrality (same number of positives and negatives in all body compartments). But, in the CF sweat gland, because of the missing or blocked CFTR (see Chapter 1, *The Basic Defect*), chloride cannot leave. Since chloride can't leave, it holds the sodium back too, and the fluid that emerges from the skin as sweat has a much higher concentration of sodium and chloride than normal.

Sweat Glands in Cystic Fibrosis

It has been known for many years that people with cystic fibrosis (CF) have an extremely high salt content in their sweat. You've seen in Chapter 1, *The Basic Defect,* that CF cells set up a roadblock to chloride trying to pass through their membranes. This block in the cells of the sweat duct means that chloride is stranded within the duct fluid. Because the negatively charged chloride can't leave, it holds sodium and its positive charge back as well. This means the fluid that emerges from the skin surface as sweat has abnormally large concentrations of sodium and chloride (salt).

The sweat abnormality is important for two reasons: (1) It allows the diagnosis of CF to be made through the sweat test, and (2) it means that some patients, especially babies, may become sick by losing more salt than they take in during the summer (see the section *Salt Loss* below).

Over 99% of people with CF have abnormal sweat. They sweat the same amount of sweat, but there is an excess of salt (sodium and chloride) in it. People without CF have less than 40 milliequivalents per liter (mEq/l) of chloride in their sweat (and a similar concentration of sodium), whereas people with CF have more than 60 mEq/l (and usually more than 80 mEq/l). This means that an analysis of the sweat can tell physicians whether someone has CF or not. Once the result of a test is positive, it will always be positive (meaning that if someone has CF, he or she will always have it). Also, a "positive test" is positive. Period. There are no differences between someone whose sweat chloride concentration is 83 mEq/l and someone whose is 115 mEq/l. Both have CF. The higher number does not mean a worse case of CF.

The Sweat Test

Much of the following information can also be found in Chapter 2, *Making the Diagnosis.*

Informal sweat testing has been done for centuries. There was a folk belief in Europe in the Middle Ages that "a child who tastes salty from a kiss on the brow . . . is hexed, and soon must die." Modern-day parents of children with CF frequently notice that their babies taste salty when they are kissed and that their older children have salt crystals on their faces and in their hair when they are active in the summertime. However, not everyone's taste buds are sensitive enough to distinguish between CF sweat and non-CF sweat. Fortunately, although a positive result of a sweat test means a child has CF, it is no longer true that he or she "soon must die." (Nor do we believe that he or she is "hexed"!)

Since the 1950s, a more accurate method of sweat testing has been available. The **Gibson-Cooke** method is a sweat test that is highly accurate. When sweat testing is done by any almost other method, mistakes frequently arise, resulting in *false positives* (children who *do not* have CF but whose tests indicate that they *do* have it) and in *false negatives* (children who *do* have CF but whose tests indicate that they *do not* have it). The correct method is the Gibson-Cooke method of sweat testing by *pilocarpine iontophoresis with quantitative analysis of sodium and/or chloride.* Here's what all that means:

The Gibson-Cooke method employs the chemical *pilocarpine* to stimulate the sweat glands to produce sweat. Pilocarpine reaches the working part of the sweat gland by first being placed on the skin, and then directed into the sweat gland by a small electrical current; this process is called *iontophoresis*. The sweat is then collected on a cloth or paper pad, or in a tiny coiled tube. It is then weighed carefully, and the sodium and/or chloride concentrations are measured very precisely (*quantitatively*).

To perform the test and collect the sweat takes 30–60 minutes. The laboratory analysis takes another 30 minutes or so. Therefore, it's usually several hours between the time someone comes into the laboratory and the time the results are ready.

The first step in the test is that the forearm (or occasionally, in a small baby, the lower leg, or even the back) is washed off, to remove any salt that might be on the skin. Then some *pilocarpine* is placed on the skin. Pilocarpine is colorless and odorless, and looks and feels like water. Two flat metal electrodes are placed on the skin and connected to a small box that sends a slight electrical current (approximately 2–5 milliamperes) into the skin, driving the pilocarpine into the vicinity of the sweat gland, where it can "turn on" the sweat gland. The electrical current is usually not felt at all, but some people feel a mild tingling, and a few may even feel a harsher tingling or burning. It should not burn, and if it does, you should tell the technician, so that the current can be turned down.

After about 5 minutes with the electrodes in place, they are removed, the arm (or leg or back) is again wiped off, and a piece of absorbent material (gauze or filter paper) or a tiny coiled tube is placed on the skin. The technician then wraps the arm, covering the gauze with a dressing that is airtight and watertight, so that no sweat will evaporate or leak out. During the next 30–60 minutes, the dressing is left in place while the "revved up" sweat glands are making sweat. The technician then removes the dressing with tweezers or forceps, taking care not to touch the gauze or filter paper with his or her fingers, puts the paper (now soaked with sweat) into a bottle, and takes it to the laboratory. In the laboratory, the technician weighs the bottle to see how much sweat there is, rinses the sweat out of the paper or gauze or squirts it out of the coiled tubing into a container, and then puts it through the chemical analyzers to find out precisely how much sodium and/or chloride is in the sweat. Some laboratories measure the chloride, some measure the sodium, and some measure both. As long as the sweat is obtained by this method, it doesn't matter which part of the salt is measured.

When the test is performed by this method, *by a laboratory experienced in performing this test*, the result should enable the physician to make a definite and accurate diagnosis.

One other method of sweat testing is also acceptable, one that is not very widely used; that method is the *Macroduct Sweat Collection System*®, whose use is mostly confined to a "screening" test in doctors' offices or hospitals that are not near a CF center. Positive tests from this method should then be confirmed with a test by the Gibson-Cooke method.

Problems with Sweat Testing

In an experienced laboratory, not getting enough sweat is the only major problem that can interfere with obtaining a reliable result. Most laboratory experts say that they must have 100 mg of sweat in order to be able to do an accurate analysis. Some people, especially some very young babies (under 1 month old) may not make enough sweat to analyze. There is a common (incorrect) belief that sweat testing cannot be done in very young babies. However, it **can** be done, and **should** be done in any baby for whom the possibility of CF has been raised. If enough sweat is collected—as it will be for the majority of babies—the results will be valid, even within the first weeks of life, and even in a premature infant.

Adults have higher sweat sodium and chloride levels than children, but even in adults, a sweat chloride concentration greater than 60 mEq/l is abnormal.

There are a very few conditions which give elevated sweat chloride or sodium levels, and these are usually readily distinguished from CF. Similarly, there are very few people with CF whose sweat sodium and chloride concentrations are below 60 mEq/l. Finally, there are very few people whose sweat sodium and chloride concentrations are between 40 and 60 mEq/l. These few people are said to have test results in "the gray zone," or the "intermediate range," meaning neither definitely positive nor definitely negative. Tests in this range are discussed in the *Introduction* to Chapter 2, *Making the Diagnosis*.

That a hospital or laboratory *says* they can perform a sweat test is not adequate assurance that they can do it correctly. *Nearly one-half of all patients who come to CF centers having had sweat tests done in outlying hospitals have received incorrect results from these tests.*

Salt Loss

In addition to making the sweat test possible, the sweat abnormality can also affect the health of some people with CF. For each drop of sweat made, considerably more sodium and chloride are lost from the body than would be lost in someone without CF. In most children and adults with CF, the body is able to regulate the amount of salt in the bloodstream amazingly well. When more salt is lost, people want and take in more salt, and the kidneys reduce the amount of salt lost through the urine. Under most circumstances, even including active exercise in hot weather, if adequate salt is available, children and adults with CF will take in the proper amounts. Pretzel sticks and other salty snacks may be available for toddlers, whereas older children and adults can have access to the salt shaker, and no further supplements are needed. Salt tablets are not needed.

Infants with CF may lose too much salt in their sweat, and are not able to let their parents know that they feel like having a pickle or pretzel or other salty food. Each year, especially during summer months, some infants with CF become ill because of having lost too much salt. They become lethargic, their appetite falls off, and they seem sickly. If this happens, they may require hospitalization and intravenous fluids containing replacement sodium and chloride. In order to prevent this problem, it's advisable for infants to be given a tiny bit of salt in their bottles during hot summer months. An amount as small as $^1/_8$ teaspoon, once or twice a day, is probably adequate. Since too much salt can cause problems, it's best to provide *moderate,* regular supplements.

Some older children and adults who are very active during hot weather will need to be careful about replacing lost fluid and salt. The only immediate danger for a teenager under extreme exertion, such as marathon running or a long, tough football practice in full uniform in hot weather, is fluid loss. Athletes should drink more water than they feel they need, since thirst is not as sensitive a guide as is the taste for salt. All children underestimate their need for fluid when they exercise in the heat, and young people with CF underestimate their fluid needs even more than other children. Salt replacement does not need to be immediate, and will be accurately guided by taste.

REPRODUCTIVE SYSTEM IN CYSTIC FIBROSIS

Although the reproductive systems of people with CF are basically normal, the thick mucus found in so many other places in the body also affects this system. (The reproductive system is discussed at greater length in Chapter 14, *Cystic Fibrosis and Adulthood.*)

The Male Reproductive System in Cystic Fibrosis

In boys and men with CF, the reproductive system is completely normal, with one exception. In 98% of boys and men with CF, the **vas deferens** is incompletely formed or totally blocked. The vas deferens is the tube that carries sperm from the testicles to the penis. This is the tube that is cut and tied when a man has a vasectomy. The sperm are formed normally in the testicles, but because of the blockage, they cannot be released. Men with CF have completely normal sex lives, but the 98% of these men who have this blockage are sterile. (It is very much as though everything had been normal, and they had gotten a vasectomy.) A small proportion of men with CF (about 2%) are not sterile, and some have fathered children.

It is possible to test whether a teenager or adult with CF is one of the 98% who are sterile, or one of the 2% who are not. The patient simply gives a semen specimen to the laboratory, where it is analyzed for sperm.

The Female Reproductive System in Cystic Fibrosis

In women with CF, the problems related to the reproductive system are more subtle than in men. The main problem is that the mucus lining the cervix (the opening to the uterus, or womb) is thick, just like mucus elsewhere. As a result it is harder for women with CF to get pregnant than for women without CF. It certainly is possible though, and several hundred women with CF have gotten pregnant, and many of these women have delivered babies.

Women whose lungs are in excellent shape when they get pregnant usually do well with the pregnancy. Women whose lungs are at all involved with CF lung disease may have a very hard time with the pregnancy. There are many women with CF who have been in fairly good health before they became pregnant, but whose health deteriorated during the pregnancy.

Delayed Physical Development

Both boys and girls with CF may go through puberty 1–2 years later than their classmates. This occurs as an indirect result of CF, and is likely to be a direct result of poor nutrition or of chronic lung infection. Delayed development can be a problem in any chronic illness, for energy expended to fight the illness depletes the body's energy reserve for growth. This can be difficult emotionally for young people, too, if all their friends are shooting up in height, and filling out, growing into physical adulthood, and they are left behind, with the body of a small child. It may soften the blow somewhat if they know that the majority of young people with CF eventually go through puberty, although it may be a year or two behind their friends. The treatment for this problem is directed at the underlying causes, and in CF that means treating the lungs and improving the nutrition.

6

Nutrition

THE BASICS

1. Nutrition is important for people with CF for growth and overall health, including the health of their lungs.
2. Good nutrition for CF patients has 3 parts:
   a. High-calorie diet
   b. Pancreatic enzymes with every meal and most snacks
   c. Vitamins
3. If someone can't gain weight on a regular diet, tube feedings may be very helpful.

THE IMPORTANCE OF NUTRITION IN CYSTIC FIBROSIS

Malnourished people do not grow well, and often they do not feel well. Malnutrition damages the immune system, which is the body's defense against infection, and, in someone with cystic fibrosis (CF), may contribute to the pulmonary disease and hasten death. Cystic fibrosis patients who are better nourished grow better, have better pulmonary function, and live longer than patients with poor nutrition.

MONITORING GROWTH AND NUTRITION

In an adult, generalized malnutrition shows up first as weight loss. In children, who should grow and gain weight actively, a slowing down of the normal weight gain may be the first sign of malnutrition. This is most easily detected by plotting a child's weight on a growth chart (Figure 6.1 on page 112), which compares an individual's growth to that of other children of the same age and sex. If the child's growth does not keep up with the curves, malnutrition may be the cause. This growth curve should not be used as a "grade" where you strive to attain a high number, but as a form of tracking a child's growth over time. The growth curve shows the child's individual growth pattern over the years and is an indication of how the child is doing nutritionally.

When malnutrition affects growth, it usually affects weight first. When weight has been severely affected, the poor nutrition can affect height in a similar fashion, and a child may begin to show signs of falling behind in the height curves (that is, he or she may not grow taller as fast as a healthy child of the same age). Finally, if severe malnutrition affects a very young child at a time when the brain is actively growing (up to about 36 months old), the head circumference may grow more slowly than normal. These three measurements (weight, height, and head circumference) should be plotted regularly for babies, and height and weight for all children and adolescents, in order to identify signs of malnutrition or other health problems when they begin, before you might notice them in the children's appearance.

Another method of assessing a person's nutritional state is called *anthropo-metrics* ("measuring people"). Measurements are taken, such as skinfold thickness, which gives an estimate as to how much fat is stored in the body, and mid-arm circumference, which gives an estimate of the amount of muscle protein the body has. It is important to have both fat and muscle protein: when someone is not eating well, fat stores can be broken down to be used for energy, sparing the muscle protein, so that the person does not become too weak. When the fat stores run out, the body is forced to use protein for energy, and muscle wasting takes place. Low muscle mass may also result from lack of use. By comparing annual measurements of muscle and fat mass, the nutritionist and physician can determine the adequacy of the fat and muscle mass. Diet and exercise recommendations can be made when these measurements need improvement.

Many aspects of a person's nutritional state can also be measured by blood tests such as albumin, total protein, triglycerides, cholesterol, carotene, glucose, and hemoglobin.

CAUSES OF MALNUTRITION IN CYSTIC FIBROSIS

At one time it was assumed that the malnutrition that affects so many children and adults with CF was entirely due to the poor digestion of food, which, in turn, was due to the lack of pancreatic enzymes and bile salts, as was discussed in Chapter 4, *The Gastrointestinal Tract*. Though enzyme deficiency is a major cause of malnutrition in CF, there are additional contributing factors to malnutrition: (1) enzyme supplements do not work perfectly, (2) people with CF may not take in enough calories, even for someone with normal needs, and (3) there are increased caloric needs in CF.

Enzyme Deficiency

Although oral enzyme supplements help a great deal, they do not work perfectly; and despite taking every prescribed capsule, most CF patients' digestion is still not complete, and some degree of malabsorption of foods still occurs. (Remember that digestion is the process of breaking down food into particles tiny enough for them to be absorbed into the bloodstream from the intestines; enzymes are needed for digestion; digestion is needed for absorption; and absorption of food is needed for growth and energy.) The imperfection of oral enzyme supplements is due to the difficulty of mimicking perfectly the body's finely tuned system for trickling the pancreatic enzymes into the duodenum just as the food arrives from the stomach. When pancreatic enzyme capsules are swallowed with the meals, they may not arrive in the duodenum at the precise time to meet up with the food. The oral enzyme supplements can also be inactivated in the stomach by the stomach acids. We do not usually supplement bile salts (similar to those naturally produced in the gallbladder), and the possible lack of bile salts may also prevent the oral enzymes from acting optimally. Finally, with CF, the secretion of bicarbonate from the pancreas is also limited, causing incomplete neutralization of stomach acid, which may prevent the enteric coating on the oral enzymes from dissolving. All of these factors may contribute to malabsorption and poor nutrition, even in patients who take all of their enzymes as prescribed. Not taking the prescribed enzymes can also be a problem, and it is not unheard of for CF patients to "forget" to take enzymes because of not wanting their classmates to see them.

In addition to interfering with good nutrition, malabsorption of food can also cause bothersome side effects. Some signs of malabsorption include:

- Gas and bloating
- Stomach cramps
- Frequent stools
- Greasy or floating stools
- Larger and looser, bulky stools
- Malodorous stools
- Lighter brown or yellow stools

Often, malabsorption can cause the child's appetite to become bigger to make up for the food he or she is not absorbing. In fact, the "textbook picture" of a baby or child with untreated CF is someone with a voracious (huge) appetite, but poor weight gain. If you see a large increase in your child's appetite, you should watch for other signs of malabsorption listed above. If you suspect malabsorption, discuss with the CF team how to adjust the oral enzyme supplements.

Intestinal infections can cause diarrhea with an increase in number of stools that become watery instead of bulky. Diarrhea is different from malabsorption in that it is not treated by adjusting oral enzymes. To treat diarrhea that persists for more than one day, contact your doctor. A common approach is to eliminate milk products and switching to a bland or "BRAT" diet (bananas, rice cereal, apple-sauce, and toast).

Inadequate Caloric Intake

It is commonly believed that people with CF have a large appetite, and some do. But many children, teenagers, and adults with CF actually eat less food than their friends. Malnutrition itself may decrease a person's appetite (this is called the "anorexia of malnutrition"). Feeling sick and coughing a lot can also decrease a person's appetite. In the past, patients with CF were prescribed a low-fat diet, because it resulted in less fat in the stools. Having less fat in the diet meant less fat in the stools; unfortunately, it also meant fewer calories for the body to grow. The low-fat diet attempted to make up for the lost fat calories by increasing calories from carbohydrates. However, an ounce of fat has more than twice as many calories as an ounce of carbohydrate; so if you are on a low-fat diet, you have to eat a lot more to get the same number of calories for growth. On the low-fat diets, many people with CF were unable to eat enough calories and became malnour-ished. With the right amount of oral enzymes, even a high-fat diet can be digest-ed and absorbed, giving more calories with less food. *A low-fat diet is no longer recommended* except under very special circumstances. Instead, a high-fat, high-protein diet is recommended for all patients with CF unless otherwise instructed. Even so, it simply may be impossible for some CF patients—try though they will—to eat enough to supply their needs. In this case, it still is possible to re-establish good growth, with one or more of the available additions to a well-rounded diet (see below, after the section on enzymes).

Increased Caloric Demands

The third main reason for malnutrition in CF is an increased use of calories. Coughing, breathing hard, and fighting an infection all require additional calo-ries. If you are using more calories in these ways all day long, the need for extra calories accumulates. It may be difficult for the person with CF to keep up with this high calorie demand. The caloric intake required to maintain good growth in someone with CF is usually $1\frac{1}{3}$ to $1\frac{1}{2}$ times that required for a person of the same age and sex without CF.

SPECIAL DEFICIENCIES IN CYSTIC FIBROSIS

Hypoalbuminemia (Low Blood Albumin Levels)

Albumin is the main body protein in blood. One of its primary roles in the blood is to keep water in the arteries and veins. If there is not enough albumin in the blood (hypoalbuminemia), water leaks out into the skin and other organs, and produces skin puffiness called **edema**. Hypoalbuminemia and edema may occur in infants with CF before they are diagnosed, and may be the clue that leads to the diagnosis of CF. It can show up earlier in undiagnosed infants fed with soy milk formula, because the protein in soy formulas may not be as good as the protein in human milk or cow milk formulas. Hypoalbuminemia is treated by giving pancreatic enzymes and plenty of protein in the diet. Some infants with very low blood albumin also benefit from several intravenous injections of albumin, which increases their albumin level before they are able to begin making their own through the diet.

Essential Fatty Acid Deficiency

Fatty acids are the parts of the fat (triglyceride) molecule. Essential fatty acids are fatty acids that the body needs and which it cannot make from other nutrients. Two essential fatty acids, linoleic acid and linolenic acid, are found in all dietary fats and are also abundant in plant oils such as safflower and sunflower oils. These are used for a number of complex and necessary functions, including the manufacture of cell membranes. They also appear to be needed for optimal lung function. The difficulties in fat digestion and absorption in untreated CF patients can show up early in life as deficiencies of these essential fatty acids, since the body's need for them cannot be met by making them out of other nutrients. In addition, the essential fatty acids that do get absorbed may get used for other caloric needs: for example, they may get "burned up" to supply energy for breathing. Essential fatty acid deficiency can be treated by increasing the caloric intake, and by adding special supplements such as safflower oil to the diet. With infants being diagnosed and started on enzymes at a younger age, fewer infants have this problem now than used to in the past.

Iron Deficiency

Iron is concentrated in the blood, but some is present in every living cell of the body. Iron's main function is to carry oxygen and carbon dioxide from one body tissue to another via the blood. The majority of iron is present in the *hemoglobin* molecule of the red blood cell. Any more than very mild iron deficiency will lead to low hemoglobin levels and to anemia (low red blood cell concentration). Symptoms of iron deficiency include easy fatigue, decreased resistance to infection, and soreness in the mouth. To screen for iron deficiency the hemoglobin levels are measured.

Good dietary sources of iron are fortified cereals, meats, dried fruits, and deep green vegetables. Iron in meat, poultry, and fish is absorbed better than the iron from vegetables. Iron-deficiency anemia is the most common nutritional deficiency in children in North America, affecting almost 40% of young children. It is most common after one year of age (between 12 and 36 months) when children stop taking breast milk or iron-fortified formulas, and start whole milk, which is low in iron. It also occurs in adolescent males, and females from adolescence through adulthood. Iron deficiency may occur from inadequate iron intake, impaired absorption, or blood loss. It is important during times of higher iron needs to encourage the intake of iron-rich food sources, or to supplement the diet with a multivitamin with iron. These times of high-iron needs include times of blood loss, either through healthy causes (especially menstruation), bleeding from injury or disease, or times of multiple blood tests.

If anemia is detected, an oral iron supplement will be prescribed. When taking iron supplements, it is important to remember to take them **without** pancreatic enzymes because (unlike the case for fat or protein, where enzymes help absorption) the enzymes interfere with the iron absorption. To improve iron absorption take the oral iron supplements with a beverage that contains vitamin C (orange or grapefruit juice).

Fat-Soluble Vitamins (Vitamins A, D, E, and K)

Vitamins A, D, E, and K require fat to be absorbed and, since CF patients have trouble digesting and absorbing fat, the bloodstream levels of these vitamins are often low in patients with CF. As part of their daily medical therapy, CF patients are put on a "standard CF dose" of vitamins, based on age. This dose is higher than that recommended for people without CF. It is important that the vitamins prescribed are taken daily to prevent deficiency of those vitamins. To make vitamins easier to absorb they can be taken with meals when oral enzymes and food are supplied. A physical examination and blood tests can then tell if more vitamins are required.

Some people may want to take more vitamins and minerals than have been prescribed, thinking that more may be better. Actually the body uses only a certain amount of each vitamin and mineral and a large excess cannot be used. For some vitamins (water-soluble vitamins), the extra amount just ends up in the urine (some public health experts who laugh at Americans' overzealous use of vitamins say that "Americans have the most nutritious urine in the world!"). The fat-soluble vitamins are not excreted in the urine, and taking an excessive amount can be dangerous.

Vitamin A

Vitamin A is needed for fighting infections, preventing night blindness, and general growth and maintenance of the body. Retinol and carotene are two types of vitamin A. Vitamin A is found in animal products, particularly liver, egg yolks, and fortified milk. Carotene is found in dark green and deep yellow and orange vegetables and fruits, and is converted to active vitamin A in the body. Vitamin A is normally absorbed from the intestine and then stored in the liver to be used when it is needed. Two proteins made by the liver—prealbumin and retinol-binding protein—are needed to extract the vitamin A from the liver. Blood levels of vitamin A have been found to be below normal in some people with CF, even when supplemental enzymes and vitamins are given, but actual symptoms of vitamin A deficiency are rare. The abnormal fat digestion is part of the problem with vitamin A in CF, but even when vitamin A is absorbed and stored in the liver, it will not be available to the body if there are low levels of prealbumin and retinol-binding protein (two forms of albumin). Zinc is a mineral that helps retinol-binding protein extract vitamin A from the liver, so it is important that patients receive zinc in their multivitamins.

Vitamin D

Vitamin D is needed for growth of strong bones and teeth, and for normal functioning of many other organs. It is important for the absorption of calcium and phosphorus from the diet into the bloodstream. Vitamin D deficiency causes a bone disease called *rickets,* in which the bones are abnormally soft. Vitamin D is found in fortified milk and dairy products. It is also made in the skin by the action of sunlight. Vitamin D from the diet or skin must be activated by the liver and kidneys, which means that people with liver disease or kidney disease are more susceptible to vitamin D deficiency. Rickets or other evidence of vitamin D deficiency is rare in CF, particularly when patients are given oral enzymes and a multivitamin with vitamin D. If deficiency does occur, it can be detected by blood tests and treated with special supplemental vitamin and mineral preparations. Plenty of sunshine is also helpful to keep an adequate amount of vitamin D in the body.

Vitamin E

Vitamin E is important for the functioning of a number of important body parts, especially nerves. Good sources of vitamin E are vegetable oil, wheat germ, and dried beans and peas. Symptoms of vitamin E deficiency may include unsteadiness while walking. Vitamin E deficiency also causes an abnormal knee-jerk reflex, which the doctor checks by hitting the knee with the rubber reflex hammer.

Vitamin E deficiency can be detected by blood tests. This is the most common fat-soluble vitamin to be low in CF patients, mainly because people do not eat a lot of foods that are rich in vitamin E, and amounts of vitamin E tend to be low in standard multivitamin preparations. It is important for CF patients to take extra vitamin E daily. If blood tests indicate a deficiency, a higher dose of vitamin E can be prescribed. Water-soluble forms of vitamin E are more easily absorbed than the more expensive health food store preparations of vitamin E.

Vitamin K

Vitamin K is needed by the liver for making some of the clotting factors that stop bleeding. Green leafy vegetables and cauliflower are good food sources of vitamin K, and it is also found in dairy products. The average diet contains plenty of vitamin K. In addition, bacteria that normally live in the intestines make vitamin K, so for most people no vitamin K supplements are needed. People with CF may need extra vitamin K, though, because both dietary and intestinal sources of bacteria may be less than normal: first, vitamin K may not be well absorbed by the patient with CF. A second problem that someone with CF might have is that antibiotics given to treat infection in the lungs may kill the bacteria in the intestines, cutting down on the number of intestinal bacteria available to make vitamin K. This means that some people with CF who take a lot of antibiotics may need additional vitamin K. Vitamin K deficiency more often occurs during infancy (before diagnosis) or with the onset of CF liver disease.

Low blood levels of vitamin K can lead to very serious bleeding. There are two blood tests for clotting factors to estimate vitamin K levels. These are the "PT" test (prothrombin time) and the "PTT" test (partial thromboplastin time). The PT becomes abnormal if levels of vitamin K are too low, and in more severe deficiencies, the PTT may also become abnormal. Vitamin K deficiency can be corrected by adding oral or injected vitamin K supplements. Since the liver is needed to make the clotting factors, even vitamin K given by injection may not provide enough if the liver is failing to work (as in severe cirrhosis, discussed in Chapter 4). In this case, the already-made clotting factors may be administered by giving a transfusion of "fresh-frozen plasma."

Hypomagnesemia (Low Blood Magnesium)

Magnesium, like calcium, phosphorus, sodium, and chloride, is one of the minerals the body needs. Good food sources of magnesium include whole grains, dark green leafy vegetables, milk, soybeans, and molasses. Normally, magnesium is absorbed from the diet, and the kidneys get rid of any extra through the urine. When there is too little magnesium in the blood (hypomagnesemia) the signs include weakness, shakiness, and muscle cramps. In CF, there are a number of causes for hypomagnesemia. Maldigestion and malabsorption may prevent the magnesium from being absorbed from the intestine. Some antibiotics given for lung infections (especially the ones ending in "-micin" or "-mycin"), and diuretics given for heart or liver problems may cause too much magnesium to be lost in the urine. During a physical examination hypomagnesemia can be checked for by assessing the knee-jerk reflex. If the knee-jerk reflexes are too brisk (the opposite of what happens with vitamin E deficiency) then this could indicate low magnesium levels. The hands and face muscles can be evaluated for muscle spasms. Blood measurements of magnesium can confirm the diagnosis of hypomagnesemia. The treatment is by oral or intravenous magnesium supplements. Sometimes a large amount is needed in order to correct a deficiency.

Hypoelectrolytemia

The main chemicals in the bloodstream that carry an electrical charge, such as sodium, chloride, and potassium, are called *electrolytes*. People with CF lose a lot of salt in their sweat, and since salt consists of sodium and chloride, they may lose enough sodium and chloride to lower the blood levels of these electrolytes. This is especially likely to happen during exertion (exercise) in hot weather, or in infants whose diet is low in salt, and who can't tell us they feel like having something salty to eat.

Once CF is diagnosed, the problem can usually be prevented, and most CF experts advise adding extra salt to the diet. Infants receiving formula and plain baby foods that are low in salt should have a small amount of salt ($^1/_8$ teaspoon) added to each 8 ounces of formula. This small amount of salt should prevent any problems from developing and will also avoid the serious problems that could be caused by giving too much salt at one time. During hot weather or times of increased sweating, this amount of salt may need to be increased. Older children need no special treatment, other than free access to salty foods or the salt shaker. Their taste will tell them how much salt they need. This is discussed more in Chapter 5, *Other Systems*.

NUTRITIONAL TREATMENT

Basic dietary treatment in CF consists of a well-rounded diet with plenty of fat, protein, and carbohydrate, taken with enough pancreatic enzymes to provide maximum absorption. Tables 6.1 and 6.2 contain guidelines and suggestions for maintaining good nutritional intake. There is a whole section later in this chapter devoted to how to use pancreatic enzymes.

NUTRITION THROUGH THE YEARS

For infants, either formula or breast milk is recommended. If formula is used, a milk-based formula fortified with iron is advised until one year of age. Since pancreatic enzymes are often given in baby fruit at a young age, it is OK for babies to start baby foods as early as 3–4 months of age. Remember, though, before going overboard with solids, ounce-for-ounce, formula usually has more calories than solid baby foods, so you want to avoid filling up with foods that are lower in calories than regular infant formula. If the infant needs to "catch up" on the weight curve, special recipes can be given by the dietician to concentrate formulas or breast milk for higher calories (see Table 6.3 for examples). Babies who are tiny

TABLE 6.1. *Suggestions for Improving Your Child's Nutrition*

1. Plan a definite eating schedule with three well-balanced meals and at least two snacks daily. Try to have the meals around the same time each day.
2. Meals should last 20–30 minutes. Young children have short attention spans and usually lose interest in eating after spending this amount of time at the table.
3. If the child refuses to eat for more than 10 minutes, remove him or her from the table and offer nothing to eat until the next scheduled meal or snack.
4. Scheduled snacks are important, but all day snacking or "grazing" should be avoided. Grazing keeps the child full and he or she never really feels hungry.
5. Give a large, high-calorie snack at bedtime, unless the child has reflux (see Chapter 4).
6. Keep food offered simple. Children can be overwhelmed by too many foods at one meal.
7. Try to make foods attractive and appealing. Offer foods that the child can easily manage (cut-up meats, etc.).
8. Make the child's eating environment comfortable. Children should sit in sturdy chairs with their feet supported. The table and food should be easily reached.
9. Avoid distractions at meal time, such as TV. TV provides too much stimulus and the child does not focus on eating.
10. Be sure the child is not filling up on fluids. Do not give any beverage 30–60 minutes before a meal.
11. Reward positive behavior with verbal praise. Sticker charts may work well with younger children.
12. Parents should set good examples by eating nutritious meals *with* their children. If you don't eat well, you can't expect your child to eat well.

TABLE 6.2. *Ways to Increase Calories*

1. Add margarine to the bread of sandwiches; grill sandwiches. Melt margarine on vegetables, waffles, potatoes.
2. Add grated Parmesan cheese to spaghetti, casseroles, popcorn, and salads.
3. Melt cheese with scrambled eggs, casseroles, and add to sandwiches. Order extra cheese on pizza.
4. Chopped nuts add lots of calories; add to cookie dough, breads and pancakes. Buy breakfast cereals with nuts and dried fruit for higher calories a serving.
5. Drink whole milk instead of 2% or skim milk. Use whole milk cheeses instead of skim milk cheeses.
6. Add powdered nonfat dry milk to whole milk to increase the calories ($1/4$ cup powder milk to 8 ounces whole milk). Use the high-protein milk in cooking.
7. Use cheese sauce on vegetables, potatoes, pretzels, nachos, and french fries.
8. Use gravy on meats, potatoes, rice, noodles, and french fries.
9. Top hot chocolate, pudding, gelatin, milkshakes with whip topping.
10. Use extra eggs in pancake, waffle or french toast batter.
11. Add a package of vanilla instant breakfast to instant pudding mix.
12. Choose glazed doughnuts instead of cake doughnuts (275 calories vs 105 calories), or chocolate-covered sandwich cookies instead of vanilla wafers (90 calories vs 10 calories).

TABLE 6.3. *Ways to Increase Calories for Infants*

1. If your baby seems thirsty, feed formula, rather than juice or water, since the formula has more calories and nutrition.
2. Regular infant formula has 20 calories per ounce. You can use several different kinds of supplements to increase that to 24 calories per ounce. Here are some examples (DO NOT USE ANY OF THESE FORMULAS WITHOUT CHECKING FIRST WITH A CF DIETICIAN OR PHYSICIAN—WHILE THESE ARE SAFE AND EFFECTIVE FOR MOST BABIES, SOME COULD BE HARMFUL FOR INDIVIDUAL BABIES):
   a. Concentrated formula: The usual recipe for 8 ounces of 20-calorie-per-ounce formula is 4 scoops of powder and 8 ounces of water. By using 5 scoops of powder and 8 ounces of water, you can increase the calories to 24 calories per ounce.
   b. Polycose powder (a special sugar): add 4 teaspoons of Polycose powder to 8 oz of 20-calorie formula to make 24 calories per ounce.
   c. Corn oil or safflower oil is a very inexpensive way to add extra calories: add 3/4 tsp of corn oil to 8 oz of 20-calorie formula to make 24 cal/oz formula.
3. MCT (medium chain triglyceride) oil is more readily absorbed fat than corn or safflower oil, but is more expensive: add 1 teaspoon of MCT oil to 8 oz of 20-calorie formula to give 24-calorie formula.
4. Baby rice cereal: add 2 tablespoons to 8 oz of 20-calorie formula to give 24-calorie formula.

and cannot put on weight before they are diagnosed often catch up on their growth curve and begin to look much healthier very soon after starting their oral enzymes and general CF care (see Figure 6.1).

Toddlers and preschool age children with CF should use whole milk (4% fat). Continual snacking or "grazing" is discouraged because it makes it harder to time the oral enzymes accurately, and hard to make the diet nutritious. Three meals and two to three snacks a day work well for most children with CF.

Feeding problems are common in all children, with meals often becoming battlegrounds, and the problem can be worse in someone with CF: The parents know the importance of nutrition, and the child senses how important this is to the parent. Further, it is one area of a child's life where he or she can exert a lot of control: you cannot force a child to eat if he or she truly does not want to. The parents' responsibility is to offer their children nutritious foods at mealtimes and snacks and encourage them to eat, but in the end, it is up to the child how much he or she will eat. Avoid force-feeding your child. By making the mealtime enjoyable you can keep eating a pleasant part of CF care. A child may enjoy a picnic lunch outside, eating with a friend, or in another room of the house for a change. If you have a picky eater who is eating just a small amount of food, the goal is to make that small amount as high in calories as possible. Children at this age will start learning the importance of taking oral enzymes, and some will start swallowing the capsules.

School-age children with CF will be learning to take more responsibility for their care as they start spending more time away from home. They will be responsible for deciding what foods to eat and when to take their enzymes. The frequent smelly stools caused by malabsorption can be embarrassing for school-age children. They may find it hard to discuss their stools and symptoms, but it is im-

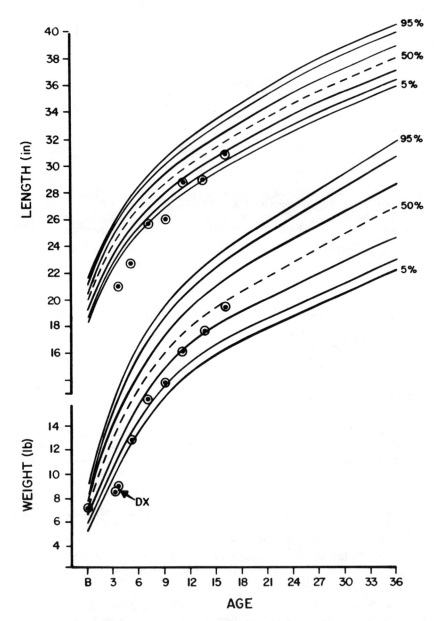

Figure 6.1. Growth chart. The *solid lines* represent the length and weight growth curves for normal children at various ages (in months). The "5%" line refers to the length and weight of healthy children in the lowest 5% for their age; that is, 5% of healthy children will have a weight that falls on or below the 5% line, whereas 95% will be heavier. The "50%" *dotted lines* represent the 50th percentile, or the average length and weight for healthy children. The *circles* represent the specific measurements for one youngster with CF. This child's weight was near average at birth (**B**), and fell below the 5th percentile by the time of diagnosis (*Dx*). Treatment began after diagnosis, and the child's weight reached just below the average for age by 18 months.

portant that they overcome this embarrassment so they can learn to take care of themselves. The wish that most children have to be the same as all their friends is difficult to fulfill with the CF diet and enzyme capsules required for each meal. The routine of taking enzymes needs to be continued no matter where they eat, at home or away. With sports and other physical activities, children with CF will need to use extra salt and drink more fluids than their friends.

HOW TO USE PANCREATIC ENZYMES

See also Appendix B, *Medications*.

Remember from the previous discussion of how pancreatic enzymes work that, normally, these digestive chemicals are released from the pancreas into the duodenum (the part of the intestine right after the stomach) just as the food passes into the duodenum from the stomach. We try to duplicate this process by using oral pancreatic enzyme supplements. These enzymes should ideally mix with the food in the duodenum, just as happens in people without CF. This means several things. First, **enzymes need to be taken with meals (and with *each* meal)**: these are not a once-a-day or a three-times-a-day medication. If someone has two meals, the enzymes should be taken twice; if someone has three meals and two snacks, the enzymes need to be taken five times, directly with the food. Some physicians recommend taking the whole enzyme dose at the beginning of each meal, while others think it's better to take one half the enzymes at the beginning and the rest halfway through the meal. Once you take the oral enzymes, they are effective for about 45 minutes to 1 hour. This means that if you are a slow eater, or are eating over a long period of time, then the dose should be split, and some enzyme given later in the meal. If you finish eating, and have a snack 5 minutes later, no more enzymes are needed, but if you have a snack 1½ hours after your last enzyme capsule, you need to take more enzymes.

Enzymes come in two main types: enteric-coated (the most common) and non-enteric-coated. The enteric-coated enzymes come in capsules with little beads inside (these beads are called "microspheres" by some drug companies, and "microtablets" by others). These beads are a bit like an M&M: there's a thin coating, and the good stuff (in this case, the enzyme itself) is inside the coating. The coating protects the enzymes from stomach acid, since acid destroys the enzymes. The coating is designed to dissolve when it's in a nonacid environment, which is usually the case in the duodenum (the part of the intestine right after the stomach). So it "melts in your duodenum, not in your stomach," like the M&M melts in your mouth and not your hand. This works beautifully, because it means that when the system works as designed (most of the time), the coating dissolves, and the enzymes are released in the duodenum, exactly where the body's own pancreatic enzymes are designed to enter the intestine and mix with the food to begin digesting fat and protein. When enteric-coated enzymes were introduced in the 1970s, they provided a revolutionary change in CF patients' ability to digest and absorb food.

TABLE 6.4. *Pancreatic Enzymes Comparison Guide*

Product	Manufacturer	Lipase[a]	Protease[b]	Amylase[c]	Special Features
Cotazym	Organon	8,000	3,000	3,000	Capsules, no enteric coating
Cotazym S	Organon	5,000	20,000	20,000	Capsules, enteric-coated spheres
Creon 5	Solvay	5,000	18,750	16,600	Capsules, enteric-coated minimicrospheres
Creon 10	Solvay	10,000	37,500	33,200	Capsules, enteric-coated minimicrospheres
Creon 20	Solvay	20,000	75,000	66,400	Capsules, enteric-coated minimicrospheres
Pancrease	McNeil	4,500	25,000	20,000	Capsules, enteric-coated microtablets, dye-free
Pancrease MT4	McNeil	4,000	12,000	12,000	Capsules, enteric-coated microtablets, dye-free
Pancrease MT10	McNeil	10,000	30,000	30,000	Capsules, enteric-coated microtablets, dye-free
Pancrease MT16	McNeil	16,000	48,000	48,000	Capsules, enteric-coated microtablets, dye-free
Pancrease MT20	McNeil	20,000	44,000	56,000	Capsules, enteric-coated microtablets, dye-free
Ultrase	Scandipharm	4,500	25,000	20,000	Capsules, enteric-coated microspheres
Ultrase MT12	Scandipharm	12,000	39,000	39,000	Capsules, enteric-coated microtablets
Ultrase MT18	Scandipharm	18,000	58,500	58,500	Capsules, enteric-coated microtablets
Ultrase MT20	Scandipharm	20,000	65,000	65,000	Capsules, enteric-coated microtablets
Viokase tablet	Robins	8,000	30,000	30,000	No enteric coating
Viokase powder	Robins	16,800	70,000	70,000	Amount per ¼ teaspoon, no enteric coating
Zymase	Organon	12,000	24,000	24,000	Enteric-coated spheres in capsules

Note: Numbers refer to content in USP units.

[a]Lipase, fat-digesting enzyme; most important for CF patients; one capsule with 8,000 units of lipase is roughly equivalent to two 4,000-unit capsules of lipase (if all are enteric-coated or all non-enteric-coated).

[b]Protease, protein-digesting enzyme.

[c]Amylase, starch-digesting enzyme.

The older, non-enteric-coated enzymes are still available, and are useful in a few situations. These enzymes come as a powder, tablet, or capsule (with powder in it).

The enzyme capsules can be swallowed whole (that's the most convenient way, once a child is old enough to swallow capsules), or opened up and the beads taken separately. The beads can be mixed with some soft food, such as applesauce. This is the most common way for babies to take the enzymes. Applesauce is a good food to mix the beads in, because applesauce is acid, and therefore the enzyme's coating will not dissolve while it's sitting in the food waiting to be eaten. The applesauce or other food should not be heated, since the heat will dissolve the coating. Even with cool applesauce, the beads should not be allowed to sit in the applesauce (or other food) for long: they should be mixed in just before the meal. If they sit too long and the coating does dissolve, the enzyme will start to digest the food, and may make it less tasty. It won't be dangerous, but it just won't be quite as attractive or effective. The beads can also be just placed on a baby's tongue, and rinsed right down with a bottle or breast-feeding. For older children and adults, beads can be taken alone, in their capsules, or mixed with most any foods, but it's important that they not be chewed, for that will break the protective coating, with two bad results: the patient will get a bitter taste (and possibly some lip or mouth irritation), and the enzymes will likely be destroyed by acid once they get to the stomach.

It's a good idea for anyone using enzymes to practice good mouth care, and be sure that all the beads are out of the mouth at least by the end of the meal. For people (usually this is little people: babies) using the powdered enzymes, this is essential in order to prevent irritation from the raw enzyme. Breast feeding mothers will need to clean their breasts carefully to avoid nipple irritation. In some babies, enzymes passing out with the stools can cause a burn to the buttocks if the diapers are not changed frequently or the bottom not cleaned thoroughly.

The enteric-coated enzymes come in many different strengths, based on how much fat-digesting enzyme (lipase) they contain. These different preparations (Table 6.4) are labeled by their strength with numbers representing how many thousand units of lipase are in each capsule: An MT4 is a capsule of *Micro*T*ablets* containing 4,000 units of lipase, while an MT20 has 20,000 units. The high-dose capsules are convenient for people who need a lot of enzyme, since one MT20 is easier to swallow than five MT4's. But it's harder to make small adjustments in dosage: if someone taking two MT4's needs a little more enzyme, it's easy to increase by one capsule per meal. If you take MT20's, and increase by one capsule, it's like increasing by 5 standard MT4 caps. The high-dose capsules also cost much more than the low-dose caps (although the cost is roughly the same unit-for-unit of lipase).

Who Needs Enzymes?

Most people with CF (85–90% of all patients) need to take enzymes with their food in order to digest that food. As many as one-half of all newborn babies with CF do not need to take enzymes, but most of these babies will gradually develop a need for enzymes over the first months or years.

How Much Enzyme Is Needed?

There is no rule for how much enzyme a patient will need, and the amount varies tremendously among patients, and even changes a bit for each patient depending on what is in the particular meal or snack. The amount of enzyme needed for a particular meal depends on several things, including:

1. The person's age and size
2. Amount of pancreatic blockage
3. Amount of fat in the meal or snack

A tiny snack, or one with no fat, will require no enzymes, while enzymes will be needed for a meal or snack with fat in it, and more enzymes will be needed for an extra large meal, or for one with a lot of fat. A plain potato is virtually all carbohydrate, and therefore doesn't require enzymes for digestion. However, if you eat your baked potato loaded with butter and sour cream, then you would need to take enzymes with it. Many patients know that for pizza or their dad's chili they will need more enzymes than for most meals.

How Do You Know How Much Enzyme to Take?

At first, it seems that it will be very difficult to learn how to adjust the enzyme doses, but most families become experts very quickly. Here's how: Some people say that the digestive system is a long tube that leads from the kitchen to the bathroom (food in the top, bowel movements out the bottom). There is a certain truth here, and it's the key to knowing how much enzyme you need. Undigested fat ends up in the stool, making for frequent, bulky, smelly bowel movements that will sometimes have oil or grease droplets visible in them or leave an oily film on the toilet water. If you see bowel movements like that, you know that more enzymes are needed. Be careful not to make changes in the usual enzyme dose based on one messy stool; instead, make sure that there is a pattern. Everyone—CF or no— has a sloppy stool on occasion, whether it's because of a little virus, some bad food, a medication, or other cause. These common sloppy stools are nothing to worry about, and will get better on their own. Frequently, patients with CF get so used to increasing their enzymes for "sloppy" stools that they see a messy bowel movement, increase the enzymes, and find that the stools become normal quickly (which they might have anyway if it wasn't an enzyme problem that caused the one abnormal bowel movement in the first place). Then, since the stools have become normal, they keep the enzymes at the new higher dose. The next time there's another single abnormal stool, they increase the dose again, and so on. In this way, many patients with CF end up taking much larger doses of enzymes than they really need. So what? In most cases, the only problem with taking too much enzyme is the minor bother of swallowing extra pills, and cost: you're paying for more medicines than you need. For some people taking very high enzyme doses, however, there is a small chance of a dangerous complication, with scarring of the colon (the large intestine), with the scary name *fibrosing colonopathy*. This condition almost always requires surgery (and is discussed in Chapter 4, *The Gastrointestinal Tract*). This problem almost never occurs in anyone taking less than 2,500 units of lipase each meal for each pound they weigh. A 25-pound child who takes 5 MT20's with each meal is probably taking too much:

$$5 \times MT20 = 100,000 \text{ units of lipase}$$
100,000 units for 25 pounds of body weight:
$$100,000 \div 25 = 4,000 \text{ units of lipase per pound}$$

Most people can get by with much, much less. A reasonable starting dose of enzymes is more like 250–500 units of lipase per pound of body weight. For the same 25-pound child, this would be between:

$$25 \times 250 = 6,250 \text{ units of lipase, and}$$
$$25 \times 500 = 12,500 \text{ units of lipase}$$

This is between $1\frac{1}{2}$ and 3 MT4's.

(For those of you who prefer the metric system—the language most physicians and nutritionists speak—the guidelines we just gave have been translated from the original: a good starting dose of enzymes is 500–1,000 units of lipase per *kilogram* (kg) of body weight, and there have never been cases of colon scarring in people taking less than 5,000 units of lipase per *kg* of body weight. The child in the example above weighs 11.3 kg, and was taking 8,850 units of lipase per kg of body weight.)

Even people whose enzyme dose has crept up over the years to what might be a dangerous dose can do well with a greatly decreased dose.

Poor Response to Enzymes

There are several reasons that someone may not get the appropriate benefit from a usual dose of enzymes. If stools continue to be loose, you should contact the CF center staff. Some causes of loose stools have to do with enzymes not working well, while others don't have anything to do with the enzymes. Some causes of loose stools are as follows:

- Excessive juice intake (very common with toddlers, no relation to enzymes)
- Introduction of solid foods to an infant (may need more enzymes)
- "Grazing" eating makes enzyme dosing difficult
- Not taking extra enzymes with "fast foods" or other high-fat meals
- Not taking extra enzymes with milk or other beverages with fat
- Not taking enzymes with snacks that contain fat (candy bars and peanuts are high in fat, for example)
- Lactose intolerance (inability to digest the sugar in milk) can cause malabsorption
- Chewing enzymes
- Excessive stomach acid
- Not taking enzymes

HIGH-CALORIE NUTRITIONAL SUPPLEMENTS

Milkshakes and commercial high-calorie nutritional supplements can be pre-scribed if routine nutritional measures are not sufficient. Sometimes people who cannot eat enough calories in their regular diet can drink the supplements for enough extra calories to start gaining weight. Busy teenagers and active adults find the ready-to-drink nutritional supplements very convenient when away from home or in place of a meal. Examples of high-calorie supplements are presented

TABLE 6.5. High-Calorie Oral Supplements

Product Name	Serving Size	Calories per Serving
Boost	8 ounce can	240
Calories Plus	1 pkg & 6 ounces milk	562
Carnation Breakfast	1 pkg & 8 ounces milk	300
Deliver 2.0	8 ounce can	480
Ensure	8 ounce can	250
Ensure Plus	8 ounce can	355
Ensure Pudding	5 ounce can	240
Jevity	8 ounce can	254
Kindercal	8 ounce can	240
Lipasorb	8 ounce can	324
Magnacal	8 ounce can	480
Nutren 1.5	8 ounce carton	355
Pediasure	8 ounce can	240
Peptamen	8 ounce can	240
Polycose Powder	As desired	30 per Tbsp
Pulmocare	8 ounce can	360
Respalor	8 ounce can	365
Resource Plus	8 ounce carton	355
Scandishake	1 pkg & 8 ounces milk	600
Sustacal	8 ounce can	250
Sustacal Plus	8 ounce can	365
Sustacal Pudding	5 ounce can	240

in Table 6.5. Special high-calorie recipes are presented in Appendix D: *High-Calorie Recipes*.

TUBE FEEDINGS

A few patients cannot take in enough calories by mouth to gain weight or to maintain weight. For these special patients, calories (in the form of liquid formulas) can be given by tube feeding while they sleep. The tube used reaches directly into the stomach or intestine. This has been done for CF patients in a number of different ways. Some patients have used a **nasogastric** tube (or NG-tube) that passes in through the nose, down the throat, and into the stomach. Some young children who found this idea repellent at first have quickly become used to the tube, and older children have learned to insert the tube themselves each night before bed. The improvement in growth and appearance and feeling of well-being has made this extra effort worth it to them.

A second method of tube feeding is through a **gastrostomy** (or G-tube). In this method a tube is placed through the skin of the upper abdomen and into the stomach during a minor operation. In some centers, it can even be done in the radiology department with the patient sedated, but not under general anesthesia. After the tube is placed, the patient is usually not allowed to eat large amounts for the first few weeks, while the small surgical wound heals. Once it has healed, the patient can eat as much regular food as he or she wants, and additional calories are fed through the tube while the patients sleeps. As with the NG-tube, results from this type of feeding have been dramatic. This tube has the advantage of not having to be replaced each night, and it does not involve the discomfort of a tube that goes through the nose. It also does not interfere with breathing or coughing. It is invisible under the clothes when it is not being used, and can be hooked up to the supplemental feeding at night. When it is no longer needed it can simply be removed without an operation.

Jejunostomy (or J-tube) feeding is similar to gastrostomy feeding, except the tube goes into the second part of the intestine instead of the stomach. It is less commonly used, but has the advantage of protecting against gastroesophageal reflux of the tube feeding (see Chapter 4). Predigested formulas are often used for the gastrostomy and jejunostomy feedings. These formulas do not need enzymes for digestion or absorption.

No one likes the idea of tube feeding when they first hear about it. But many people with CF have been "converted" when they see the dramatic growth that is often achieved with these tube feeds. Many patients have also felt a big burden has been taken off them: they have usually been *trying* to eat enough to gain weight, and their parents have certanly been "on their case" continuously to eat more; now with the food coming in by tube feeds, they don't have to force themselves to eat. It is important not to wait too long if tube feeds are to be tried: someone whose nutrition and overall health are **too** bad may not benefit.

Problems with Tube Feeds

Tube feeds require either the discomfort of placing the tube each night and removing it each morning, or the discomfort and risks of a minor surgical procedure. Many people feel "full"—uncomfortably so for a few—in the morning after a night of tube feeds, and they may not want to eat breakfast. Some may even vomit from being overfull. These problems can usually be taken care of by slowing down the feeds toward morning. Occasionally the tubes will leak, causing some wetness and mess. This leaking can usually be taken care of by changing the tube. Finally, for many people, the weight gain is very good only while they get the tube feeding, and the benefits are lost if the feeds are stopped.

INTRAVENOUS NUTRITION

Intravenous nutrition is rarely required, because nutritional supplements or tube feeding is usually sufficient to improve nutrition. Intravenous nutrition (also called *parenteral* nutrition) can be given through a long-term IV into a large vein, usually in the upper chest. As with the supplemental nutrition by mouth and by tube, intravenous nutrition can be given at home, so that a person's life can be continued normally. This is a very expensive form of nutrition and should only be used if the patient is unable to tolerate tube feedings into the stomach or intestine. There is a slight risk of serious infection of the intravenous line. If the line does become infected, it needs to be removed, and another placed.

SUMMARY

In summary, there are three components of CF nutrition (high-calorie diet, oral pancreatic enzymes, and vitamin supplements). With aggressive application of all three components, most people with CF should be able to grow well, and maintain nutrition that is adequate to support their overall health.

7

Hospitalization and Other Special Treatments

THE BASICS

1. Some patients need to be in the hospital, especially to treat worsened lung infection.
2. These hospitalizations usually last 2 weeks, but can be shorter or longer.
3. During the hospitalization, patients get antibiotics through an IV, and have some blood tests.
4. There are ways to make the hospitalization less scary than it might otherwise be. Your CF center staff can help.
5. Some patients can get IVs at home.

HOSPITALIZATION

In a given year, about 35% of CF patients will have to be hospitalized. The most common reason for a hospital admission for someone with cystic fibrosis (CF) is for treatment of worsened lung infection (commonly referred to as a *pulmonary exacerbation* (see Chapter 3, *The Respiratory System*). The time needed in the hospital is the time it takes to get back to your usual state of health, most commonly about two weeks. This chapter reviews what happens during such a hospitalization, and includes general information about hospital routines and procedures, an explanation of the various treatments and tests, and an introduction to the different health professionals you'll see in the hospital.

Preparing for Hospitalization

Admission to the hospital upsets the daily routine of a family, and, in effect, creates a crisis. The family members must draw on new resources to cope with this stress; healthy coping patterns help the child and family learn something from the experience and come away from it as stronger, more mature individuals. However, in order to accomplish this, the family must be able to rely on new resources and must be well-informed about what to expect.

Parents should ask questions they may wonder about in order to know what to expect in the hospital. Here are some examples:

- What are the visiting hours?
- May I stay overnight with my child?
- May brothers and sisters visit?
- Is a "pass" allowed, so I can take my child out of the hospital for a break?
- Can I assist with my child's care (baths, feeding, treatments) if I would like to do so?
- Which doctor is in charge of my child's care? What other doctors will be working with him or her?
- Who are the other members of the health care team?

The child who is old enough to understand should be prepared for the hospital with simple, honest information. Questions he or she may want answered include:

- How long will I be in the hospital?
- When will I go into the hospital?
- When will I come home?
- Will I get any needle "sticks"?
- What will the other kids be like?
- Can mom and dad stay with me?

As you answer these questions you will acknowledge that there will be some painful procedures (IVs, blood tests). These things need to be mentioned, but do not need to be dwelt on. Similarly, you can and should point out the "neat" things about the hospital (playrooms, etc.), without implying that all will be wonderful fun. Some children may not ask their parents questions about the hospital. They may choose to discuss their worries with another trusted adult in an effort to spare their parents additional concern. Developing relationships outside the family circle is a normal part of growing up and this should be fostered as it occurs.

It is helpful for children to have descriptions of what the hospital rooms look like, and how daily life will differ from what they are used to. A prehospitalization tour is especially helpful so the children can see for themselves, and see that things may not be quite a scary as they feared, and some things can even be fun. These tours can be usually be arranged through the CF staff (especially nurses and social workers).

Encourage your child to pack personal items from home (toys, blanket, clothes, pajamas, school books, cassette tapes and tape player) and perhaps pictures of family members. In most cases, the children should dress in their regular clothes, and should be out of bed most of the day.

When leaving the hospital it is important to get written instructions about home care and whom to call with questions and when to return for a checkup.

Parents may notice some temporary changes in their child's behavior after hospitalization. Children may have nightmares, fear of strangers, fear of the parent's absence, become aggressive or rebellious, have tantrums, or try to avoid returning to school. Some children have "regressive behavior"—that is, they act babyish even though they had been quite "grown up" for their age before the hospitalization. These reactions are not unexpected but should be brought to the attention of the pediatrician or cystic fibrosis center team for recommendations.

Admission: Checking In

The following events occur just preceding most admissions to the hospital: the hospital admissions office will be notified by your physician of the date and reason for your hospitalization. The people in the admissions office will need to ask some general questions and get your insurance information. This is done over the phone before you come in, or in the admissions office on the day of your arrival. After you "check in," in the admission office, you will be sent to one of the in-patient floors. A member of the staff will orient you to the floor (show you how to call for a nurse, how the bed, phone, and TV work, inform you of the usual floor rules and schedules, etc.).

Soon after you arrive on the floor, a nurse or patient care assistant will check your "vital signs" (pulse—how fast your heart is beating, respiratory rate—how fast you're breathing, blood pressure, and temperature), and will weigh and measure you. This person will usually ask you about what medicines you take at home, and whether you are allergic to any medications or foods. He or she will ask things like nicknames, food preferences, and where parents can be reached. These things will enable him or her to help plan for your care during your hospital stay.

The next step is usually to meet a doctor who will ask more extensive questions about your medical history and then perform a physical examination. In a small community hospital, the doctor may be your own physician; in a large university hospital, the doctor is likely to be an intern or resident (see below for an explanation of the "cast of characters"). After the questions and exam, the physician will write orders for treatment and the necessary treatment will begin.

Teaching hospitals, in which many cystic fibrosis centers are located, have the advantage of providing highly skilled care by a group of specialized professionals (the "cast of characters" is discussed later in this chapter). However, families may find the system frustrating because of the many staff members involved in their child's care. They find themselves repeating their child's medical history several times for medical students, interns, and residents. These physicians-in-training often have limited experience with CF, and the parents can become upset at their lack of knowledge. Young staff members may feel threatened when faced with a knowledgeable, articulate parent and find it difficult to care for the child. Although some aspects can be trying, this is a superb opportunity for you to help the community: the more exposure young nurses and physicians-in-training have to CF, the more knowledgeable they will become. Since they soon will be the doctors and nurses in the community, it is essential that they be as aware of CF as possible.

Parents play an important part in their child's health care and contribute their intimate knowledge of their child. Health care providers have experience with many different children over a span of years. Together, in a cooperative, positive attitude, parents and health care providers can educate one another about the needs of *this* child and effectively plan and carry out hospital care.

Daily Life in the Hospital

Most often when CF patients are admitted to the hospital for treatment of a pulmonary exacerbation, they are not terribly sick or disabled. The reason for these hospitalizations is to *keep someone relatively well*, and not to cure someone who is dreadfully ill. Some people, including young doctors or nurses, may not understand that and may even say, "you don't look sick enough to be in the hospital." They miss the point that your health is suffering and that the reason for the hospitalization is to get you back to your normal state of good health. While you probably won't be so sick that you need to be in bed all day, it is important to remember that you are in the hospital to improve your present and future health.

Most children's hospitals, and many general hospitals, encourage parents to participate in their child's care but to take care to remain *parents*, not *nurses* or *doctors* in the eyes of their child. Bathing, feeding, play and bedtime stories, and maintaining normal discipline standards are activities that promote normalcy in the hospital. While parents may want to be present as a source of support and consultation during painful or frightening procedures, some experts feel that they should avoid being enlisted to assist directly with such procedures (such as stabilizing an arm for blood test or injection). When this does happen, it may seem that the parent has given up his or her job as *protector*.

Hospitalized children need different things from their parents at different ages. The infant and toddler are too young to understand what is occurring and cannot fully comprehend the parents' explanation. For an infant, the parents' trusted, nurturing presence can be comforting. Cuddling, rocking and singing, and playing are all familiar activities that bring security to a new, frightening environment.

As children advance to the toddler and preschool years they begin to understand more of what is occurring. Their primary fears in the hospital are abandonment and lack of mobility. They benefit from regular contact with parents and the presence of a stable group of caretakers when their parents cannot be there. They also enjoy active play, despite their IV lines!

Children in this age group have many fantasies and develop their own reasons for why things happen. They may interpret hospitalization as a punishment. New signs, smells, and sounds may be particularly frightening. They benefit from simple, concrete explanations immediately before the procedure about what they will *sense* (see, hear, feel, smell) during a new experience. They may also attempt to stall a nurse or doctor who is about to perform a painful procedure: as a general rule it is best to provide a simple explanation and then allow the staff member to proceed quickly and with confidence.

Preschool and school-age children have an even greater understanding of events and benefit from explanations. They also benefit from participating in planning their daily care and being provided with choices about their schedules, meals, and therapy where applicable. They should be encouraged to maintain contacts with friends while in the hospital and to develop new friendships with other patients.

Teenagers with CF are faced with the complications of a chronic illness at a time when they are most concerned with a changing body, achieving independence from the family, and establishing relationships with the opposite sex. Cystic fibrosis may thwart many of these goals by slowing growth and delaying puberty and by imposing a home-care regimen that perpetuates dependence on the parents. In addition, no teenager wants to be different from others, and the young man or woman with CF may appear different or have different needs, making it more difficult to establish new relationships. In the hospital, teenagers benefit from many of the same practices as their younger counterparts: explanations of what to expect, opportunity to participate in planning their care, making choices about some flexible areas of care, and contact with school friends. This assistance should be provided in the context of the special needs of the changing, developing adolescent who is seeking to establish some measure of independence.

What to Wear

You will probably be up and around most of the day, so you should wear regular clothes. You might need to be sure you have roomy, loose sleeves to fit over IVs.

Activity

You should try not to let being in the hospital decrease your activity. Most hospitals, especially children's hospitals, will have playrooms and teen lounges, and you should take advantage of these facilities. You may be able to use a physical therapy gym, or even to leave the hospital (on a pass) to get even more activity. This may be a chance to visit museums or other favorite places. You may be a bit tired, particularly at first, and you shouldn't push yourself *too* much, but you should try to be up and around most of the day. If you lie in bed all day, you will definitely get out of shape, and will soon be unable to do much at all.

School Work

Two or three weeks is a lot of time to miss from the school year, so it is very important to try to keep up with your school work. Your doctor can help you arrange for work to be sent or brought to you in the hospital. Some hospitals have a schoolteacher on their staff to help students keep up with work. Some school systems have arrangements for home (or hospital) tutors for anyone who will be out of school a certain amount of time. It is very important that you do whatever is necessary to keep up with school work while you're in the hospital.

Infection Control

Lung infection is of course one of the main things that cause deterioration of the health of people with CF. Worsened infection—particularly with bacteria like *Pseudomonas aeruginosa, Burkholderia cepacia,* and *Staphylococcus aureus*— is the main reason for hospital admission. We are not sure yet how people with CF become infected with these different bacteria (this topic is discussed at greater length in Chapter 3, *The Respiratory System*), but increasing evidence shows that *one way* is "person-to-person" transmission, meaning you can get some bacteria from other people. These other people include other CF patients who might already have a particular kind of bacteria, and could also include health care workers. Because of the possible risks of getting new—and perhaps more dangerous and difficult-to-treat—bacteria from other patients, many hospitals and clinics now have rules that separate CF patients from each other. These rules may include:

- No rooming together
- No visiting in one another's rooms during chest PT sessions or other times with heavy coughing
- The necessity to cover mouth and nose during coughing spells
- Careful disposal of tissues that have mucus in them
- No touching other CF patients
- Perhaps requiring wearing masks
- Etc.

Some hospitals have set aside separate floors of the hospital for patients with and without certain specific bacteria (especially *cepacia*). These restrictions can be annoying, and perhaps even frightening, but they seem to keep to a minimum the number of cases where patients come down with new bacteria, and therefore should be followed. In fact, you can help, by suggesting good hygiene to other people coming into your room: ask other patients to cover their mouths when they are coughing and to wash their hands after coughing spells. Demonstrate that you're not "picking on" anyone else by doing the same things yourself. And don't be shy about suggesting to your nurses, respiratory therapists, or doctors to wash their hands before they touch you.

Treatments and Test

Intravenous (IV) Antibiotics

One of the main reasons for being admitted to the hospital is to get powerful antibiotics (especially those that kill *Pseudomonas*) that are effective only when given directly into the bloodstream. A short soft plastic tube or catheter is inserted in the vein with a needle; the needle is then removed, leaving the soft catheter in place. (Some children seem to like to know that the dreaded "N-word"—needle—will be thrown away, leaving just a tiny strawlike tube in.) The end of the catheter is taped to the skin, and its end is closed off with a rubber cap, or attached to more tubing through which fluid can be administered. When the needle is first inserted, it will hurt a little as it pierces the skin, but once it is removed, leaving the plastic catheter in place, it is rarely painful. Babies, children, and older patients alike can usually carry on their daily activities with an IV in place. There is a medicated cream (EMLA® cream) that can be used to numb the skin where the IV will go. The only problem with this cream is that it needs to be in place for 45 minutes for it to work, so putting it on will delay things a bit while you wait for it to take effect.

The veins that are most often used are those on the back of the hands and on the forearms, but if these veins are difficult to find in an infant (as is often the case with a chubby baby), foot veins or veins in the scalp may be used. Foot veins should not be used in anyone who can walk unless there is no other choice. Scalp vein IVs look as though they'd be very uncomfortable, and most parents are bothered by the idea of them at first, but they are no more painful than an arm vein IV and have the advantage of not requiring the immobilization of an arm. If a hand or arm vein is used, an arm-board (which looks like a splint) helps to keep the hand or forearm stable, which in turn helps keep the IV within the vein. A plastic or cardboard cup may be taped over the needle to protect it and prevent it from being bumped.

When the IV is about to be started, it's a good idea to tell the person starting it if you have preferences about which hand or arm to use: If someone is right-handed, it's better to leave the right hand alone, so it can be used for writing, playing Ping-Pong, etc. Similarly, it's better to pick a spot that will leave the elbow free to bend. If a baby has favorite fingers or thumb to suck, he or she will be much happier if those fingers or that thumb is not taped out of mouth's reach.

Once the IV is in place, the medicines can be given through it. The medications are mixed with saline (salt water) or dextrose (sugar) water and then either allowed to drip through tubing into the IV under the force of gravity, or are pushed through the tubing by electric pumps that regulate precisely how much goes in and how fast. It usually takes 30–60 minutes for antibiotics to run into the vein. When the medications have finished going into the vein, the IV may then be connected to tubing through which simple saline or dextrose mixtures are passed until it is time for the next antibiotic. A much more convenient procedure is to flush the IV with a small amount of saline and heparin (a drug that prevents blood clots from blocking the needle) and then to leave a cap on the end of the IV. Once the IV line is flushed with heparin and capped, it can safely be left alone for many hours and will be ready for use when it's time to give the next dose of antibiotics. This means that the person does not have to be tied continually to the IV pumps, tubing, and bottles, and will be free to move about.

IVs last only for a limited period, for they eventually go bad ("infiltrate") and need to be replaced: antibiotics are powerful chemicals, and may irritate the vein, eventually weakening its wall so that it starts to leak, making the arm swell and become tender. When this happens, it is time for a new IV. Although IVs may occasionally last a couple of weeks, a few days is closer to the average.

Two different antibiotics are commonly used. Each of the antibiotics must be given on its own schedule. Schedules range from every 4 hours to every 12 hours, with the most common intervals being every 6 or 8 hours. If blood levels are checked, they may indicate that the dosage or schedule needs to be changed, for example, from every 8 hours to every 6 hours. "Central lines" (see later in this chapter) generally do not go bad, and many patients and physicians prefer them, even though they may be a little harder to put in.

The effectiveness of these medicines probably relates to the peak level of the drug (the highest level that is reached), and their toxicity (harmful effects) most likely relates to the "trough" (lowest level). Since the peak usually occurs within 30–60 minutes after the medication enters the vein, and the trough is hours later (just before the next dose), careful monitoring of drug levels will necessitate a double test, one just after the drug has gone in, and one just before the next dose. If the levels are too low or too high, the physicians will know that they must adjust the dose. In this way, it is possible to get the maximum benefit from the medications and the minimum toxicity. This is good, but at the same time it's a bother, since blood levels may need to be checked again with the new dose. (An idea that occurs to a lot of patients is: "Why not draw my blood from my IV, so you don't have to stick me?" This *can* be done for some tests, but not for antibiotic levels. The reason it can't be done for the antibiotic levels is that, since the antibiotics were given through the tubing, there is often some extra left within the IV tubing itself, so the level within the tiny length of tubing will be higher than the *real* level in the rest of the bloodstream.) Once the right dose is found, it is not necessary to recheck the levels frequently.

Length of IV Antibiotic Treatment

The ideal length of time to get IV antibiotics to fight bronchial infection is the time it takes to get you back to your baseline pulmonary function, that is, the amount of time needed to get you back to your usual state of health. Most often, this is about 2 weeks, but it can easily take 3 weeks. It is rarely more than 3 weeks or less than 2. Most CF experts feel that it is a mistake to let the calendar determine the length of treatment without regard to the patient's progress; rather, it is the patient's response to treatment that should dictate the length of hospitalization. Pulmonary function tests (PFTs) and a physical examination can often help in determining the length of stay, but often it is the patients themselves and their families who contribute most to this decision. They are the people who know best, for example, just how much the patient is coughing. The observations of the patient and family are very important in this regard. While several weeks in the hospital can seem like a very long time, and it may be tempting to try to arrange discharge as early as possible, it is wise to remember that the time invested in achieving good health is time well spent. It is quite possible that a few extra days at the end of a hospitalization may mean several more weeks or months of good health.

Other Treatments and Tests

Other aspects of the treatment will vary at different CF centers, but will often include chest physical therapy (postural drainage or other form of airway clearance; see Chapter 3,) two to four times a day (or even more), aerosol treatments (with bronchodilators, antibiotics, or both—also discussed in Chapter 3), vitamins, pancreatic enzymes, and plenty of calories. It is not unusual for a patient (especially a teenaged patient) to get a bit cranky when he or she is awakened in the morning for an aerosol or chest PT. It's important to remember that these treatments are a big part of the reason for the hospitalization, and the people who are giving you the treatments are trying to help you get better. Anti-inflammatory medications (e.g., prednisone) may be included in the treatment. Exercise may or may not be prescribed, and on admission patients may be feeling a bit "under the weather," and need more rest than usual. In most cases, after the first few days, patients should be up and out of bed most of the day. In some hospitals, you may be able to attend school (your own school or an in-hospital school room) or work, on an altered schedule built around the medication schedules.

Nutrition is also an important part of in-hospital treatment. Food can sometimes be an issue, since the hospital food is seldom as good as home cooking. Most hospitals give a choice of foods, and many even allow inpatients to order from a hospital cafeteria menu if they don't see something they want on the regular patient menu.

Other Blood Tests

When someone is admitted to the hospital, several kinds of blood tests are usually done. Almost always, these admission tests can be done with one needle stick, even if several tubes of blood are needed (the total amount of blood needed will seldom be more than one tablespoon). Different tests may be done, including blood counts and measurement of blood electrolytes (chemicals such as sodium, chloride, and potassium). It is also common to check the blood levels of chemicals that reflect kidney function, since many antibiotics can affect kidney function.

Some of the tests are done only at admission, but others are repeated periodically through the hospitalization. For example, kidney function tests might be repeated once or twice a week to make sure that the drugs have not caused a problem. As we've already discussed, blood may be taken several times to measure antibiotic levels.

Other Tests

Chest x-rays and pulmonary function tests, perhaps including a blood gas test, may also be done shortly after admission and at intervals during the hospitalization, in order to monitor the progress you are making (see Chapter 3, *The Respiratory System,* for a discussion of these tests). Electrocardiograms (ECGs) and echocardiograms are often performed in order to determine the heart's condition and see if it's showing evidence of having to do extra work. Other tests might also be done, depending on the circumstances. A hearing test might be performed if drugs are being used that might affect hearing. As always, if you do not understand what a test is, or why it's being done, ask.

The Cast of Characters

You will meet many different people in the hospital in addition to other patients, and it can be confusing as you try to figure out who everybody is. Remember, with any problems or major questions, your doctor is in charge.

Nurses and Patient Care Assistants

Hospitals could not run without nurses and patient care assistants. They will check you in, check your vital signs, administer medications, help you to communicate your needs and concerns to the appropriate staff, and in general help to make your stay successful and pleasant. They may be able to answer many of the questions that arise regarding treatments, schedules, etc.

Physicians

You are likely to see a number of different physicians in addition to your own doctor. Especially if you are in a children's hospital and/or a teaching hospital (one that has students, interns, and residents), you will also be meeting a number of people at the various levels of medical training. It is helpful to know the different stages of medical training.

Medical students have gone to college for four years and are now enrolled in a four-year medical school. The first two years consist of classroom and laboratory learning. In the third and fourth years, students spend time in the hospital, learning the various specialties such as pediatrics, general internal medicine, and surgery. After completing four years of medical school, students graduate and get their doctoral degree (M.D. or D.O.). They are now doctors.

The first step after becoming a doctor is internship. An *intern* is a doctor who is beginning to train in one specialty—pediatrics, internal medicine, family medicine, surgery, psychiatry, or obstetrics/gynecology. After the internship year, the specialty training continues with 2–4 years of "residency." (Most programs no longer call first-year trainees "interns," but rather, "first-year *residents*.") After a resident has finished the three-year residency, he or she is qualified to set up practice as a specialist (family doctor, pediatrician, etc.).

Some physicians choose to get even more specialized training, and take 2- or 3-year subspecialty *fellowships.* Subspecialties include pulmonology (respiratory problems, including CF), cardiology (heart), and neurosurgery (brain and nervous system surgery). Some of the "trainees" you meet might be young students, whereas others may have had 4 years of college, 4 years of medical school, 3 years of pediatric or medicine residencies, and several years of fellowship.

As we've already mentioned, interacting with many different people at various levels of training and understanding can be difficult for patients and families, especially when several people ask you the same questions. It may also be frustrating to realize that you know more about CF than some of the nurses and physicians who will be taking care of you or your child. Remember, though, that your own physician is knowledgeable about CF and is in charge of your (or your child's) treatment.

In addition, you can view this as an opportunity to help in the education of the people who will be the nurses and physicians in the community. Many families with a child with CF have had the very frustrating experience of going from doctor to doctor trying to find out what was wrong until they found one who knew about CF. One of the best things that anyone can do to help future children with CF is to make a contribution to the education of physicians who will be seeing those children, so that eventually all family doctors, pediatricians, and even adult medical specialists will be knowledgeable about CF, will be able to recognize it, and will have an idea of how to begin treatment.

Consultants

Occasionally, your physician may ask a colleague to give an opinion about a problem or a possible treatment. The other physician will probably look through your chart, ask some questions, and do a physical exam. This colleague is likely to be a specialist or subspecialist, possibly, a gastroenterologist (stomach, liver, and digestive system specialist), surgeon, or cardiologist. These colleagues who are called in to give an opinion about one part of the treatment plan are called *consultants*. It is the job of the consultant to give an opinion and perhaps make suggestions. It is not the consultant's job to carry out treatments or order tests without your physician's approval.

Other Health Professionals

In addition to nurses and physicians, you are likely to have contact with other professionals, including physical therapists and respiratory therapists, who may be involved with your aerosols and postural drainage treatments. Some hospitals will have child-life workers to help make the hospitalization a more positive experience. These people are trained in child development principles, and are frequently clever at finding just the right kind of entertainment for a child in the strange environment of the hospital. More importantly, they are sensitive to the signals children give through their play and talk about things that are upsetting or threatening to them. Child-life workers and child development specialists often can give parents, nurses, and physicians important insights into what is going on in the minds of hospitalized children.

Nutritionists or dieticians may help with menu selection, recommendations about high-calorie supplements, special diets that might be needed (for example, for someone with diabetes), adjustments to enzymes. Social workers will be available to help with a variety of problems, from very tough family adjustment problems (these are discussed in Chapter 12, *The Family*) to the day-to-day worries of insurance and transportation expenses. Other people you may come in contact with include people from a TV service, hospital maintenance people, and janitors.

BRINGING THE HOSPITAL HOME

There are many ways that complex kinds of treatment can be carried out at home, thus avoiding prolonged hospitalization. These include home IVs, various kinds of tube feedings, and different ways of giving oxygen.

Home IVs

Intravenous treatments are usually done in the hospital, but in some cases, once it is clear that progress is being made, can be completed at home, and in some cases, even be started at home. Whether you can do these treatments at home will be determined by your physician, in consultation with you. Insurance companies and HMOs (health maintenance organizations) are putting increasing pressure on families and physicians to use home IVs instead of the hospital, since it may be cheaper for these companies, whether or not it is as effective as the hospital. Several things must be taken care of before someone can be sent home with an IV: there must be someone at home to take care of the IV—to connect the tubing to the needle for infusing the antibiotics, to flush the tubing after the antibiotics have run in, to keep the IV from clogging. The medications must be mixed and stored properly, and they must be run in at the right speed. Someone must be available who knows what to do if the IV comes out or goes bad. Arrangements also have to be made for regular checkups, including blood tests (antibiotic levels, etc., as would be necessary in the hospital) and physician exams. This can be extremely tiring, and—depending on how well the IV is working, and what schedule is needed for the particular antibiotics—time-consuming. For example, a common combination of two antibiotics includes one that needs to be given every 6 hours and another that is given every 8 hours. This is a schedule that leaves little time or energy for the parent (or adult patient) to do anything else, including good chest PT for airway clearance.

Who Takes Care of the IV?

In many metropolitan areas, home medical care companies or IV infusion companies have taken on many of the tasks of visiting homes, helping to restart IVs when necessary, working with families to run the IV medications, supplying electric pumps to regulate the speed at which the medication is run in, drawing blood for tests, working with pharmacies to supply the medications, and so on. If such a service is not available, public health organizations, such as Visiting Nurses, may help with these details. In other cases, families and physicians have been able to piece together a team of people to do the various things. Some emergency room nurses have volunteered to restart IVs when necessary, and helpful pharmacists may take care of preparing the antibiotics. Your CF center staff can help you make these arrangements. It is very important to check whether home IVs will be covered by your insurance.

Checking Up

Once someone is freed from the constraints of the hospital, by being sent home on IVs, it is easy to forget that if he or she were in the hospital, there would be physicians to monitor the progress of the treatment and to check for evidence of drug toxicity at least once a day. It is important to maintain close contact with your physician after hospitalization, particularly if you're still taking the powerful drugs that traditionally have been given only under supervision in a hospital. Checkups once a week, or more or less frequently, may be necessary.

IVs for Prolonged Use: The Central Line

In some patients, IV antibiotics (or rarely, other IV treatment) may be needed very frequently or for a prolonged time. In these cases, and, in fact, in patients who are getting the standard two or three weeks of IVs, it is not convenient or comfortable to keep using regular hand or arm vein IVs, which only last a few days before they have to be changed. In these cases, a "long line," or a "central line," can be lifesaving, or at least much more convenient. These lines are a special kind of IV that has its end in a very large vein, or in the heart. When this IV is used, the medication runs into an area of very large blood flow, so that even powerful chemicals will be diluted quickly and will not irritate the veins the way they do with a hand vein. Long lines are usually tunneled under the skin (and in some cases, placed *entirely* under the skin) so that they will not accidentally become dislodged.

The three main types of central lines are Broviac and Hickman catheters (permanent—or very long-lasting—central lines, with exit tubing tunneled under the skin, exiting through the skin on the chest), Mediports®, Infusaports®, and Portacaths® (also permanent—or very long-lasting—central lines that are totally under the skin), and "PICC" lines (*p*ercutaneously *i*nserted *c*entral *c*atheters, which are designed for temporary use for up to several weeks). The Hickman and Broviac catheters are similar, and are lines that are inserted through a small incision, usually in the skin of the neck or by the collarbone, with one end being placed in one of the large veins in the neck, and threaded down into the *superior vena cava* (the largest vein bringing blood back to the heart from the upper part of the body) or into the heart itself, while the other end may be tunneled under the skin of the chest. In this way, the only part of the catheter that is in contact with the external environment (air, clothes, bath water, etc.) is the tip, which comes out from under the skin on the front or side of the chest. Once the original incisions have healed completely, it's safe to bathe, play sports, and pursue normal activities with the line in place. You should avoid getting hit directly in the chest, and some surgeons prefer that you not swim with one of these long lines in place, but everyone agrees that most normal activities are perfectly safe.

Mediports®, Portacaths®, and Infusaports® are used much more commonly nowadays than the Hickmans and Broviacs, mostly because of their greater safety and convenience: They are inserted similarly to the Hickmans and Broviacs, with the tip ending in the *superior vena cava* or the heart, but the end through which medicines are infused is under the skin, with no tubing sticking out. This means any activity (other than those in which the area would be hit hard) is safe with these devices, and the risks of infection are much less, since the end is not exposed. These totally implanted devices have a small *reservoir* just under the skin. It's the rubber tip of this reservoir that is punctured with the needle for hooking up to antibiotic infusions. For most of the time, these devices, which can be placed under the skin of the chest, upper leg/groin, or arm, are just left in place, and are out of the way. When antibiotics are needed, a small needle can be put into the rubber cap at the beginning of the 2- or 3-week antibiotic course, and the infusion tubing hooked to it. The skin does not need to be punctured for each dose of antibiotics. The skin will need to be punctured about once a month for flushing the tubing with saline and heparin, to make sure the line does not become blocked with blood clots.

PICC lines are very similar to regular IVs except that the tubing is much longer, and can be pushed into the vein far enough that it follows the vein back to the large veins in the chest (such as the *superior vena cava*) or even back to the heart. These lines can stay in for weeks at a time.

Placement of Long-Line IVs

Most of the long lines are placed by surgeons; but some particularly skillful pediatricians, internists, or radiologists might also do the line placement. Depending on the patient's age and level of anxiety, either a sedative or general anesthesia is given, and if the patient is awake, the areas of incisions will be numbed with injections of local anesthetics (e.g., Novocain®). Most often, these procedures are performed while the patient is in the hospital. Recovery from the procedure is very rapid. For PICC lines, general anesthesia is virtually never needed, since their placement is not very much different from a regular IV; they just are longer, get gently pushed farther into the vein, and last much longer than a regular IV.

Equipment

Some special equipment is needed for the proper care and use of the central lines, especially when they are used out of the hospital. Supplies for keeping them sterile are essential. Special pumps are helpful to push medications in at the proper rate, since problems could develop with medications running in too fast or too slowly. Special needles and tubing are needed to attach the central lines to the bottle or plastic bag holding the medication. For Hickman and Broviac catheters, the needles pierce the rubber cap at the end of the line, but for the Infusaports®, Portacaths®·and Mediports®, special needles are required to pierce the skin and stay firmly in the reservoir under the skin for the days or weeks of the course of antibiotics. Solutions must be on hand to flush the lines after use (these typically contain saline and heparin to keep blood clots from forming in the line while it's not being used).

Care of Central Lines

Exquisite care must be taken so that these lines do not become infected. Infection in these lines nearly always means that they must be removed. If they need to be replaced, another procedure is required and perhaps another session under general anesthesia, entailing additional risks. More importantly, these lines are in the heart or close to it, and infection in the lines means serious bloodstream infection in the patient. People can get extremely ill from bloodstream infection. Fortunately, with proper care, these lines seldom become infected, even out of the hospital, perhaps because the people who take care of the lines at home are usually the patients themselves or a close family member. Whenever the small dressing (often little more than a Band-Aid) is changed, and medications begun, the technique used must be sterile (allowing no germs to enter). Sterile gloves are worn, the area is cleaned according to strict guidelines, using strong antiseptic solutions, and all tubing ends that would touch the end of the central line are kept scrupulously clean.

Care must also be taken to see that the lines are not pulled out or bumped hard. This protection is easy to provide: the tubes are quite thin and only a short portion sticks out of the skin, so the tubing can be coiled and covered with a small amount of gauze and taped in place. Care of the central lines that are totally under the skin (Mediports®, Infusaports®, Portacaths®) is much easier between courses of medication than care of the lines with ends sticking out from under the skin. In fact, other than avoiding direct hits to the site of the implanted device, very few precautions need be taken; it's fine to swim, surf, etc. Unfortunately, every course of antibiotics does require that a needle pierce the skin to enter the central line whose reservoir lies just beneath the skin, and such a needle stick is also needed about once a month *between* courses of antibiotics, to keep the tubing open. Usually, people with these central lines do not mind the inconvenience of these few needle sticks, particularly compared to the many sticks they would have had with traditional IVs.

In deciding whether to have one of these lines, you have to decide *where* you'd like to have it. As with so many things, each location has advantages and disadvantages: on the chest, the reservoir is probably the most stable, and easiest to enter with the needle, but may interfere with chest PT treatments. In young women, the surgeon must take care to avoid breast tissue when he or she places a reservoir under the skin on the chest. The upper leg has been a convenient place for many patients, and a few young women have given the surgeons strict instructions that it be hidden by a bikini-bottom for their time on the beach. Some patients are a little shy with the placement meaning that any manipulations of the reservoir (like the every-month "flushing" of the line), done by a stranger, are in what is usually a private part of their body. Many others have liked the fact that lines placed in the upper leg are hidden from public view virtually all of the time. One patient couldn't have this kind of line because it would have hit on the lower "uneven bar" when she did her vigorous gymnastics practice and competitions. Some patients have liked the convenience—despite a small lump—of having these ports (reservoirs) in their arm.

Complications

Infection is the most common serious complication that can occur with a central line. A central line infection can be a medical emergency, and at best usually means removing the infected line and replacing it with another one. There is a limit to the number of times this can be done, because once a long line has been in a particular vein, it can be difficult to put another line back through the same vein.

A very rare complication, *air embolism,* can be fatal. This happens when the central line has been opened to the air (rather than clamping it before connecting it to the medication tubing) and the patient takes a big breath, allowing air to rush into the line, and then into the heart. A small amount of air in the line will do no harm, but a large amount can be extremely dangerous. This can be guarded against by not leaving the line open to air; older children and adults can be careful to hold their breath for the short period of time that the line might be open. The danger of air accidentally entering a central line does not exist with the Mediport®, Portacath®, or Infusaport® systems, since they are not uncapped when hooked to the bottle or bag of medication.

Bleeding from accidentally uncapping the central line can be serious, since the tip of the line is in an area of very high blood flow.

Fortunately, most of these complications are quite uncommon when central lines are taken good care of.

Nutritional Treatment Aids

Some patients who need nutritional supplements can be helped by special procedures and devices (see Chapter 6, *Nutrition*). These may include central lines for the administration of high-calorie intravenous feeding, the so-called "hyperalimentation" (or *TPN—total parenteral nutrition*) solutions. The procedures, care, and risks for central lines used for hyperalimentation are the same as those used for antibiotics.

Extra calories can also be given through the normal digestive tract, with three different types of tube feedings.

Nasogastric Tubes

"NG-tubes" go through the nose (*naso-*) and pass down the throat into the stomach (*gastric*). If a thin tube is passed this way just before bedtime, a person can sleep while high-calorie formula is slowly pumped through it overnight. As discussed in Chapter 6, *Nutrition*, this method of feeding has been successful for a small number of people with CF. It has the disadvantage of having to insert the tube through the nose and swallow it each night and remove it each morning, and although this is not a painful procedure, it is uncomfortable. A great advantage of this method of tube feeding compared with the two other methods (discussed below) is that the tube is out during the day.

Gastrostomy

A gastrostomy tube ("G-tube") passes directly into the stomach through a hole ("stoma") made in the abdominal wall by a surgeon, specially trained radiologist, or gastroenterologist. This tube is very safe, and provides a direct route for high-calorie formulas to be fed (usually at night, while the patient sleeps). There are several disadvantages:

1. It requires a procedure, with general anesthesia or IV sedation, and makes the patient quite sore for the first few days after the procedure, and not able to eat regularly for a few weeks while it heals.
2. The tube is always present, even during the day when it's not being used. (The reason it must be there even when it's not being used is that the hole would close, and heal shut within hours if the tube weren't there to keep it open.) Having the tube in is not uncomfortable, but many people don't like wearing a bathing suit if they have a tube sticking out of their abdomen. (A device called a "button" is available which has solved this problem: it is a very short tube that can go in the stoma and keep it open, but while barely extending beyond the skin. It can easily be covered with a small Band-Aid.)
3. If someone has a tendency toward gastroesophageal reflux (see Chapter 4, *The Gastrointestinal Tract*), filling the stomach during sleep may worsen that problem.

However, the advantages are also considerable:

1. It works: This method has been very successful for a large number of CF patients.
2. It avoids the discomfort of passing a nasogastric tube each evening and morning.
3. If the tube falls out, it can just be put back in (if it's replaced within a few hours).
4. It does not interfere with any activities (except for the embarrassment); it is safe to go swimming or play any sports with it in place.
5. If and when you get to where you no longer want or need to use it, it can simply be taken out.

Jejunostomy

The "J-tube" is very similar to the gastrostomy tube, except that the surgical opening is made in the jejunum (the second part of the small intestine) rather than in the stomach. It has one main advantage over the gastrostomy tube, namely, that it avoids the problem of gastroesophageal reflux. Since the formula doesn't go into the stomach, it can't back up into the esophagus. A minor advantage is that the tube used is smaller than most gastrostomy tubes, and therefore is more readily coiled up flat against the abdomen out of the way.

There are several disadvantages to the J-tube: (1) Placing it initially is more difficult than placing the G-tube. (2) If the tube falls out, it is somewhat more difficult to replace than the G-tube, especially if it falls out within the first weeks after it's been placed. Replacing it may even require another operation. Once it's been in for a few weeks or months, though, a track is well established and if the tube falls out or gets pulled out accidentally, it can be replaced readily by just putting it back in (no surgery is necessary).

Complications of Gastrostomy and Jejunostomy Tubes

Both G-tubes and J-tubes are relatively trouble-free, but some complications can occur. The first isn't really a complication, since it is to be expected, namely, the discomfort for the first few days after they are placed. Any surgery on the abdomen will make someone uncomfortable, perhaps very uncomfortable, for a few days, and placing these tubes is no exception. Occasionally, the tubes may leak, especially when someone coughs. In most circumstances, the leaking can be taken care of by pulling the tube more tightly against the abdominal wall. Some people may develop tender scar (*granulation*) tissue at the site of the stoma. This can be removed painlessly in the surgeon's office.

Oxygen-Delivery Systems

In most patients who need oxygen, the simplest way to deliver the oxygen to the patient is through nasal cannulas (this is discussed more fully in Appendix B: *Medications*), with the source of oxygen being metal canisters of oxygen. If you need oxygen a lot of the time, and/or want to be able to move around while you use it, there are some convenient systems that you can read about in Appendix B: *Medications*. These include oxygen *extractors* or *concentrators* (machines that take oxygen from the air in the room, without having to buy tanks of oxygen), reservoirs of liquid oxygen (these are tanks that store oxygen in liquid form, which takes much less space than the oxygen gas tanks, and from which small portable tanks can be filled), and some small, lightweight portable tanks.

8

Transplantation

THE BASICS

1. Transplantation is taking a healthy organ from one person and putting it in another person, usually to replace a damaged organ. This has been done with the lungs for a few hundred people with CF. (It has also been done rarely with the liver.)
2. Transplantation is very difficult and expensive, and requires as much or more care afterward than CF itself. Getting a transplant is much like trading one disease for another.
3. Some CF patients have done very well after lung transplants, and some have had months or years of problems; some have died.
4. Medicines to prevent the body from attacking the transplanted organ are important after transplantation; getting too little of this type of medicine can cause rejection, while too much can allow infection to set in.
5. About 75% of CF patients who get a lung transplant will be alive 1 year later, about 50–60% after 2 years. Longer survival is certainly possible. More than 80% of children with CF who receive liver transplants will be alive 3 to 5 years later.

INTRODUCTION

The term "transplantation" is commonly used in the daily newspapers as well as in the medical literature. Transplantation is surgically removing an organ from one person and placing it in another person. The person receiving the transplanted organ is known as the *recipient.* The person from whom the organ is obtained is known as the *donor.* In virtually all cases, transplantation is designed to replace severely damaged organs with organs that are healthier. In almost every case, the damaged organs are removed from the recipient at the time the new organs are put in.

The donor organ is removed from someone who doesn't need it. In the case of a kidney or a bone marrow transplant, this is often a living relative of the recipient. We have two kidneys, but can live healthy lives with only one kidney. Part of the bone marrow can be removed and the remaining marrow will grow back with no harm to the donor. In each case, the living donor can spare the transplanted organ for a sick relative. In most cases, though, the organ needed for transplantation is one we can't live without—such as the heart, lung, or liver. In this case, the person from whom the donor organ comes is most often someone who is dead, particularly someone who has had severe brain damage from trauma (car crash, etc.), but whose lung (or liver or heart) has not been damaged. Later on, we'll discuss this further.

Several different types of organ transplants have been performed, dating back as far as 1906 when the first attempt was made to transplant a pig's kidney into a person. The first human-to-human kidney transplant was done in 1936, and the first successful kidney transplant was done in France in the early 1950s. (Some of the organs for these early transplants in France came from prisoners right after they had been executed by guillotine.) Since then, attempts have been made—with varying degrees of success—to transplant the liver, heart, pancreas, intestines, bone marrow, and lung.

The first human liver transplant was performed by a team directed by Dr. Thomas Starzl on March 1, 1963. At that time, there were only a few drugs available to prevent rejection of a transplanted organ. Dr. Starzl persisted in his pursuit of liver transplantation, despite the fact that it was not until 1969, some 6 years after the first attempt (!), that a patient lived for more than 1 year after a liver transplant. In June 1963, only three months after the first liver transplant, the first human lung transplant was carried out. That first patient survived less than one month after the transplant. Rejection of the transplanted organ and infection were both major problems in the early days of transplantation. They still are formidable challenges to successful transplantation today and will be discussed later in this chapter.

A major advance in transplantation was the discovery of the powerful antirejection drug cyclosporine in 1978, which improved the ability of physicians to prevent rejection of transplanted organs. Recognizing this new drug as one that would be useful for organ transplants, Dr. Bruce Reitz of Stanford University successfully carried out the first combined heart-lung transplant in 1981. Only a couple of years later, in 1983, the first heart-lung transplant in a CF patient was performed at the University of Pittsburgh by a team headed by Dr. Bartley Griffith.

The number of successful liver, lung, and heart-lung transplants increases every year, but there are many more people awaiting transplants than there are available organs.

Some patients with CF may be faced with the possibility of a transplant because of their disease. In most of these cases, it will be a lung transplant; in a very few cases, it will be a liver transplant. In 1994, of the 20,000 patients who were seen in accredited CF centers, 97 received a lung transplant, and 8 received a liver transplant. That means less than $\frac{1}{2}$ of 1 percent of all CF patients got a lung or liver transplant in 1994. Adding in the transplants done in previous years brings the number up to 317 patients who had received new lungs and 51 with new livers, for a total of about 2 percent of all CF patients seen in CF centers in 1994.

In this chapter, we'll describe transplantation, explain the reasons some people with CF might benefit from a transplant, and identify some of the more important problems with transplantation. In addition, we'll try to explain why transplants may sometimes have to be considered even if the patients don't feel sick enough to think they need a transplant. First, we'll discuss transplants in general, then, matters that are specific to lung transplants, and, finally, matters that pertain especially to liver transplants.

WHO NEEDS A TRANSPLANT?

With a treatment as new and hazardous as transplanting an organ, it is difficult to say that anybody needs it. With a broken arm, it's easy to say, "you need to have that bone set, and the arm put in a cast," because we know that you will have much less pain, suffering, and long-term disability if the break is treated that way. With organ transplantation, particularly lung (or liver) transplantation for someone with CF, it's much harder to be certain of the outcome with or without the treatment. This uncertainty is related to the difficulty in predicting what will happen to CF patients who do and don't get transplants. We will discuss this later in this chapter. Despite the uncertainties, most CF doctors agree on some broad guidelines for which patients should be considered for transplantation. These guidelines assume that in order to be a "good candidate" for a transplant, you need to be sick enough, but not too sick. If you're not very sick, it doesn't make sense to get a transplant because your chances of doing well for a long time are better without a transplant, and you would be using organs that could otherwise be used for someone who might die without them. On the other hand, if you are too sick, or have certain medical conditions that we'll discuss later, the chances of success with the transplant are small, and you and your family will have been put through a very hard (and expensive) ordeal, again using organs that would have had a better chance of helping someone else.

LUNG TRANSPLANTATION

Who Should Be Considered for Lung Transplantation?

For lung transplantation to be worth the risks, most experts feel that the patient's quality of life must be intolerable, with difficulty breathing and an inability to carry out the daily tasks of living (school, work, recreation activities). The experts also feel that lung transplantation should not be done if the person is likely to survive for more than two years without a transplant. One difficulty here is that there are no good tests to tell us when someone's life is intolerable or when someone with CF will die. People are amazingly different from each other in their ability to function under what seem to be the same circumstances. This is certainly true for people with CF and their lung function. Two CF patients with equally good (or bad) lungs, as measured by their PFTs (pulmonary function tests: see Chapter 3, *The Respiratory System*) may have very different lifestyles: one may be nearly bedridden, while the other carries a full load of college courses and works part-time in a pizza shop. So, the PFTs cannot tell us if someone's quality of life is good or bad. One yardstick that is sometimes used is that if someone needs to use oxygen all the time in order not to feel short of breath, he should consider lung transplantation.

What about knowing when someone with CF will die from her lung disease? Just as the PFTs don't tell us exactly how well someone feels or what she can do, they also can't tell us how long she will live. As is discussed in Chapter 15, *Death and Cystic Fibrosis,* there are some rough statistics that say someone with CF with a PFT (specifically, the FEV_1) below 30% of what it should be has a 50–50 chance of being alive in two years. Many physicians have taken this information to mean that if someone has PFTs that low, she should consider lung transplantation. Later in this chapter, we'll talk about how to make the final decision about whether or not to go for lung transplantation.

Who Should Not Be Considered for Lung Transplantation?

Just because certain organs, such as the liver or the lungs, can be transplanted, it does not mean that every patient will benefit from a transplant. For some people, the modern medical approach of "if it's possible, we should do it!" does not fit with their view of the world. For these people, the very high-tech (and high-cost) modern medical procedures are not appealing, especially if it means that they might lose control of their own destinies. Some patients have felt that, although a transplant might be the only way to prevent dying within the next few years, dying may not be the worst thing possible. There is no question that the possibility of transplants has changed the way people with CF die. In the past (or now, if someone is not considering transplantation) when patients' lungs had reacjed a certain point, and it was likely that a patient would die in the near future, and all the physicians', patient's, and family's efforts were directed at trying to keep the patient comfortable while providing care that might help make the patient better if that were possible. If there were ever a conflict between patient comfort and a treatment, the treatment would be skipped, patient comfort emphasized. Now, if someone is waiting for an organ to become available, there is often a level of desperation: we need to wait for the organ, to keep alive at all cost!! So a patient and family may not be able to deal with their own thoughts of losing each other, and may not be able to say or do things that need to be done. Instead, all efforts are put into survival at all cost until the call comes saying that lungs are available. Losing the little peacefulness and calmness that previously was possible in contemplating death seems too high a price for some patients, and they choose not to consider transplantation. Patients, families, and physicians also now realize that getting new lungs does not guarantee that everything will be perfect afterward. Instead, many patients have as much trouble, and spend as much time in the hospital after transplant as they did before transplant. So, some patients and families choose not to be considered for new lungs.

In some other situations, the likelihood of success of transplantation is very small and the known risk of the procedure is quite large. Such situations are known as *contraindications* to (reasons not to do) transplantation. Physicians must take into account all such factors before deciding whether or not a transplant procedure is indicated. Certain factors are associated with such a poor outcome that they are considered *absolute* contraindications to transplantation. Other factors may be associated with an increased risk, but this risk may be acceptable in a sick patient; these factors are considered *relative* contraindications to transplantation. A single relative contraindication usually does not prohibit transplantation, but the presence of several relative contraindications may be adequate to disqualify a patient from receiving a transplant. Not all transplant centers agree on relative or absolute contraindications, although all transplant physicians must confront such issues in each patient they see. The decision to "list" someone for transplantation (see below for more on the transplant list) is often made by a group of physicians, and their view of the relative or absolute contraindications in each patient becomes the basis for their final decision to proceed or not proceed with transplantation.

There are several absolute contraindications to lung transplantation. A severe infection that has spread into the bloodstream and caused alterations in the function of other organs, such as the kidney, heart, and brain, is one of the most important contraindications to transplant. A cancer that is not confined to the organ for transplantation is a second absolute contraindication. In many centers, severe kidney or liver disease are contraindications to lung transplantation.

Because patients with CF commonly have bacteria such as *Pseudomonas* or *Staphylococcus* in their airways, the mere presence of these bacteria is not a contraindication to transplantation. However, as will be discussed in the next section, bacterial infection of the transplanted lung is a common complication in CF patients. Over the years, several transplant centers have reported that airway bacteria that are resistant to antibiotics are a problem following lung transplantation.

In several of these reports, a specific type of *Pseudomonas* known as *Pseudomonas cepacia* (recently renamed *Burkholderia cepacia*), which is often resistant to all antibiotics ("panresistant"), was associated with a very high mortality. More recent studies have shown that the bacteria present in CF sputum before lung transplantation are the same organisms that cause lung infections following transplantation. This means that if a patient with CF has panresistant organisms (*B. cepacia* or others) before transplantation, then the infections after transplant will be very difficult to treat. Because of the risk for severe and untreatable infections following transplantation, many centers now consider the presence of panresistant strains of bacteria in the airway an absolute contraindication to lung transplantation.

There are numerous relative contraindications to lung transplantation. These include previous chest surgery or pleurodesis (discussed in Chapter 3, *The Respiratory System*), poorly controlled diabetes, or a history of a psychiatric disorder. Malnutrition is a relative contraindication to transplantation, and many transplant centers are unwilling to consider transplanting a patient who is too thin. As you will see, the surgery involved in transplantation is very extensive and there is a long recovery period. Patients who are weak because of malnutrition may not have the physical strength to recover from the operation. Most transplant centers suggest feeding tubes such as NG (nasogastric), gastrostomy, or jejunostomy tubes to provide enough nutrition to allow the patient to be strong enough to survive the surgery.

Another relative contraindication is a past history of what is referred to as "noncompliance." This means not taking prescribed therapy such as antibiotics or pancreatic enzymes, or not doing regular chest physiotherapy, or of failing to be seen regularly by a CF physician. The importance of a patient and family being able to take medications, do treatments, and show up regularly for their appointments cannot be overstated. Transplantation is a complex process, and the treatments and medications following transplantation must be done exactly as prescribed. Because there are many more people who need new lungs than there are lungs available, it is important that the organs be transplanted into patients who will take care of them. Patients and families must be able to cooperate with the transplant team, in order to maintain good function of the transplanted lungs; and transplant physicians are less likely to believe that a patient will do what he's told after transplant if he is unable (or unwilling) to follow instructions before transplant.

The Transplant List

There is no shortage of people whose doctors feel they need a transplant. There is, however, a big shortage of donor organs to use for these patients. There are several reasons for the shortage, beginning with the fact that most donor organs have to come from people who have died—and died in a way that has not damaged the organ in question (for CF patients, this means lungs or liver). In some circumstances, the donors have decided while they were alive that in the event of their death they wished to be organ donors. They may have signed a "donor card" and informed their families and clergy. Unfortunately, there are relatively few people who have expressed such a desire. More often, the families of potential donors must be approached at the tragic and upsetting time when their loved one is dying. It is difficult for many families to agree to organ donation at such a time, and therefore many organs that would have been suitable for transplant are not made available.

Organs must be taken for transplantation before they are too damaged to help the transplant recipient. Once the heart stops beating and blood is no longer flowing into organs such as the lungs or liver, those organs become rapidly damaged. For this reason, organs are removed from the donor before the donor's heart has stopped beating. Many of us were taught from childhood that the heartbeat is the true sign of life, and life continues until the heart actually stops beating. Medicine, however, has advanced to the point of having ventilators to breathe for us and medications to stimulate the heart to beat strongly. The availability of transplantation as a science has raised the question of what constitutes life and what constitutes death. Most physicians and scientists now feel that the true measure of life lies not in the heart beating or in breathing, as these can be artificially stimulated, but in the presence of brain function. Now, people with severe brain injuries, who are being kept alive with machines such as ventilators, can be tested to see if they have any brain function. If they don't have brain function and are not receiving medications that affect brain function, they can be considered "brain dead." This term means that their brain will not recover any function and, although the machines may keep them "alive," they are not experiencing life, are not thinking, and have no brain function. (It may be more appropriate to think of the machines that keep air moving in and out of their lungs, and blood circulating, etc. to be "organ support," and not what they're usually called, "life support.") Such patients could serve as donors of organs for transplantation if those organs (heart, lung, liver, etc.) still function normally. This is the reason for the timing of when organs are taken from donors. It also helps to explain why many families find it difficult to agree to organ donation: their loved one appears asleep, rather than dead.

Once the organs are removed from the body of a donor, they are cleared of all blood by washing a salt solution through the blood vessels that go to the organ. This preparatory phase before transplantation is known as preservation. A liver can be preserved for up to 24 hours after it is removed from the body, while lungs become hopelessly damaged within 4 to 8 hours. So even if there is no difficulty with a family's agreeing to donate the organs from their family member, the organs do not keep very long at all. If they are to be transplanted, it needs to be within a matter of hours. You can't call central supply to order up a lung or liver.

Soon after transplantation became a widespread medical technique, it was apparent that there were many more people who were waiting for transplants than there were organs available. Because physicians and politicians were worried that organs might actually be sold or not given to the most needy recipient, The Transplant Act of 1984 was passed by Congress to make sure that organ donation is fair and equitable. A private nonprofit national organization known as the United Network for Organ Sharing (UNOS) was set up to keep track of transplant recipients and donors. As a part of their job, UNOS maintains a computerized list of patients awaiting transplantation and matches donor organs with appropriate recipients. In the UNOS system, the country is divided into regions served by local Organ Procurement Organizations (OPOs), which in turn are responsible for helping local physicians identify potential organ donors and helping transplant centers obtain the organs for transplantation.

Getting on the Transplant List

The first step in being considered for transplantation and getting on the transplant list is being referred to a transplant center by your regular physician. In the case of patients with CF, this physician would most likely be your CF physician. The referring physician sends information about you to the transplant center, and the transplant physicians then decide whether or not you should be seen and evaluated. The information your physician will send to the center will include your recent PFTs, chest x-rays, and results of your sputum cultures. In addition, your physician will usually speak with one of the transplant physicians about your illness, how many hospitalizations you've had, and how well you follow the physician's advice. The transplant physicians will look at the information, including the sputum culture results, and decide whether you should be evaluated more fully to see if you should be listed for transplantation. If the decision is made to evaluate you, then you travel to the transplant center and undergo more tests (x-rays, blood tests, exercise tests, etc.). You are seen by a number of physicians, usually including a transplant surgeon, a pulmonary specialist, and an infectious disease specialist. You and your family are interviewed by social workers and, in many centers, a pediatric psychiatrist. This latter point is important, and emphasizes the fact that transplantation is not only a difficult surgical and medical procedure, but also a highly stressful circumstance for patient and family. If all the members of the transplant team agree that you are sick enough to require a transplant and that you do not have one of the absolute contraindications to the procedure (such as the presence of panresistant *Burkholderia cepacia* in your sputum), then you are "listed" on UNOS's computer as an "active" candidate for transplantation.

Your Spot on the List

The main reasons for UNOS to keep a transplant list are that there are more people waiting for transplants than there are organs to go around, and it is necessary to decide as fairly as possible who should get an organ when it becomes available. There are separate lists for different organs, and, although it may seem a bit odd, the "rules" governing the different lists are different.

The List for Lung Transplants

Where you are on the list waiting for lungs depends on very few things: your size (since lungs that are either too big or too little are more difficult to transplant successfully), your blood type, and, most importantly, the length of time you've been on the list. If two people on the list are the same size and blood type, and one has been on the list for 2 years and the other has been on for 1½ years, the one with the 2-year wait will be offered the next set of lungs, even if she is not as sick as the other one. In some ways this system seems unfair, but UNOS decided that anyone who was sick enough to be accepted onto the list was sick enough to deserve organs, and the fairest way to allot available organs is on the basis of the total waiting time a potential recipient has acccumulated.

The assignment of lungs solely on the basis of waiting time has had an unexpected effect. The wait for lungs now is often 2 years or longer in most U.S. transplant centers, and this has led to the earlier "listing" of patients. In other words, the long wait for lungs means that in order to get a set of lungs when you need them, it's probably necessary to get on the list before you're actually sick enough to need them. So, if you're not sick enough now to need new lungs, but might be that sick in two years, now is the time to start the evaluation process to get on the list. Another problem that has arisen because of the long wait for lungs is that patients who delay being considered for lung transplantation may find themselves very sick and not able to receive lungs. One of the painful lessons learned at many lung transplant centers is that between one-fourth and one-third of the patients waiting for lungs will die before lungs become available.

Waiting on the List

Once the patient is "listed" for transplantation, he must wait until he has moved to the top of the list and until an organ becomes available. As we've just discussed, this can be as long as two or more years for patients waiting for lung transplants. In most cases, routine follow-up care is done by the referring physician (your usual CF physician and family physician), but the transplant physicians will often want to see you at their center at regular intervals (usually every 6–12 months). The visits to the transplant center will allow the transplant physicians to examine you, to look at your sputum cultures, PFTs, and x-rays, and to get an idea of how sick you are.

Some transplant centers require candidates for transplantation to become involved in specific exercise and nutrition programs, which are designed to strengthen the patient and improve his ability to withstand the stresses of surgery and recovery during the postoperative period. Several centers require that patients and their families move to the city where the transplant will take place. Some of these demands on patients may improve their chances of surviving until the transplant can be done, and some of the demands placed on both patients and their families will show the transplant team that these prospective recipients are able to follow directions, take medications, and comply with all therapeutic measures. While this may seem unfair, we should remember that organs for transplantation are a rare and valuable commodity. There are many more patients who seek transplantation than there are available organs. A patient who does not take care of himself after transplantation not only hurts himself, but has also "taken" a donated organ away from someone else—someone who might take better care of himself (and the new organ). Many centers doing transplantation are less willing to transplant organs into patients who have shown that they are not able to take care of themselves properly before transplantation.

"Active" and "Inactive" Patients on the List

The list of candidates awaiting transplantation is divided into *active* and *inactive* status. Being active or inactive is referred to as the status of the candidate. The status of any candidate can be changed from active to inactive (or vice versa) depending on a variety of factors that we'll discuss below. People who are "active" move up toward the top of the list as people ahead of them go off the list (because of getting a transplant, dying, deciding against transplant, or becoming inactive). Once he reaches the top of the list, the active candidate will be offered the next organ that becomes available.

People who are inactive will not be offered an organ (even if they are at the top of the list), nor will they be given credit for the time they are waiting as long as their status is inactive. They can move up the list as people ahead of them come off the list, but other active candidates can pass them on the list as the active candidates receive credit for the time they are waiting for organs. However, candidates who change their status from active to inactive do not lose credit for the time they've waited as active candidates. So, if someone has been an active candidate on the list for 22 months and then becomes inactive, he still has 22 months of waiting time to his credit if he goes back on the active list later.

There are several reasons that a patient might change from active to inactive on the list. First, a candidate may be at the top of the list and receive a call to be transplanted at a time that she doesn't feel sick enough to have the transplant, or she might be too frightened. She may then turn down the offered organ. The lung will then be offered to the next person on the list, and the first candidate will not be penalized. If this happens several times, however, the transplant team can suggest that the candidate be changed to inactive for a while. If some time later she is ready to be considered for a transplant, she will become "active" again and her place on the list will be determined by the amount of time she had accumulated waiting while she had been on the active list.

A second major reason for changing a candidate from active to inactive may be a change in the candidate that is an absolute contraindication to transplantation. An example of this might be the finding of a major new infection outside of the lungs, such as an infection in a Mediport® central line (see Chapter 7, *Hospi-*

talization and Other Special Treatments). This would have to be treated before the patient could get a transplant. Most of the time, the patient is not put on the inactive list while such an infection is being treated, but if organs became available during the treatment of the infection, those organs would have to go to the next person on the list. If the infection proved difficult to treat, the candidate might have to change his status to inactive at that time.

Sometimes the problem may not be in the patient's overall health, but in his sputum cultures. As we've already discussed, some centers will not transplant patients who have panresistant bacteria in their sputum. An example of this would be a patient who starts to grow *Burkholderia cepacia* in his sputum after being listed as active. If someone's culture begins to show those bacteria, the patient may be inactivated until the culture clears up. In many centers, such patients are not inactivated, but they will not be transplanted. This allows them to continue to move to the top of the list while efforts are made to get rid of the resistant bacteria in their sputum.

In some instances, candidates have been made inactive when they have not been able to follow through with their medical therapy. For example, patients who refuse to do prescribed chest physiotherapy treatments or who fail to be seen regularly by their CF physician are more likely to be inactivated by a transplant center. Most transplant teams feel that if patients cannot do prescribed treatments *before* transplant, they are hurting themselves and showing that they probably won't do prescribed treatments *after* the transplant. If patients can't follow the directions of their physicians after they receive a transplant, they are not only hurting themselves but also are punishing a patient who might have received their organ and taken better care of themselves (and the donated organ, too).

The Technique of Lung Transplantation

General Considerations

Transplantation surgery is complicated and difficult. It is done in specialized medical centers by highly skilled surgeons and anesthesiologists. The surgery involved in lung transplantation requires large incisions (cuts) through the skin and other tissues that make up the wall of the chest, which permit the surgeons to inspect, remove, and replace the damaged organs. The removal of the organ from the recipient must be done carefully, leaving the arteries, veins, and (in the case of the lung) airway (trachea and main bronchi: see Chapter 3, *The Respiratory System*) in place, for these must be attached to the donor organs in such a way as will allow the new organ to function normally. These new attachments, in which a donor artery, vein, or airway is joined to the *native* (recipient's) artery, vein, or airway, is known as an *anastomosis* (pronounced a-*nass*-to-*mo*-sis), and is a crucial part of the surgery. The site of the anastomosis may be weaker than the rest of the donated organ and can come apart more easily. This breakdown of an anastomosis, known as *dehiscence* (pronounced de-*hiss*-sense), can result in severe bleeding or (in the case of the airway) sudden respiratory difficulty. Another problem that anastomoses are subject to is narrowing, known as *stricture* or *stenosis*. In blood vessels, this can lead to blood clots at the site of stricture. Stenosis of the anastomosis in an airway can result in difficulty in breathing.

Although the transplant surgery is done while the patient is deeply anesthetized, there is a lot of pain and discomfort during recovery from these operations. While many patients do very well right after lung transplant surgery, full recovery from these procedures may take weeks or even months.

Specifics of Lung Transplantation Procedures

Until the late 1980s, most lung or heart-lung transplants were done through what is called a median sternotomy, in which the breast bone is cut from top to bottom and the chest is opened by pulling the cut sides apart. Now, most lung transplant operations are done using what is known as an *anterior-inferior transthoracic incision,* also known as the "clamshell" approach. This means the surgeon cuts across the lower part of the chest wall from one side to the other, allowing the entire upper part of the chest wall to be lifted up, much as you would raise the hood of a car (or open a clamshell). This gives the surgeon a better look at both lungs and makes the surgery somewhat easier. A good view inside the chest is especially important if the recipient has CF, because CF patients often have scarring of the thin membrane (the *pleura*) that covers the surface of the lung. This scarring may also involve the lining of the chest wall, which is also a thin membrane and is also called the pleura. Normally, the space between these two membranes (called the *pleural space*) is lined only with a tiny amount of fluid, and the lungs can be pulled out of the chest cavity relatively easily, but in CF, there can be a lot of scar tissue between the pleural surfaces, making it difficult to remove the lungs. Furthermore, scar tissue bleeds easily when it's pulled apart.

The earliest operations for lung (and heart-lung) transplantation involved removing the donor lungs together, still attached to the lower part of the donor trachea. (In the case of heart-lung transplantation, the lungs still had their attachments to the heart, and the heart and lungs together, known as the "heart-lung block," were removed from the donor.) For those early lung transplants, the recipient lungs were also removed together, leaving behind most of the recipient's trachea, along with the pulmonary arteries coming from the right side of the heart and the pulmonary veins leading back to the left side of the heart. The top of the donor trachea was attached to the lower part of the recipient trachea and the donor and recipient arteries and veins were joined. This is known as double lung transplantation, because the two lungs are placed into the donor as a single unit.

As you can imagine, this is very exacting, tedious, time-consuming work. The surgeons must use many tiny stitches in these delicate tissues, making sure there is not even a small hole left behind that would allow blood to leak out of the veins or arteries being sewn together, or air to leak out of the ends of the trachea which were sewn together. The surgery takes hours, during which time the patient has no functioning lungs (and in the case of heart-lung transplantation, no beating heart). In order for this surgery to be possible, the patient's blood must be rerouted outside the body through plastic tubing to a "heart-lung machine," also called "cardiopulmonary bypass." This machine takes blood and oxygenates it, then pumps it back into the body. Blood going through cardiopulmonary bypass machines has the danger of clotting within the plastic tubing, or in the patient when it returns, so it needs to be treated with "anticoagulants," drugs that interfere with clotting. Like so many other things done in medicine, this can be a double-edged sword: along with preventing the bad clotting that might take place within the bypass machine or the patient's blood vessels, these medicines can also prevent good clotting that is needed to stop the bleeding of surgical wounds. Some of the early CF patients who had this kind of surgery for lung transplantation had a lot of bleeding into the pleural space around their new lungs and many of them died because the bleeding would not stop. This is one of the reasons that previous pleurodesis (see Chapter 3, *The Respiratory System*) is considered a contraindication to lung transplantation at many centers. Another problem with this form of double lung transplantation is that the anastomosis of the trachea may not receive good blood supply and the tissue may die, leading to dehiscence of the anastomosis, which can lead to sudden respiratory difficulty and death. In addition, the tracheal anastomosis is more likely to become narrowed (stenosed) if the tissue is damaged at the junction.

There is a newer technique for lung transplantation that has become more widely used. It is called "sequential single lung transplantation." In this technique, each donor lung is removed as a separate entity, with its attached artery, vein, and airway. Each recipient lung is also removed one at a time, leaving small lengths of the artery and airway that can be joined to the corresponding donor artery, vein, and airway. One donor lung is transplanted into the recipient while the patient is breathing with the remaining lung. Once the first lung is transplanted, the recipient breathes with that new lung while the second lung is removed and the second donor lung is transplanted into position. The technique of sequential single lung transplantation is considered safer and has a better survival record than double lung transplantation. In many cases, cardiopulmonary bypass is not needed during sequential single lung transplantation, so the risk of bleeding during and after the transplant surgery is much less. (A few patients with especially poor lung function may still have to go on bypass during the surgery, because they don't have enough functioning lung tissue left in one lung to support them with that lung alone while the other lung is being removed and replaced.) By reattaching each airway near the lung instead of reattaching both lungs as a unit to the trachea, this technique leads to a lowered risk of dehiscence of the airway anastomosis. However, the risk of stenosis of the airway with sequential single lung transplantation is increased, because the airway near the lung is smaller than the trachea.

At the time of surgery, several plastic drainage tubes are placed through the skin into each side of the chest. These tubes will drain any air or fluid around the transplanted lungs and will help keep them inflated. They are usually removed within the first two weeks after surgery.

"Living Related" Lobar Transplantation

A relatively new and exciting development is the technique of "living related" transplantation for lung recipients. This procedure uses two live donors, each of whom donates a part of one lung. The donors are usually family members of the recipient. The part donated is one of the sections of the lung known as a *lobe* and serves as an entire lung for the recipient. Living related lobar transplantation offers several potential advantages over transplantation using organs from people who are unrelated and who have died. First, since the donor organs are being given specifically to the recipient, there is no competition for those particular organs, and therefore no need to be on a waiting list. This means that someone who is too sick to survive the long waiting list time might be able to get a transplant anyway. Second, the operation can be *scheduled,* and can be done during the day with everything relatively calm and prepared. All too often, organs for the usual lung transplant recipient arrive on very short notice, in the middle of the night, perhaps when the chief surgeon is out of town, or when the patient and family are not fully prepared to take the huge leap necessary for transplantation. Yet decisions must be made within minutes or hours to "go" or not. Finally, if the donors are closely related to the recipient, there may be a lowered risk for severe rejection. While the risk for rejection is always present (unless an organ is transplanted from an identical twin), living related transplantation may mean that the recipient will require lower doses of immunosuppressive medications.

There are, however, several potential disadvantages to living related donation. First, it involves three people who have major chest surgery: the recipient and two donors. All surgical procedures have some risk involved, and although the risk is greatest for the recipient, there is some risk to the donors. Second, there is the possibility that a donor might feel undue pressure to donate part of his lung even though he is not sure he wants to do it. In families with more than one CF patient, the decision to consider living related lobar transplantation can be agonizing: if you donate a lobe to one patient, you will *not* be able to do so for anyone else.

PROBLEMS (COMPLICATIONS) ASSOCIATED WITH
TRANSPLANTATION

General Considerations

Transplantation is a science that is still in its infancy. There are many problems associated with organ transplantation, and complications of transplant procedures are common. Several of these complications can occur with any type of transplant, and we shall discuss these, and the care necessary to prevent and treat them, in this section. Specific problems with lung or liver transplantation will be discussed separately.

One problem that many people with CF wonder about is whether their transplanted lungs will develop CF. *They will not.* CF is a part of the cells that make up the actual tissue of each organ, and if you get a new organ, that organ will not develop CF. There are many other problems that can develop, some of which are related to the fact that the patient still has CF, even though the transplanted organ does not. Patients with CF who receive a new lung or liver will still have to be seen regularly by their CF doctor in addition to their transplant doctor. Many other problems are complications of the transplant itself, and we will be discuss these problems now.

Immunosuppression: Too Much or Too Little (Infection or Rejection)

The saying: "Each one of us is unique," has special importance in relation to transplantation. Each of us has built-in systems designed to protect our body from attack from bacteria, viruses, and fungi. These complex defense systems, known as our immune system, work together to kill invading germs and keep them from harming us.

But our immune system can do more than protect us from germs that may try to invade our bodies, for it can recognize and destroy cells or organs from another person. When a new organ is transplanted into someone, the immune cells of the recipient will know that the new organ is from someone else, and they will set about to destroy it. This destruction of the transplanted organ is known as *rejection.*

Rejection is one of the major problems following transplantation, and medical researchers have struggled for years to understand it and try to prevent it from destroying transplanted organs. There are a couple of ways to do this. The first way is to transplant an organ or tissue that is not foreign. That can be done if the organ comes from oneself (as can be done with bone marrow transplants in some cases of cancer treatment: a person donates some of his or her own bone marrow for storage, and then that same bone marrow is transplanted back into the person after the cancer treatment). It can also be done if the organ comes from the recipient's identical twin, since these two people are immunologically identical. Such transplants have been done very successfully; but of course this option is open to very few people, since most of us don't have an identical twin, and the bone marrow, a kidney, or a single lobe of a lung is about the only tissue or organs that a living donor can safely contribute.

For people who don't have an identical twin to donate an organ, or need an organ (like lungs or liver) that a living twin can't do without, we must interfere with the immune system's ability to recognize and attack foreign tissue. In other words, we must suppress the immune system. The most common way of doing this is by giving the recipient medicines that weaken the immune system, making it incapable of rejecting the transplant. Such drugs are known as *immunosuppressive* agents (or immunosuppressive drugs or *immunosuppressants*) (see Table 8.1).

TABLE 8.1. *Immunosuppressive Medications*

Type of Drug	Brand Name	Generic Name	How It's Given	How It Works
Corticosteroids *Decrease inflammation and can treat or prevent acute rejection.* The exact mechanism of action of corticosteroids is not understood. They are able to directly decrease lymphocytes, the cells that are involved in rejection. Corticosteroids enter cells where they attach to a protein called a receptor. This steroid-plus-receptor goes into the nucleus of the cell where it affects the activities of the cell. Corticosteroids also interfere with the activation of lymphocytes by other cells of the immune system.	Deltasone (and others Medrol, Solu-medrol	Prednisone Methylprednisolone	Oral I.V.	See Column 1. See Column 1.
	Prelone	Prednisolone	Oral	See Column 1.
Lymphochyte-specific drugs *Decrease the ability of lymphocytes known as T-helper cells to function properly.* These T-helper lymphocytes are central to the immune system's ability to reject foreign tissue such as a transplanted lung or liver.	Sandimmune	Cyclosporine	I.V./Oral	Attaches to a protein called cyclophilin inside lymphocytes. This inhibits the ability of the lymphocyte to make proteins called interleukins, which stimulate other cells to attack the graft.
	Neoral	Cyclosporine/microemulsion	Oral	Works like cyclosporine, but may be absorbed better from the gastrointestinal tract.
	Prograf	Tacrolimus	I.V./Oral	Similar to cyclosporine, except that it has a different binding protein and is more potent in its action.

Antimetabolites
Interfere with the ability of cells to manufacture normal DNA, which is essential for cell division. This will decrease the number of cells available to reject foreign tissue.

Imuran	Azathioprine	I.V./Oral	Metabolized in the body to a compound called 6-mercaptopurine, which interferes with normal DNA production.
CellCept	Mycophenolate Mofetil	Oral	Metabolized in the body to mycophenolic acid, which interferes with DNA production.

Antilymphocyte antibodies
Preparations of antibodies that can bind to and attack proteins on the surface of lymphocytes. This will inactivate and/or destroy those lymphocytes.

Atgam	Anti-Thymocyte Globulin	I.V. (7–14 days)	See Column 1. This antibody preparation is derived from horse serum. The horses are "immunized" with human cells.
Orthoclone OKT3	Muromonab-CD3	I.V. (7–14 days)	See Column 1. This antibody is "bioengineered": it is produced by mouse cells in culture.

Few immunosuppressive drugs were available at the time of the first transplants. Steroids, such as prednisone, were used to decrease the function of certain white blood cells known as lymphocytes. An anticancer drug known as Imuran® (azathioprine) was used. It works by interfering with the ability of any cell to divide. Unfortunately, it decreases the production of good cells as well as potentially harmful cells. Steroids and anticancer drugs like Imuran® were somewhat effective, but they could not prevent rejection completely without causing severe side effects.

With an improvement in our understanding of the mechanisms involved in rejection came the development of new immunosuppressants that were more powerful in their actions on the immune system, yet didn't have as many side effects. Table 8.1 describes the major types of immunosuppressive medications now in use at most transplant centers, how they work, and what major side effects they have. We will discuss them in the next several paragraphs.

A revolution in transplantation occurred in the early 1980s with the development of a drug called cyclosporine, which was the first of these more specific and powerful agents. The improved success of liver and lung transplantation is a direct result of the development of new antirejection drugs like cyclosporine. Cyclosporine and other modern immunosuppressive drugs (including FK506, which is now known as *tacrolimus*, or Prograf®) are more effective than earlier drugs, and have fewer side effects. Unfortunately, fewer side effects does not mean *no* side effects, for all drugs (even aspirin) have side effects. We'll discuss several of the more important side effects of each class of immunosuppressive drugs in the next section (see also Appendix B: *Medications*).

Probably the most important "side effect" of the immunosuppressive drugs is that they might work too well. Remember, the immune system's primary job is to protect us from infections, and weakening it too much with immunosuppressants will result in an increased risk of developing infections. As we might expect, transplant recipients who take immunosuppressive agents are at increased risk for developing infections, either in the transplanted organ or elsewhere. Some of these infections may be life-threatening. Infections can be caused by bacteria, such as *Pseudomonas,* by viruses, or fungi. Viral infections can be particularly difficult to treat and may have further complications, which will be discussed later.

Two particular viral infections deserve special mention here. These are *cy*tomegalo*virus*, known as *CMV*, and *E*pstein-*B*arr *v*irus, called *EBV*. CMV is a common virus, which many of us have been exposed to (often without realizing it) by the time we are adults. If we've been exposed to CMV, we have built up an immunity to it and don't usually get sick if we are reexposed to it, even if we take immunosuppressive drugs. CMV is a very clever virus, however, and seems to be able to hide in lungs, liver, or blood of people who have had the virus. It can stay there, not causing any trouble as long as the person's immune function is normal. If the lungs of a donor who had CMV in the past are transplanted into someone who has never had CMV (and therefore doesn't have any immunity to CMV), and then the recipient has to get immunosuppressive drugs, the CMV can cause serious disease in the transplanted lung as well as in other sites such as the eye, the intestines, or the liver. There is another situation that can lead to CMV disease in a transplant recipient: If neither the recipient nor the donor has ever had CMV, the recipient can still be exposed to CMV after the transplant. This can happen simply by coming into contact with someone who has CMV (remember, a lot of healthy people have CMV and don't know it) or—as was common up until recently—through blood transfusions from someone who has had CMV. Transplant recipients now get blood only from people who have no evidence of ever having had CMV. Children may not have had CMV disease (and therefore have no CMV immunity), and if they have a transplant and are exposed to CMV while they receive immunosuppressive medicines, they may become quite ill. Fortunately, there are new medicines to treat CMV, but it is still a major problem, particularly in lung transplant recipients, and we shall discuss this a little more, below.

EBV is the virus associated with mononucleosis ("mono"). Like CMV, it seems to have the ability to "hide" in the tissues (and possibly blood) and cause severe problems in people who receive immunosuppressive drugs. Also like CMV, many adults have had EBV, even though they may not have had an illness like mononucleosis. Children, however, are less likely to have had EBV. They may become infected with EBV after transplantation and become ill with a disease that is similar to mononucleosis. Of more concern, however, is the association of EBV infection in transplant recipients with a special complication, which is a tumor of the lymph glands (lymphoma). This lymphoma is called *post*transplant *l*ymphoproliferative *d*isease, or PTLD. If PTLD occurs following transplantation, it usually is treated by decreasing the immunosuppressive medications. On rare occasions, PTLD may require other special forms of therapy. Although PTLD often does respond to treatment, it doesn't always, and can be fatal.

Another problem with immunosuppressive drugs is that they may not work well enough. When this happens the immune system recognizes the transplanted organ as being foreign and tries to destroy it, leading to rejection. There are two major "types" of rejection: acute and chronic. Rejection, along with infection, remains a major problem for transplant recipients, and is discussed later in this chapter.

In summary, the transplant doctors try to use immunosuppressive drugs in just the right amount. Too little immunosuppression leads to the threat of rejection; too much immunosuppression leads to the risk of infection or PTLD. Transplant physicians and scientists are constantly trying to widen the distance between the extremes of rejection and infection that can cause severe illness in the recipient. As more research is done, it is likely that safer yet more powerful immunosuppressive drugs will be discovered, allowing for better control of both rejection and infection.

Side Effects of Immunosuppressive Drugs

As we've already said, the major "side effect" of immunosuppressive drugs is either having too much immunosuppression, which leads to infection or PTLD, or too little, which leads to organ rejection. Immunosuppressives are medicines that can have other true side effects, that is, effects that are unrelated to the main reason you take them in the first place.

The main side effects of cyclosporine, tacrolimus, and similar drugs are kidney damage, high blood pressure, diabetes, seizures, increased growth of the gums in the mouth, and excessive body hair. Despite this long list of possible side effects, many of the most serious ones can be minimized by measuring the blood levels of the immunosuppressive drugs and adjusting the dose as required. In some cases, however, where the immunosuppressives are harming the kidneys, it may not be possible to lower the drug without causing or worsening lung rejection. In those few cases, it comes down to a choice between saving the lungs and saving the kidneys. The lungs always win, because you can live (with treatments several times a week from a kidney dialysis machine) without kidneys, but you cannot live without lungs. Some patients have even received kidney transplants after a heart or lung transplant because of the kidney damage caused by the immunosuppressive drugs. Some of the recipients who develop diabetes from the immunosuppressive medications may need to receive insulin shots.

The other immunosuppressants that have been used for the prevention of rejection also have side effects. Imuran® (azathioprine), as we've already discussed, interferes with the development of blood cells. Because of this, anemia and a low white blood cell count, which can increase the risk of infection, are the main side effects of Imuran®. In addition, nausea and diarrhea are fairly common with the use of this drug. Steroids such as prednisone may lead to high blood pressure, diabetes, obesity, cataracts, ulcers of the stomach and bowel, excessive bruising, and some decrease in our ability to fight off infections. Our body normally makes its own steroids similar to prednisone, and these naturally occurring steroids are important in helping us withstand stresses like infection, surgery, or exposure to cold temperature. Taking prednisone for a long time can decrease the body's ability to make these natural steroids and lead to an increased risk if we encounter any of these stresses.

Surgical Complications

Transplantation—as we've seen—involves very complex surgery. During any such procedure, it is possible that something (a blood vessel, nerves, the organ itself, etc.) could get cut that shouldn't get cut. This can cause problems after surgery.

Complications of Lung Transplantation

Aside from the general complications of transplantation we've mentioned already (as "side effects" of the immunosuppresive drugs), most importantly, infection and rejection, there are several complications specific to lung transplantation. These complications include organ failure, bleeding in the chest, blood clots in the veins going from the lung to the heart, and narrowing of the airway where the donor lung is attached to the recipient. Some of these complications happen soon after transplantation (*early complications*), while others happen later (*late complications*).

Early Complications of Lung Transplantation (Hours-to-Days After Transplant)

Organ Failure

Any organ that does not have a good healthy blood supply can be damaged. This can happen to a donor lung when it is removed from the donor, or when it is still in the donor, if the donor's illness or injury has interfered with the blood supply to the lung (or harmed it in any other way). Once the organ has been removed from the donor, it is washed free of blood with a special solution designed to keep it healthy for the trip to the operating room where it will be put into the recipient. If the trip takes too long, or if the preservative solution doesn't work perfectly, there can be damage to the organ. Any one or combination of these factors can damage the transplanted organ badly enough that it may not be able to function. This kind of problem shows up in the early hours or days after transplant, and is referred to as *preservation injury*. This injury is felt to be the result of inadequate blood supply to the lung for too long a time. A severe form of this injury results in damage to the air sacs throughout the lung and can lead to respiratory failure soon after transplantation. While this injury may resolve, it may leave scarring in the lung that will limit the amount of recovery.

Bleeding in the Chest

The surgery for lung transplantation involves opening the chest by making an incision across the front of the chest wall (the "clamshell incision"). As we've already mentioned, one of the important reasons this incision was developed was because of the problem of bleeding from the lining of the chest wall (pleura) following surgery, bleeding that is common in patients with CF because of frequent scarring of the pleural space that has resulted from chronic lung infections. This can be a problem when a surgeon tries to remove the lungs from a CF patient in order to put new lungs in. The clamshell incision, by allowing better access to the lungs, helps the surgeon find and stop the bleeding, but bleeding after surgery (after the chest is closed again) is still a problem in CF patients following transplantation, particularly in those patients who had to go on heart-lung bypass during their surgery.

Blood Clots

Blood clots can form in the veins leading from the transplanted lungs to the left side of the heart, and can greatly interfere with heart and lung function right after a transplant procedure. In order to find such clots, the physicians usually use a technique known as *transesophageal echocardiography*. In this technique, a plastic probe about as big around as a finger is passed through the mouth, down the back of the throat and into the esophagus. The probe contains a miniature echocardiograph machine, similar to the machines used for ultrasound. Because the esophagus is behind the heart and because the veins from the lungs enter the back side of the heart, the physicians can see them better with this approach. Transesophageal echocardiography is usually done with the patient heavily sedated.

Rejection

Despite the use of immunosuppressive drugs, rejection remains a major problem following lung transplantation. Rejection, which is the result of the recipient's cells trying to destroy the "foreign" lung tissue from the donor, takes two major forms, called *acute* and *chronic* rejection.

Acute rejection is especially common in the first weeks to months following transplantation, but may occur years after transplant. Episodes of acute rejection tend to occur fairly abruptly and cause breathing difficulties, cough, lowered blood oxygen levels, and changes in the chest x-ray. If acute rejection is diagnosed and treated promptly and aggressively, it usually responds well to treatment, and the patient improves. The usual treatment of acute rejection is with high doses of steroids given through an IV. The other immunosuppressive drugs, such as cyclosporine or tacrolimus, are often given in higher doses to prevent acute rejection from coming back. If the steroids don't work (*they usually do*), some other treatments may be used and are often effective. These more specialized treatments are designed to attack the specific kind of blood cells (lymphocytes) that are causing the acute rejection. The two major treatments are known as OKT3 and ATG (which stands for "*a*nti-*t*hymocyte globulin"). Both of these must be given, in the hospital, by IV over several days.

Chronic rejection is less well understood than acute rejection, and it is more difficult to treat. It tends to have a slower onset, and last longer, with more subtle symptoms of shortness of breath with exercise, cough, or a fall in PFTs. We will discuss chronic rejection in more detail under the section that deals with the late complications of lung transplantation.

The diagnosis of rejection is made with certainty only by examining a piece of lung tissue under the microscope. The piece of tissue, known as a *biopsy* specimen, is usually obtained with a procedure called *bronchoscopy*, which will be discussed later in this chapter. Acute rejection is easier to diagnose than is chronic rejection with this type of biopsy. At times, the biopsy specimen must be fairly big to diagnose chronic rejection, and this may lead the transplant physicians to recommend an "open" biopsy, in which the chest is opened surgically and a piece of lung removed by a surgeon.

Infection

As we've seen, immunosuppressive medicines increase the risk of infection in transplant recipients. This risk is greatly increased in the lungs of CF patients. In fact, the major cause of death following lung transplantation in CF patients is infection. The CF patient's windpipe (trachea) and sinuses still "have" CF, even though the new lungs don't. Bacteria such as *Pseudomonas* or *staph* will remain in the airways (sinuses, trachea, and bronchi) of these patients and can cause infection in the transplanted lung. The combination of immunosuppression and *Pseudomonas,* particularly if the *Pseudomonas* is resistant to antibiotics, can prove deadly for the recipient. Because of this risk, some centers decrease the immunosuppression as much as possible in CF lung transplant recipients. More importantly, virtually all transplant centers look closely at the bacteria in their CF patients before transplantation. As we've already discussed, organisms that are resistant to all antibiotics are considered by many centers to be a contraindication to transplantation. Infections can be an early or late complication of lung transplantation. Infections can occur in the transplanted lungs, or elsewhere.

The new lungs are the most common target for infections after transplantation, for several reasons. First, the lungs are the only major transplanted organ in direct contact with the outside world after transplantation. Every time we breathe, air enters our lungs; the very air we breathe is often contaminated with materials that can harm us. Bacteria, viruses, small particles of dust or dirt, or certain toxic gases may be in that air. Our lungs normally have a set of barriers or ways to deal with a lot of these dangerous materials. Scientists and physicians refer to these as the *lung defenses.* Transplanting lungs directly affects lung defenses, and this makes the lungs more susceptible to infection. Some of these have been discussed in Chapter 3, *The Respiratory System,* but we'll review the affected lung defenses in the next few paragraphs.

Since the nerves supplying the lungs are cut and not reattached during a transplant, the new lungs do not have any sensation. One important sensation that we all normally have in our lungs is what we call the *cough reflex,* which is the stimulation to cough that is brought about when any material like increased mucus builds up in the airways. This urge to cough is lost at least for the first months after transplant, meaning that mucus can build up in the new lung without the recipient's feeling the need to cough. Of course, some people—who have coughed all of their lives up to the time of the transplant—might think that the lack of cough was wonderful. But we must remember that cough is one of the lung's most effective ways of getting rid of bacteria and excess mucus. So this loss of the cough reflex adds to the risk of developing infections in the lung. Lung transplant recipients can still cough, but they must actually *decide* to cough because, without the cough reflex, coughing won't happen on its own.

Another of the lung's usual defenses which is altered by a transplant is *mucociliary clearance.* Normally, secretions such as mucus help to trap unwanted small particles such as bacteria and keep them from damaging the lung. Because the airway cells are continuously making mucus, a way to move the mucus out of the lung is needed. This movement is the responsibility of the cilia, which are very small hairlike tufts that project out from airway cells and are in contact with the mucus. Normally, these cilia move in a regular way that slowly but surely moves the mucus up the airways to the trachea, from which it can be coughed out, or to the back of the throat, where it can be swallowed. For unknown reasons, even though the cilia are still present on the airway cells following a transplant, they just don't move as well, allowing mucus to build up in the lung.

Finally, for reasons that we don't yet understand, the white blood cells that fight infection in the lungs do not seem to be able to get into the lung as well as they should following a lung transplant. All of these defenses and their status following lung transplantation are the subject of intense scientific experimentation. It's likely that we'll have better ideas on how to improve the lung defenses and decrease the risk of infection following lung transplantation as we learn more about the way the lungs defend themselves normally.

Narrowing (Stenosis) of the Airway

It sometimes happens that the one or both of the main bronchi can become narrowed following transplantation. This is most often right where the donor and recipient airways are joined (the bronchial anastomosis). If the narrowing is severe, it can be hard to breathe, and hard to move mucus past it, setting the stage for hard-to-control infection. The narrowing can be caused by the surgeon's having sewn the bronchi too tightly, by the bronchi simply being too small, or (and this is by far the most common) by the formation of scar tissue at the anastomosis.

Late Complications of Lung Transplantation (Weeks-to-Months After Transplant)

Infection

As we just mentioned, infection can be an early or late complication of lung transplantation. Infection can be caused by bacteria like *staph* and *Pseudomonas* that the CF patient has had in the sinuses and trachea for months or years before transplant. These bacteria can infect the new lungs at any time.

Although we discussed it earlier, the problem of cytomegalovirus (CMV) infection deserves special mention when discussing the late complications of lung transplantation. Once CMV has infected a person, that individual will make antibodies to CMV, which is one of the body's ways to try to fight off infection: antibodies attack specific targets; antibody to CMV fights CMV. The virus is a clever one, however, and it may not be entirely eliminated from the body, and instead may lie dormant in the lung, intestines, kidney, or liver, temporarily not causing trouble. We can determine whether antibodies to CMV are present in the blood of a lung donor and a lung recipient. If the donor is positive for the antibodies (meaning the donor at one time had a CMV infection), then CMV may be lying dormant in the donated lung. The immunosuppression given to the recipient will allow the CMV that has been lurking in the donor lung to become free to cause a new infection, particularly if the recipient is negative for the antibodies (meaning that the recipient has probably not ever been infected with CMV, and has no antibodies to help fight CMV). CMV infection in this setting can be an especially bad infection, causing fever, sore throat, or other symptoms. In addition, it now seems that CMV disease in the lung recipient may be a partial cause of chronic rejection, which we mentioned briefly before and will discuss further below.

Several approaches have been used to try to prevent and/or treat CMV disease and chronic rejection in lung transplant recipients. In some transplant centers, recipients and donors are now "matched" whenever possible, so that lungs from CMV-positive donors are transplanted into CMV-positive recipients, while lungs from CMV-negative donors are reserved for CMV-negative recipients. Another approach is to treat CMV-positive recipients and CMV-negative recipients who have received CMV-positive lungs with an anti-CMV medication known as ganciclovir. A third approach is to give CMV-negative recipients a special antibody preparation that is high in antibodies directed against CMV. These approaches are not all always feasible (particularly the method of "matching" donors and recipients) or completely effective. Physicians and scientists are working on new approaches to try to minimize the effects of CMV in transplant recipients.

Rejection

Chronic (long-lasting) rejection, which was mentioned earlier, is a poorly understood form of lung rejection. While it is clear that chronic rejection is a way that the recipient's cells try to attack and destroy the new lung, the part of the lung that is attacked is usually the small airways. This leads to a very serious form of airway damage known as *bronchiolitis obliterans*, which is characterized by scarring of the small airways. We don't yet know the reason for this pattern and the exact cause of chronic rejection. Chronic lung rejection is sometimes associated with CMV infection in lung transplant recipients. Several other factors, including recurrent episodes of acute rejection, especially severe episodes of acute rejection, and stenosis of the airway anastomosis, have also been associated with chronic rejection. Approximately 25% to 35% of all lung recipients develop some form of chronic rejection, and it remains a major cause of death in transplant recipients. Of those lung recipients who develop chronic rejection, approximately 35% to 50% will die, and the majority of the remaining 50% to 65% of patients will have some degree of compromise of their airway function. As is the case for acute rejection, steroids as well as medications like OKT3 and ATG have been suggested for the treatment of chronic rejection. There are several experimental treatments that are currently being tested for the treatment of chronic rejection. We hope that as more is learned about chronic rejection, we will get better at preventing and treating it in lung transplant recipients.

Other Late Complications of Lung Transplantation

Although infection and rejection are the most common and usually most serious complications of transplantation, there are some others as well.

Narrowing (stenosis) of the airway was discussed under the section *Early Complications* above, but actually is more likely to be a problem weeks-to-months after the transplant. A little bit of narrowing of the airway usually causes no problems. More severe narrowing can cause difficulty in breathing, difficulty moving mucus, and therefore worse problems with infection beyond the narrowed area. Sometimes the physician can open the stenosis with bronchoscopy (we'll describe bronchoscopy later in this chapter). This can happen in several ways: Sometimes just pushing the bronchoscope through the narrowed area can stretch it open. Instead of a bronchoscope, surgeons or radiologists may be able to pass a special deflated balloon to the narrowed anastomosis, inflate the balloon with a lot of pressure, making the now-rigid balloon stretch open the stenosis. Sometimes the extra scar tissue that is blocking the airway can be taken away using a very small instrument that has sharp-edged cuplike blades that can be opened and closed. Such an instrument is known as a biopsy forceps and is useful for obtaining pieces of lung to diagnose rejection. A third way of dealing with stenosis is to use a special laser beam (again during bronchoscopy) to "burn off" some of the scar tissue. Finally, in very severe cases, a surgeon or radiologist may be able to place a plastic or metal *stent* in the airway. This device is stiffer than the airway and props it open. This is a difficult procedure, and is used only when there seems to be no other choice. If the length of narrowed bronchus is short, and the stenosis is severe, in rare cases, the surgeon may reopen the chest, and cut out (*resect*) the narrowed portion, sewing the open ends of the normal-sized bronchus back to each other.

Psychological, Social, and Financial "Complications" of Transplantation

Transplantation is very expensive. Figures from one major transplant center for 1995 show that pretransplant care for a CF patient averaged $80,000. The transplant itself (and the hospital stay afterward) cost $200,000 to $250,000, and the costs for the first year after transplantation were about $100,000. Most, but not all, insurance companies will pay for transplantation, but some still consider the procedure (and some of the medications used afterward) experimental, and therefore not covered.

A lot of care is required after transplantation and, in addition to costing money, this adds to the inconvenience and discomfort of the process. Many patients will have one or more of the complications of transplantation and will require further testing and care. All this may increase the time spent in the hospital and away from work, school, family, and friends. Often these hospitalizations are at the transplant center, which may be hundreds (even thousands) of miles away from home.

Transplantation is stressful for patients, their parents, and their physicians and nurses. Even for someone who does very well, there can be emotional challenges:

it is often not easy for someone who has had trouble breathing for months or years to adjust to not needing oxygen, and to trust in his newly gained energy.

As in any new field of medicine, difficult lessons about transplantation are learned all the time. Unfortunately, many of these lessons are taught by the patients who develop problems related to the transplant or to the medications given to prevent rejection. The history of transplantation (particularly for lung transplants) is short, and the length of survival following a new lung or liver is impossible to predict. The uncertainty of the course someone will take after transplantation adds to the stress of the procedure. Transplantation is probably not a good treatment for someone who needs assurance that "everything will be fine." We'll discuss this further in the section entitled "Making the Decision."

CARE AFTER TRANSPLANTATION

General Considerations

During any transplant operation the patient is unconscious, under general anesthesia, with her breathing being done by a machine (a *ventilator*) through a tube that goes in her nose or mouth into her trachea (*endotracheal tube*). She will have other tubes in as well: drainage tubes from the chest, a urine tube in her bladder, and several different catheters in blood vessels, including IVs, sometimes a tube in an artery (an "a-line") for easy measurement of the oxygen and carbon dioxide levels in the blood, and sometimes a long tube that goes into the heart to be able to measure blood pressure very accurately. Immediately after the transplant surgery, she is cared for in the ICU until she is strong and healthy enough to breathe on her own, and to withstand the removal of the various tubes. During this time in the ICU, tests will be done to make sure that the new organs are working satisfactorily and that there haven't been any immediate problems associated with the surgery, like bleeding or formation of large blood clots. Once it seems that there are no major postoperative problems, and the patient is ready to breathe on her own, the endotracheal tube can be removed (we say the patient is "extubated"). Getting to this point usually takes a few days, but can take longer. There are a couple of different approaches to extubation of a patient after surgery: one approach is to get the tube out absolutely as soon as possible, since the tubes are very uncomfortable, and the patient cannot talk while the tubes are in place. The other approach is more conservative, and delays extubation until it is absolutely clear that the patient is ready because an extubation that is done too early can fail (if the patient isn't strong enough yet, she could tire, and must be reintubated). Reintubation may be harder for patients than a slightly longer single intubation.

In the ICU, the patient will usually need a lot of pain medication and sedatives. While a patient is on the ventilator, medications are often given that paralyze the patient, to make it easier for the ventilator to "breathe" for him. Once he is breathing on his own, and is relatively alert and not requiring large amounts of sedatives and pain medication, and all organ systems are working satisfactorily, he can be moved to a regular hospital room. This usually takes several days to a week or so, but in some cases can take weeks or even months.

After transplantation of any organ, that organ requires a lot of care and close monitoring to be sure that it continues to function well. Rejection of the organ and infection (of the transplanted organ and of other parts of the body) remain dangers forever after a transplant. The posttransplant care is at least as time-consuming, bothersome, and important as regular CF care is. Because of the health risks, and because of the care required after transplantation, we often say that getting a transplant is like trading one disease for another (the new lungs or liver don't have CF anymore, but they will have other problems that need to be treated). And of course, someone with CF who has new lungs or a new liver still has CF, even if the new organs don't. So digestive enzymes, vitamins, and so on, continue to be important. Care of the lungs remains absolutely essential after transplantation of any organ in a patient with CF.

Testing a patient for rejection is necessary on a regular basis following transplantation of any organ. Pulmonary function tests (PFTs) can give early hints that there might be a problem with the transplanted lung, but any kind of problem, not just rejection, can make these tests abnormal. The most accurate way to see if rejection is present in a transplanted organ is to examine a small piece of it under the microscope. The technique of taking a small piece of an organ is known as a *biopsy* procedure, and the small piece itself is referred to as a biopsy specimen, or sometimes just a "biopsy." For liver or lung transplant recipients, it is not uncommon for 5 to 10 biopsies to be done in the first year after transplantation.

Tests

After a lung transplant, several kinds of tests are done in the ICU, in the regular hospital room, and afterward when the patient has gone home.

The most common tests that help to monitor the health of transplanted lungs are PFTs and chest x-rays. PFTs are described more in Chapter 3, *The Respiratory System,* and are no different from the PFTs used for most people with CF who have not had a transplant. In addition to regular PFTs at the clinic, most patients are given small electronic PFT machines to take home with them, which they are supposed to use 2 or 3 times per week. If the results of these home PFTs get worse, the patient notifies the doctor for further testing. X-rays are no different from the usual chest x-rays that CF patients have had for years. The types of problems that might show up on PFTs or x-rays can be different from the pretransplant CF lung problems, and might prompt the physicians to recommend specific treatment or further testing, which will almost always mean a special test known as *bronchoscopy, bronchoalveolar lavage* (called BAL for short), and *transbronchial biopsy*. We'll describe this test, which is commonly done for lung recipients, in the next several paragraphs.

Bronchoscopy is a way of looking into the trachea and bronchi of the lung, using a tube called a *bronchoscope*. There are different kinds and sizes of bronchoscopes. In most cases, the kind used for patients who have had lung transplants is flexible, so it can be passed through the nose, bend around curves down the back of the throat, through the vocal cords, and into the trachea and bronchi. It has a light and lens at the end, so the physician doing the procedure can see into the dark bronchial tubes. In most transplant centers, the bronchoscope is hooked up to a video camera, and the physician doing the bronchoscopy (the "bronchoscopist") moves the bronchoscope while watching the TV image. (The patient can watch the procedure "live" on the TV, too, if she likes, or afterward on a video playback.) There is also a hollow suction channel running the length of the bronchoscope through which liquids can be squirted in or sucked out, and through which thin, flexible wire instruments can be passed.

Bronchoalveolar lavage (BAL) means, quite simply, that a liquid, usually saline (salt water) like that used for an IV solution, is washed ("lavaged") into an area of the lung through the thin channel of the bronchoscope and then sucked back out into a sterile container. The total amount of fluid used is often several ounces, given a small amount at a time, with suctioning done after each individual amount of fluid. As the saline washes into the lung, it mixes with the cells and fluid in the lung. When it is sucked back, it carries with it some of those cells and fluid. In addition, if there are bacteria or viruses in the airway, the suctioned saline will contain it and these can be cultured in the laboratory. Cultures of the fluid for bacteria, viruses, or fungi take several days to weeks to give definite answers, however. The number of cells taken out of the airway and the type of cells removed can be determined by the laboratory, also. These tests will help tell the physicians if there is evidence of an infection in the lung or if there might be rejection. To diagnose rejection most accurately, the physicians will also want to do a biopsy through the bronchoscope (see below).

Within the first day or so after a lung transplant, one of the physicians might perform a bronchoscopy for a quick look at the bronchial anastomoses (the places where the donor bronchi are sewed to the recipient bronchi). For this procedure, the bronchoscope can simply be passed through the endotracheal tube into the trachea and bronchi, and the procedure should not be much of a big deal for the patient.

Beyond the first days, bronchoscopies with BAL and biopsy are performed every few weeks at first, then every few months if things are going well. Bronchoscopies will also be performed if there is any hint that there is a problem. These "hints" might come from symptoms, like increased cough or sputum production, or lab tests, like lower oxygen level, worse PFTs, or some new findings on the chest x-ray.

A biopsy done through the bronchoscope is known as a *transbronchial biopsy*. There are other types of lung biopsies, and we'll describe those later in this section. For a transbronchial biopsy, the physician using the bronchoscope will pass small forceps through the bronchoscope. These forceps are at the end of a long

thin wire, and are a tool which has small jaws with tiny teeth. The jaws of the forceps can be opened and then closed to take biopsy specimens ("bites") of the small
bronchi and surrounding lung tissue. These samples are also sent to the laboratory for examination under the microscope. It usually takes a day or so for the biopsies to be prepared and examined. The biopsies can give some information about
possible infection, but their main use is to tell if there is rejection. The more pieces
of tissue the physician obtains, the better the chances that they will give a true
representation of the situation in the lungs. However, the more pieces taken, the
greater the chances of a complication of the procedure, too (see below).

Complications of Bronchoscopy

There are several important possible complications of bronchoscopy, but fortunately, complications are relatively rare. The most important of these complications are oversedation, nosebleed, cough, bleeding within the bronchi, and pneumothorax (collapsed lung). These will be discussed in the next several paragraphs.

The usual bronchoscopy procedure is done by passing the bronchoscope through
the patient's nose, down the back of the throat, through the vocal cords, and into
the trachea and bronchi. The procedure sounds brutal, but is surprisingly easy to
tolerate. The bronchoscope itself is soft and flexible, and the procedure, while a
bit uncomfortable, is not painful. To minimize the discomfort, several things are
done. Most patients are given sedatives through an IV. This will help the patient
relax and make it easier for the physician to do the bronchoscopy. Notice, we did-
n't say the patient had general anesthesia: most flexible bronchoscopies are done
with the patient sedated, but awake (or sleeping lightly) and breathing on his own.
This is important, because the patient has to breathe around the bronchoscope.
The usual bronchoscope is about as big around as a pencil, and most patients
breathe around it without any difficulty. Occasional patients don't want any IV
medications, and actually watch the procedure being done on the same TV screen
that the bronchoscopist watches. Others prefer to see the video afterward, while
others want nothing to do with the bronchoscopy, preferring to be asleep for it.
As much or as little sedation as the individual patient needs can be given.

Whenever sedative (or any other) medicines are used, there is a small chance
that dosing errors can happen, and the patient get too much. In this case, that could
cause the patient to be oversedated, and fall so deeply asleep that he doesn't breathe.
In order to prevent this complication, sedative doses are checked carefully, and
usually given in relatively small doses, with extra amounts being given as needed. Furthermore, the patient is monitored carefully for any signs of not breathing
enough (a pulse oximeter, or "pulseox," is attached to the finger to give a continuous reading of blood oxygen levels). Finally, medicines are readily at hand to reverse the effects of the sedative medicines. The sedatives are usually very effective in keeping patients comfortable, without their needing general anesthesia as
they would for painful surgical procedures. The sedatives used most often have

the added benefit of causing what is known as *retrograde amnesia,* which means the patients forget what happened while they were sedated.

As soon as the patient is comfortable, her nose and back of her throat are numbed with xylocaine drops (like the dentist uses, but not injected with a needle), and sometimes with xylocaine jelly on the end of a cotton swab, or even xylocaine aerosols. As the bronchoscope is passed through her nose and to the back of her throat, her vocal cords are also numbed with xylocaine dripped through the suction channel of the bronchoscope. The nose is the narrowest part of the patient's body that the bronchoscope has to pass through, and it can sometimes bleed from the rubbing. These nosebleeds are not serious and not common (about one of every 20 or 30 patients).

The bronchoscope is then passed through the patient's vocal cords into his trachea. The trachea also gets some xylocaine, not really to prevent pain (it doesn't hurt), but to prevent cough (the body's natural reaction to an "invader" like a pencil-sized tube at the vocal cords or in the trachea is to try to expel it with cough). In some CF patients, it is difficult to numb the vocal cords and trachea completely, and they do cough a bit during the procedure. Once the bronchoscope reaches the bronchi of the new lungs, the need for anesthetizing the airways has lessened, since the new lungs do not have nerves connected to them. The new bronchi do not have any feeling or cough reflex.

Once the bronchoscope is in the small bronchi, it is pushed so that it is firmly sealed into the airway (this is known as *wedging* the bronchoscope). When the bronchoscope is wedged into place, blocking off the bronchus, the physician performs the BAL (that is, she washes in the saline, and sucks it back out again, saving it for culture and microscopic examination). Sometimes, just pushing the bronchoscope down bronchi, especially bronchi that are inflamed because of infection or rejection, can cause bleeding. Usually this bleeding is not serious, but on occasion it can be.

After doing the BAL, the physician repositions the tip of the bronchoscope so that it's well-placed to obtain biopsies. Most often, the physician uses an x-ray screen (*fluoroscopy* or just "fluoro") to show the exact position of the bronchoscope and the forceps. The physician then passes the forces through the suction channel and takes a few "bites" of tissue for the biopsies. One would think that the taking of biopsies would be painful, but it is not. Taking bites from the lung (or any living tissue) almost always causes some bleeding, as you might expect. Usually the bleeding stops very quickly, but on occasion, particularly if the lungs are inflamed (infection or rejection), the bleeding can be difficult to control and can be dangerous. In extremely rare cases, it has even been fatal.

Taking a bite of tissue can also cause a hole in the outside of the lung, allowing air to leak outside the lungs. This air that escapes through a hole in the lung is still trapped within the chest, and can accumulate around the lung, press in on the lung, and cause it to collapse. This condition is called a pneumothorax, and is discussed a bit more in Chapter 3, *The Respiratory System.* A pneumothorax is much more likely to occur in a patient who is breathing with the help of a ventilator, since the ventilator works by blowing air into the lungs under pressure. This added air pressure can open up a small hole and prop it open, preventing it from sealing itself shut, and allowing air to escape with each breath in. If someone develops a pneumothorax, she will usually need to have a tube placed through the skin, between the ribs, and into the chest in order to let the air escape and allow the lung to reexpand. These tubes are called chest tubes, for obvious reasons. A pneumothorax is usually painful, and chest tubes are always painful, so pain medications are given if this problem develops.

There are some situations where a biopsy with the flexible bronchoscope (a transbronchial biopsy) might not be possible, but a biopsy of the lung is needed. For example, the patient may be too small to have a flexible bronchoscope, or the patient may be too sick to have flexible bronchscopy, or the physicians feel that the small bites taken with biopsy forceps are likely to be too small to give an accurate diagnosis. In these cases, an *open* lung *biopsy* might be necessary. An open biopsy is done in the operating room, under general anesthesia. The surgeon makes an incision through the chest to expose part of the lung under his direct vision, and cuts out a small piece of the lung, sews the hole, and closes the chest. This procedure is more involved, requires general anesthesia, and takes more time to recover from, but, in a very sick patient, is probably safer than the transbronchial biopsy, and guarantees a bigger piece of tissue, which is more likely to allow for a correct diagnosis.

Ongoing Care

After transplantation, as you've heard many times already, continuing care is absolutely essential and never-ending. Treatment with immunosuppressant (antirejection) medications is essential. Other CF treatments, like enzymes and nutritional supplements, are also important. Many patients will still need to do chest PT, or use their Flutter valve (or other airway clearance techniques) for clearing mucus from their new lungs. Some patients may have to have special treatment for their sinuses, if their physicians feel that infected sinuses have been causing problems in their new lungs. In most cases, care can take place at your regular CF center, but with periodic visits back to the transplant center. Your physician and the transplant team should be able to work together.

RESULTS OF LUNG TRANSPLANTATION
(PROGNOSIS AFTER TRANSPLANTATION)

Lung transplantation for CF patients is still a relatively young science and art. The first procedure, you'll recall, was in 1963; and for the first several years of lung transplantation, patients did not live more than a few weeks. Although we have improved a great deal since then, we are certainly not at the point where it's simply a matter of ordering a set of new lungs, getting them hooked up, and going on about our business. Now, and for the foreseeable future, lung transplantation, perhaps especially for CF patients, will be a very difficult procedure, with many deaths, and with much suffering for many of those who survive. In fact, as of 1994, "transplant complications" moved into second place in the list of reasons for death of CF patients (whereas CF pulmonary disease used to account for 95% of the deaths of CF patients each year, in 1994, the lungs are listed as the cause of death in 86.6%, and transplant complications in 7.2%).

Nonetheless, many patients have done spectacularly well, with full resumption of work, school, recreation, and family life, some of them 8 or 9 years after their transplant. As transplant centers gain more experience, and as scientists develop better ways to preserve lungs outside the body and better and safer immunosuppressive drugs, we can expect the results to improve. It is worth keeping in mind that the first kidney transplant patients did not survive long, and liver transplantation had *no* long-term survivors for the first several years that the procedure was performed. Now, both of those procedures are accepted as standard care for many conditions, and the outcome is excellent. As experience with lung transplantation increases, the results will almost certainly improve.

At the writing of this book, most centers report about 50–60% two-year survival after lung transplant for CF patients. That means that if 100 patients get a transplant, 50–60 will be alive two years later; 40–50 will be dead. Let's look at some other numbers that don't have anything to do with transplants: CF patients with the worst PFTs have about a 50% two-year survival (without transplant). So of 100 of those patients, 50 will be alive and 50 dead in two years. Transplantation may allow up to 10 more patients out of a hundred to survive for two years than would have survived without transplantation. Other factors need to be considered too: of those who survive, about half will develop bronchiolitis obliterans, a severe condition seen in transplanted lungs. Bronchiolitis obliterans causes progressive difficulty breathing and is ultimately fatal in about one-third to one-half of the patients who develop it.

In one recent report from England, 76 patients with CF were referred for lung transplantation. Of those 76 patients, 36 died waiting on the transplant list, and 15 were alive (still waiting for transplant) at the time of the report; 25 patients received their transplants, and of those, 10 died and 15 were still alive. So, of the original 76 patients put on the transplant list, 46 died (10 after transplant, 36 waiting for organs), and 30 were alive, 15 of them still waiting for transplant, 15 of them after getting their new lungs. Of the 15 alive after the new lungs, we can assume that 7 or 8 have bronchiolitis obliterans, and are fairly sick. The 7 or 8 others are likely to be doing very well.

MAKING THE DECISION

The decision to proceed with transplantation is always a difficult one. Most patients express disbelief when told that they should consider a transplant; often they just don't feel sick enough to require a transplant. This is especially true for lung transplant patients, because there is a long wait for lungs and patients must get on the list early if they are going to get credit for waiting time. In addition, the idea of transplantation can be frightening. It is, after all, an "unknown" procedure to the patient, and this can be especially difficult for patients (and families) who are used to a routine of treatment for CF. Deciding to have a transplant means the patient and family will have to get used to a whole new set of physicians and nurses; ways of dealing with the CF team may not be effective when dealing with a transplant team. Finally, a patient who is very sick with CF may be able to accept his illness and decide to be comfortable and in control of his destiny. Such a patient may not want the uncertainty of transplantation, and may feel it is better to die peacefully rather than be expected to fight to stay alive long enough to receive lungs that may never come. This last point is one of the most difficult aspects of a family's decision in "going for" transplant.

When your CF doctor suggests that a transplant may be the best thing to do, you must first find out why he or she feels that way. Is it because your PFTs are very bad? Have you gotten worse quickly over the preceding year? Ask your own CF physicians; they will tell you.

Your family can often help you with your decision. For a major procedure like transplantation, particularly one that will surely require lots of care after the procedure, you will need help and support. Any form of transplantation is something that should be viewed with both eyes open. The more you and your family understand the procedure and the risks involved, then the better you and your physicians will be able to deal with the consequences of transplantation.

Finally, remember that no one can really make your decision about transplantation for you. In addition, *there is no right or wrong decision when and if you are asked to consider having a transplant.* Many patients are eager to have a transplant, many others don't want to consider one under any circumstances. Both groups of patients (and all of those patients whose feelings are in between the two) are right. You must be comfortable with your decision, for you will have to live with the results of your decision.

Deciding to be considered for transplantation, however, does not mean you have to actually have a transplant. This is an extremely important point. It is possible, in other words, to be evaluated for a lung transplant, to get on the list for the transplant, to move up to the top of the list, and then decide that you really don't want a transplant. Obviously, if you do this, you will have to have the tests needed for evaluation, and you may have to go on the "inactive" transplant list if you decide not to have a transplant. On the other hand, if you decide not to have an evaluation for a lung transplant and change your mind a year later, you will have lost a year of time on the list and you will have to wait that much longer for a set of lungs. Unless you are absolutely opposed to a transplant, you should at least discuss it with your physician when it is suggested to you. After you have all the information available, it will be possible for you to make an informed and responsible decision about proceeding or not proceeding with the process of transplantation.

LIVER TRANSPLANTATION

Who Should Be Considered for a New Liver?

Liver transplantation is usually considered in two situations (see Chapter 4, *The Gastrointestinal Tract,* for more details): (1) when there is liver failure, with buildup of toxic chemicals that the liver normally clears from the body, and low levels of chemicals (including protein and factors that help blood clot properly) that the liver normally makes; and (2) when there is *uncontrollable* bleeding from esophageal varices (the details of this problem are spelled out in Chapter 4).

Who Should Not Be Considered for a New Liver?

Just as there are some people who feel that they don't want any part of the high-tech world of lung transplantation, with its many unknowns and its possible complications, some people make the same decision about liver transplantation. There also are some situations in which there are medical contraindications to (reasons not to do) liver transplantation. A widespread bloodstream infection carries such a high risk of death after transplantation that it is considered to be an absolute contraindication for any transplant, including liver, by most transplant centers. *Very severe* lung disease is also felt by many to be a contraindication to liver transplantation [even though patients with mildly or even moderately affected lungs have stayed the same or even improved after liver transplantation (see below) and even though a couple of CF patients have gotten lung-liver transplants!].

The Transplant List for Liver Transplants

The system for determining your spot on the liver transplant list takes into account the time on the list and how sick you are. Each patient is assigned a "patient status" that affects where you are on the list. The status ranges from status 1 (patients in intensive care units, on life support) to status 4 (stable, not hospitalized). Those patients who are status 1 are automatically moved to the top of the list by UNOS and receive the first available organ. In some ways, this system may seem to be fairer than the lung waiting system, which goes solely on the basis of length of time waiting, but there have been instances where patients have been hospitalized or put in an ICU, not because they were sicker, but in order to move them higher on the list. The wait for a liver is not as long as for lungs, partly because livers can be preserved longer than lungs and therefore can be brought from farther away, and partly because the liver is less delicate than the lung and more likely to have acceptable function despite the injury or illness that has killed the donor or the treatment the donor has received in attempting to save her life.

The Technique of Liver Transplantation

The liver is located in the upper portion of the right side of the abdomen, just below the diaphragm. Its blood supply comes from an artery (the hepatic artery), and a vein (the portal vein). Blood leaves the liver in a vein known as the hepatic vein. The liver is also connected to the gallbladder, which releases bile into the small intestine through the bile duct. In order to transplant a liver, the surgeons must make a very large incision across the upper part of the abdomen of the recipient, carefully remove the liver, and then attach the blood vessels to the blood vessels going to or coming from the transplanted liver. The bile duct from the new liver may not be reattached at the time of surgery, and instead is often allowed to drain directly into the small intestine. Because of the difficulty in taking out the damaged liver and replacing it with the transplanted liver, it is not unusual for a liver transplant operation to take more than 9 hours. Because of the many blood vessels that must be attached and because the liver contains a large amount of blood, many transfusions are often needed during the surgery. In addition, some patients have their blood diverted away from the abdomen using an artificial pump to take blood from the lower part of the body and return it directly to the heart while the liver is being replaced.

Because bleeding in the abdomen is fairly common after the surgery, several drainage tubes are placed in the abdomen at the time of surgery. These tubes go out through the skin into small plastic reservoirs, which can hold blood or other secretions which come out of the abdomen. This will allow the surgeons to see if there is a large amount of bleeding in the abdomen following surgery. The drainage tubes will also help with the healing process by removing excess blood from the abdomen. They are usually removed within the first two weeks after surgery.

Complications of Liver Transplantation

The most worrisome complications specific to liver transplantation are organ failure, bleeding, and blood clots in the artery or vein to the liver. As with any organ transplant, rejection of the transplanted organ and infection (of the new organ or elsewhere in the body) are also major concerns, and necessitate very careful dosing of the immunosuppressive medications.

As is the case with any transplanted organ, the liver must be obtained from a donor and then must be kept alive long enough for the surgeon to place it into the abdomen of the recipient. Over the years, the technique of organ preservation has improved, but it is still not perfect. The liver, once removed from the donor, has its blood washed out in order to prevent the donor's blood from clotting within the vessels and to prevent the donor's white blood cells from damaging it. The blood is washed out of the liver through the blood vessels, by rinsing a large amount of a special solution that contains minerals and special sugars that will allow the liver to remain alive even though the blood is gone. Sometimes, despite the best efforts to preserve the function of the liver, it is injured, either because of liver damage while still in the donor or because the preservation process is inadequate. If this occurs, then the liver will not work after transplantation, and the patient will suffer from liver failure. In some instances, the liver damage may be so severe that the patient dies as a result. In other cases, the liver may recover enough function to allow the patient to survive and ultimately do well.

As mentioned before, bleeding is a fairly common problem during the liver transplantation procedure itself. Bleeding can also be a dangerous problem in the hours and days following transplantation. The drainage tubes placed into the abdomen at the time of surgery can alert the surgeons to bleeding after surgery. Although blood and clotting factors given to the recipient after surgery may stop the bleeding, there are instances in which the only way to stop the bleeding is for the surgeon to reopen the abdomen and find the blood vessels that are bleeding and stop the bleeding directly.

Blood clots can form and block the blood vessels to the transplanted liver. In some cases, these clots can decrease blood flow to the liver, leading to liver damage. At times, such clots must be removed surgically, by opening the abdomen, locating the clot in the blood vessel, opening the blood vessel, removing the clot, and then surgically closing the blood vessel. Clotting within major blood vessels to the liver, unfortunately, does not always resolve or may lead to irreversible liver damage before the clots can be removed.

Care After Liver Transplantation

Tests

As with lung transplant recipients, liver recipients must undergo regular tests to make sure the new liver is functioning well. Blood tests of liver function (usually abbreviated as LFTs) are followed on a frequent basis, but if rejection is thought to be likely, then biopsies are necessary.

A liver biopsy is done by cleaning and numbing the skin over the liver and then inserting a special needle directly into the liver. This needle is designed to cut into the liver and hold a small piece of the liver inside the needle as the needle is removed. The biopsy can then be sent to the laboratory and examined. As with the lung biopsies, liver biopsies are usually performed after the patient has been given some sedative medication by IV.

Complications of Liver Biopsy

Most liver biopsies are performed with no ill effects. But as with any procedure, there is a small chance of problems. Beyond the risk of oversedation, the biggest risk of liver biopsy is bleeding. The liver has a rich supply of blood vessels, and it is possible to tear one of these and cause bleeding. In most cases, the bleeding isn't serious, but, particularly if the liver isn't working well and not making blood clotting factors normally, it can be difficult to control.

Ongoing Care

After liver transplantation, as with lung transplantation, continuing care is absolutely essential and never-ending. Treatment with immunosuppressant (antirejection) medications is essential. Other CF treatments, like enzymes and nutritional supplements, are also important. Patients will still need to do chest PT, or use their Flutter valve for clearing mucus from their lungs. In most cases, care can take place at your regular CF center, but with periodic visits back to the transplant center. Your physician and the transplant team should be able to work together.

Results of Liver Transplantation

The results for liver transplantation for people with CF are a little harder to know for certain than those for lung transplantation, because there have been far fewer liver transplantation procedures done in CF patients. Nonetheless, it appears that the outcome is somewhat better at this point than for lung transplantation, probably because there is more experience with liver transplantation in general (in non-CF patients) than with lung transplantation, and because the liver can survive longer out of the body. In one large CF and transplant center, approximately 80% of the CF patients who received liver transplants survived at least 2 years after the procedure.

One surprising result has been that CF patients who have received liver transplants do not have an immediate worsening of their lung infection, as many people worried they would. The reason for the worry, of course, was that these patients have to take immunosuppressive medications to prevent liver rejection. Immunosuppressive medicines decrease the body's ability to fight infection, and there already is infection in the lungs of people with CF. So most physicians assumed that lung infection would worsen as soon as someone with CF was started on immunosuppressive medicines. Instead what happens is that most CF patients' lung function either doesn't change, or actually gets a bit better in the weeks-to-months following liver transplantation. Why? It's not clear, but one possible explanation is that the immunosuppressive medicines cut down on the inflammation within the airways. As you've seen in Chapter 3, anti-inflammatory medicines, like steroids, can sometimes be helpful in patients with CF. It may be that this anti-inflammatory action of the immunosuppressives helps more than the increased risk of infection hurts.

THE FUTURE OF TRANSPLANTATION

Transplantation is a young science, and many physicians and research scientists are working to unravel its secrets and solve its many problems. With the development of newer antirejection medications as well as an improved understanding of the ways to prevent and treat the complications of transplantation, the future of transplantation is bright. It remains, however, a major medical and surgical commitment for any patient who wishes to pursue this technique. Confidence in the transplant physicians, a willingness to undergo special tests, and an ability to cooperate with the transplant team will increase the chances for any one patient to undergo a transplant successfully. It is clear that there is much to learn about transplantation, but many CF patients who are alive following liver or lung transplantation are a testimony of the promise inherent in this form of therapy.

9

Daily Life

THE BASICS

1. Most CF patients should be expected to live a very normal daily life (except for treatments): they go to school, do homework, have friends, play sports, grow up, many marry, and so on.
2. Children with CF should have the same expectations and responsibilities as other children.

There are many aspects of daily life that are altered very little by having cystic fibrosis (CF): babies cry and laugh, and children still sleep through the night, wake up, go to the bathroom, have breakfast, go to school, play with friends, play sports, do homework and chores, watch TV, and go to parties. They may go on trips with or without their families. They grow up and finish school; they take jobs; many marry, and may decide to raise a family. It is very important for a child's emotional well-being, and that of the family, that daily life be approached with these expectations. The emotional aspect of living with CF is discussed in Chapter 12, *The Family,* and the issues that relate specifically to teens and adults are addressed in Chapters 13 and 14, respectively. This chapter addresses the few areas in which CF does have an effect on the patient's (or family's) daily life.

In most stages of life, having CF requires some form of airway clearance therapy, anywhere from one to four times a day. Approximately 90% of people with CF must remember, or be reminded, to take digestive enzymes with each meal and usually with snacks. Most patients will also have to take vitamins each day, and many will need to take antibiotics by mouth fairly frequently.

Clinic visits for checkups will be required anywhere from one to eight times a year, depending on your physician's approach and your health. These visits are very important for health maintenance (see Chapter 3, *The Respiratory System*).

During periods of pulmonary exacerbation (see Chapter 3), it may be necessary to come into the hospital for 1–3 weeks, or to receive IV antibiotics at home (see Chapter 7, *Hospitalization and Other Special Treatments*). This treatment may be necessary one to three times each year for as many as one in every three or four patients.

Patients who have more severe lung disease may need to adjust the intensity of their physical exertion, and a very few may even need to wear oxygen tubing while they are up and around and perhaps during sleep, but this is a very small proportion of patients.

Mealtimes should not be too different for people with CF than it would be if they didn't have CF, except for remembering to take the enzymes. If someone has had trouble putting (or keeping) weight on, there may be meals with added fats and calories, or even night-time tube feedings to help with growth (see Chapter 6, *Nutrition*).

MEDICATIONS AND TREATMENTS: WHO'S IN CHARGE?

During a child's early years, the parents are responsible for the medication and must know which medicines should be taken when, why they are needed, and what additional treatments are required. By the time a young adult leaves home, he or she must be in charge of these areas. Most experts feel that a good time for the transition in this responsibility from the parents to the young patient is early in the teenage years. Before the teen years, many youngsters are simply not emotionally mature enough to take on these responsibilities, no matter how smart they are, no matter how well they do in school, and no matter how much their parents want them to be "grown up." Conversely, if a parent refuses to begin the peaceful transfer of control well into the child's teenage years, it can be harmful for a teen's ability to function independently later on, and it may well fuel parent–adolescent battles.

Adolescence is both a good and a bad time for accomplishing the transition in responsibility for medical care. It is a good time because the teenager is wanting very much to become independent of the parent, and is looking for ways to assert that independence. Teenagers welcome the trust that accompanies responsibility as well as the absence of nagging that results when they have learned all their medications and take them faithfully.

Adolescence can be a difficult time, however, for the transition in responsibility, because in normal teenage rebellion against authority there is a strong urge to ignore what the parents want. When the teenager has CF, what the parents want is for the teenager to take the prescribed medications and treatments in order to stay well. This may be an area where the teenager is able to exert some control, and the relatively common feeling of invulnerability ("nothing will happen to me") may just add to the appeal of not taking medications. As with so many other aspects of the teenager's life, the best solution is to encourage him or her to take full responsibility for medications and treatments, but to be aware of what is and is not being done, and to encourage the best cooperation possible. To encourage this self-care and independence, the physician may choose to meet with the patient alone, and to have the parents sit in the waiting room during clinic visits.

DAYCARE

Daycare has become very common for many families with babies, especially if both parents work. Babies in daycare get more colds than babies kept at home. Babies with CF will get neither more nor fewer colds than the other babies, but some of these colds may develop into bronchial infections (pulmonary exacerbations). This fact has made some families try to avoid daycare. For the first months of an infant's life, when the bronchi are very tiny and when infants with CF may have more trouble keeping the bronchi clear, it may be advisable to delay daycare. However, if this is financially difficult, it should not be considered a major setback. Remember that the goal of avoiding all colds is impossible to achieve, especially if there are other children in the family, and that careful attention to an infant's health, with quick treatment for any pulmonary infections, is likely to result in very good maintenance of health.

Occasionally, a misguided daycare supervisor, parent, or even physician may be concerned that the presence of an infant with CF will pose a danger to the other children in daycare. *Cystic fibrosis is not contagious.* Even if a baby with CF is coughing a lot, the bacteria in the lungs of someone with CF are not dangerous to children without CF. Of course, a baby with CF can get a regular cold, just like any other baby, and pass that cold on to anyone else, but babies with CF should not be excluded from daycare just because of having CF, or because of cough.

SCHOOL

School is very important for all children, and virtually all children with CF should be able to go to school and carry a full load, including homework and extracurricular activities. When a child has a lung infection, he or she may not feel as well as usual, but in most cases this should not interfere with education. Children should be encouraged to go to school, even if they are coughing more than their usual, as long as they are receiving the appropriate treatment (antibiotics, and increased airway clearance treatments).

Teachers may need to be educated about CF to make a very few special considerations for the child with CF. They need to be aware that the child with CF is likely to have more cough than other children, and should never be discouraged from coughing. The child with CF may also need to have more frequent bathroom privileges. Most CF centers have a very good booklet designed for teachers (see Appendix H: *Bibliography*).

Homework should be required from the child with CF, just as from his or her peers. There should be almost no exceptions to this rule. Even if a child has to be hospitalized, he or she should keep up with school work. If a child is hospitalized, the school district should provide tutoring to enable the child to keep up with the class.

Gym class is as important (or even more important) for children with CF as for other children. Physical education class should not be graded on the basis of athletic performance for any child, especially those who might have a physical reason for lower than normal performance, as a child with CF and lung disease might have.

COLLEGE

See Chapter 13, *The Teenage Years,* for a discussion of going to college—going away or staying home.

SPORTS AND EXERCISE

In general, there is no reason for children, adolescents, and adults with CF to avoid exercise. Exercise is good for most people, including people with CF. Everyone, with CF or without it, needs to adjust the amount and intensity of exercise to his or her own abilities and needs, but this can be done fairly easily. (Exercise and sports are discussed more in Chapter 10, *Exercise.*)

VISITS WITH FRIENDS

Visiting with friends, either at their house or your own, is an important part of growing up, learning to get along with others, and learning to become independent away from home. Children and adolescents with CF should have these same opportunities as anyone else. In most cases, special arrangements will have to be made to be certain that medications are being taken and that treatments are being done. In some cases, for a single overnighter for a grade-school child, it might not be a problem to skip a single day's treatment, but this should not become a habit. Adolescents who give themselves their own treatments should be able to do this anywhere. If either part of the visiting pair is sick, changes may have to be made, but this is no different from what would be done if neither child had CF. Many experts advise against close contacts (like overnights) between CF patients, to avoid the possibility of their sharing potentially harmful lung bacteria. Although the bacteria that patients with CF may cough out or have on their hands present absolutely no danger to people without CF, there is a small but real risk of harm to someone with CF (see Chapter 3, *The Respiratory System,* for more discussion of the issue of *person-to-person* transmission of CF bacteria).

SMOKING

People with any form of lung disease should not smoke, nor should they inhale other people's smoke. This is certainly true for people with CF. Smoke is harmful to children's lungs, even if the lungs are normal. Someone who has abnormal lungs, especially if asthma is part of the condition, has a greatly increased risk of complications if he or she must breathe cigarette smoke. Smoke from cigarettes can be harmful to a child's lungs even if the person smoking the cigarette loves the child very much. Parents whose child has CF should stop smoking immediately, and smoking should not be allowed in their home. Most people, including smokers, know that smoking is very harmful to the smoker; not everyone realizes that it is also harmful to the lungs of children who are forced to breathe in the second-hand smoke. It has now been shown unequivocally that being exposed to parents' cigarette smoke causes worsened lung function in children with CF.

Many parents who have been unsuccessful at stopping smoking are able to stop when they realize that it is not just for their own health but for the children's as well. If you cannot stop right away, it is essential that you stop smoking in the house. If you're smoking in the same house, the baby will get the fumes. You must especially never smoke in the car, since that is an enclosed space where smoke can get very thick and irritating. If you need help stopping, your physician may be able to help. For someone who is truly addicted to cigarettes, the addiction is every bit as serious as—and harder to break than—a heroin addiction. (Some people feel it's even worse than heroin, since with heroin it's mostly the person directly taking the drug whose health is impaired, while with cigarettes, it's also the "innocent bystanders.") Nicotine chewing gum and patches have been helpful for people who are dedicated to stopping smoking but can't do it on their own.

TRAVEL

Patients with CF can travel, just as people without CF can. There are a few practical considerations for the traveling CF patient.

Remember to take your medicines. Some medications used for CF patients (especially enzymes) may not be carried in just any pharmacy, so it may be difficult to replace medications while you're away from your regular drug store. If you travel out of state, you may find that a pharmacy won't accept your doctor's prescription if he or she is not licensed in the state you're visiting. In most cases, pharmacists are very helpful, and will do what they can to provide you with the service you need, but it's better to be prepared for a problem.

Remember to take any equipment you might need for aerosols or postural drainage treatments. If you're traveling to a different country, you may need to bring special electrical outlet adapters for whatever electrical equipment you use, since different countries use different power sources. Adapters are available to enable you to convert the power source to fit your own equipment.

High altitude. If you live at or near sea level and travel to higher altitudes, you may experience difficulty because of the lower oxygen pressures at altitude. The air in Denver, for example, has only 80% as much oxygen as that in San Diego or Boston. Someone whose lungs are in excellent condition should have no trouble in these places, but someone who has serious lung involvement may be comfortable and safe at sea level, but develop problems in the mountains. It is a good idea to discuss travel plans with your doctor before going.

Airplane travel. Commercial airlines pressurize their cabins to 5,000–8,000 feet. That means that the oxygen level inside the cabin is comparable to Denver's or a place even higher. The large majority of patients with CF and mild or even moderate lung disease can fly in commercial airliners with no problems. If you need oxygen at sea level, you will need more in an airplane, and if you are close to needing it at home, you may need it while you fly. The major airlines are used to dealing with requests for oxygen during flights, and usually are very helpful, *but most insist that you contact them well in advance* to let them know about your plans and needs (usually there is a special medical department to contact at the airline).

SUMMER CAMP

Summer camps can provide valuable experience for children and adolescents, and most children and adolescents with CF should be able to attend camp if they want to. Most children whose lungs are in good shape and whose digestion is fairly well controlled with enzymes should be able to attend any kind of camp, as long as arrangements for medications and treatments can be made with the camp physicians and nurses. Many areas have CF camps, which have some special advantages and disadvantages. The advantages of CF camp include staff who are familiar with CF and who are equipped to give regular treatments, and the opportunity for children to get to know other children with CF and share their experiences and feelings, which increase their understanding of their condition. The main disadvantage, especially for someone who is quite healthy, is the danger of limiting a child's world to the CF world.

Many communities, and virtually all CF centers, have stopped sponsoring CF camps, because of the risks of patients giving each other undesirable bacteria. Some few have continued to hold camp, but hold different sessions for those with and without *Burkholderia cepacia* on their cultures (see Chapter 3, *The Respiratory System*).

WHERE TO LIVE

People often wonder if there are areas of the country that are better than others for children (and adults) with CF. From what is known now, the answer is no. In individual patients, it is possible that they might do better in one geographic location than another, but so many factors influence how someone will do, and patients are so different from each other, that no one place has the perfect combination of factors that make for good health for all people with CF.

Cities and states differ in the amount of pollution, cold, wetness, and allergens, and in the availability of good medical care. While one might think that the cold, wet, polluted, industrial, northeastern cities (Cleveland, Pittsburgh, Boston, Toronto, etc.) would be the worst places for CF patients to live, national survival statistics, which measure how long people live, show that it is exactly these cities which have had the *best* CF survival. The explanation almost certainly lies in the fact that these cities have had excellent CF centers for the longest time. Excellent CF centers now exist in most regions of the United States, Canada, Europe, and Australia, and the survival statistics now reflect this change. Most CF physicians feel that ready access to a good CF center is important, but other than this criterion, there is very little basis for recommending one geographic area over another for someone with CF.

10

Exercise

THE BASICS

1. Exercise is good for virtually all people with CF.
2. People with CF lose more salt and drink less fluid than normal when they exercise in the heat.
3. Physically fit CF patients live longer than those who are not fit.
4. Children with CF should be encouraged to be active from a very young age, and that active lifestyle should continue all their lives.

Everyone is interested in exercise these days. People with cystic fibrosis (CF) are no exception. Exercise done properly, in the right amount, the right intensity, and with the proper safety precautions, can be fun and beneficial for nearly everyone. Again, people with CF are no exception. There is even evidence that the more physically fit people with CF are, the more likely they are to stay alive for the next eight years and beyond!

EFFECTS OF EXERCISE ON PEOPLE WITHOUT CYSTIC FIBROSIS

Single Sessions of Exercise

When someone begins muscular exercise, the body has to make some fast adaptations, most of which relate to supplying the exercising muscles with considerably more oxygen than is needed at rest. These adaptations help the muscles remove excess carbon dioxide, which is produced when they are active. Muscles are able to contract and move the body *without* oxygen, but this is much more difficult than muscular work performed *with* adequate oxygen. Work that is performed without adequate oxygen being supplied to the muscles is called *anaerobic* work;

work that is performed with enough oxygen is called *aerobic* work. Anaerobic exercise can only be carried out for a period of seconds or minutes, whereas aerobic exercise can be sustained for many minutes or even hours. Anaerobic exercise is not only more difficult and less efficient than aerobic exercise but also results in the production of lactic acid in the muscles, and in the production of considerably more carbon dioxide, which then has to be removed.

Since oxygen is supplied to the exercising muscles (and carbon dioxide is removed) by circulating blood, one of the first changes at the beginning of exercise is an increase in blood flow to the active muscle. Since the heart has to pump more blood, it has to pump faster, and the heart rate (pulse) increases. The heart rate reaches a maximum which can be predicted accurately from the person's age: maximum heart rate = 220 – age (in years). Thus, a 20-year-old person would have a predicted maximum heart rate of 220 – 20 = 200 beats per minute. It is also necessary to increase the amount of oxygen available to the blood, and, especially with anaerobic exercise, to increase the disposal of carbon dioxide. The increase in oxygen supply and carbon dioxide removal are both accomplished by increasing the amount of air that is breathed each minute. The accuracy of these adjustments is astounding, as you've already seen in Chapter 1. During heavy exercise, the heart may increase its output five- or sixfold, and the lungs may bring in (and exhale) 5 to 10 times as much air as they do during naps, and yet, the level of oxygen and carbon dioxide in the bloodstream remains nearly constant.

It takes anywhere from a few seconds to $1\frac{1}{2}$ minutes to adjust the amount of blood the heart pumps to the exercising muscles. Therefore, during the first seconds of exercise, the muscles are undersupplied with oxygen. In other words, the first seconds of any form of exercise are anaerobic exercise. Exercise that is strictly "stop-and-go," in which you exercise, rest, then exercise again (for example, racquet sports) is anaerobic exercise. Exercise is also anaerobic if it is very heavy work and the muscles demand more oxygen than can be supplied (for example, heavy weightlifting, running, or riding a bike up a steep hill). In contrast, aerobic exercise is a low intensity, rhythmic type of activity, such as walking, swimming, easy jogging, and bike riding.

Exercise in the Heat

The more someone exercises, especially in hot weather, the more heat the body produces. If the body temperature becomes too high it can be dangerous, so there has to be a way for body temperature to remain relatively constant. This is accomplished through several mechanisms. The first is that a greater amount of blood than usual is sent to the skin, especially the scalp and hands. This is a way of bringing the warmth of the body close to the surface, where it can be given off to the surrounding air (unless the air is hotter than body temperature). If all of the blood stayed in the heart and other internal organs, it would be insulated by the skin, muscles, and fat, and the heat would build up. The other way of giving off excess heat is through sweating. As sweat evaporates, it cools the surface of the body. This is why you sweat when you exercise, especially in the heat.

Exercise Tolerance

When someone is given a test on an exercise cycle, it becomes progressively more difficult to pedal and, eventually, *everyone* will get to the point where he or she can no longer pedal. In most healthy people, the point at which this occurs is determined by two factors. The first is that the heart reaches a point at which it can no longer increase the amount of blood it pumps to the muscles, so the muscles become relatively undersupplied with blood and oxygen and become fatigued. This usually happens when the heart rate has reached the maximum limit. If a 20-year-old person is exercising so hard that the heart rate is 200 beats per minute, it will not be able to go much faster, so the amount of blood being pumped out will not be able to increase any further.

The second limiting factor may be the muscles themselves: there is a limit to how much oxygen the muscles can process, so they may become fatigued even though enough oxygen has been delivered. In someone with normal lungs, the lungs are never the limiting factor in exercise. Even at total exhaustion, the lungs have considerable reserve. Recall from Chapter 3 that the maximum voluntary ventilation (MVV) is the measurement of the largest amount of air someone can move in and out of the lungs in a minute. During exercise, even at the point of total exhaustion, most people don't use any more than 70% of their MVV; that is, their lungs could still deliver another 30% effort. But this wouldn't help, since other factors would have impeded the exercise before the extra breathing reserves were needed.

Repeated Sessions of Exercise (Exercise Programs)

If you exercise each day, or at least 3 days a week, for a certain minimum time (10–30 minutes a day), and at a certain minimum intensity (hard enough to raise your heart rate to approximately 75% of its maximum, which is around 150 beats per minute for adolescents and young adults), after a few weeks (6–12 weeks), you will become more fit, that is, you will be able to do more of the same kind of exercise with less stress on your body. If the type of exercise you were doing each day was aerobic, then you will increase your *aerobic fitness*. If it was anaerobic exercise, then your anaerobic fitness will increase. Jogging 30 minutes each day will make it much easier for you to jog, but it will not make you able to lift 200 pounds, whereas lifting weights every day may make your muscles stronger (and bigger) for weightlifting tasks, but will not improve your endurance or your ability to carry out prolonged walks or bike rides.

With repeated aerobic exercise sessions, involving walking or jogging, one of the ways in which you become more fit is that your heart is able to pump more blood *with each beat,* and therefore you need fewer heart beats to deliver the same amount of blood to the muscles. You can see this change by checking your heart rate for a certain work load before you start an exercise program, then rechecking it after a few months of exercise. The easiest "work load" to check is no work at all, that is, measure your *resting* heart rate. The more fit someone is, the lower his or her resting heart rate. You may know runners who brag about having a resting heart rate of 45 or 50 beats per minute.

Another change that occurs with a training program and increased fitness is in the muscles themselves: They become able to process much more oxygen and to put that oxygen to use in performing work.

One change that *does not* occur with an exercise training program is in lung function. Most scientific studies have shown no important changes in lung function in healthy people after they train and become very fit. Since lung function doesn't have much to do with one's exercise ability if the lungs are normal, this doesn't make much difference to most people.

There is increasing evidence that people who engage in lifelong exercise live longer than sedentary people, and have lower risks for various diseases, especially heart disease and some kinds of cancer.

Exercise training programs have long been felt to be valuable to people's emotional health as well as their physical health, with decreased depression and stress levels, and increased work productivity. Many large corporations have installed impressive gym facilities for their employees because they have felt that fit employees were happier, healthier, and more productive.

Heat Training

Another change that comes with an exercise program, especially if it's been carried out in the heat, is that you become heat-acclimatized, that is, you can withstand exercise and heat stress better than you could before you got in shape. Several changes account for this improved heat tolerance. The first is just that exercise itself is easier because of being more fit (lower heart rate, etc.), without regard to the heat. But additional changes occur that are related specifically to increased heat tolerance. People who train in the heat begin to sweat earlier during an exercise session, thus cooling themselves earlier through evaporation. In addition, and quite remarkably, when someone without CF trains in the heat for several weeks, the sweat that is produced contains less salt. This may be the body's way of preserving salt, since much salt can be lost when someone sweats excessively. (People running a marathon can easily lose 5–10 pounds of sweat in 3 or 4 hours.)

EFFECTS OF EXERCISE IN PEOPLE WITH CYSTIC FIBROSIS

Single Sessions of Exercise

The responses to exercise in people with CF are generally similar to those of people who don't have CF. To meet the increased oxygen needs of exercising muscles and to remove carbon dioxide, both the heart's output and the amount of breathing are considerably increased. If the person's lung function is normal or nearly normal, he or she will have exactly the same responses to exercise as anyone else. However, there are some differences in the response to exercise in someone with CF whose pulmonary function is not normal. One difference is that people with CF frequently stop exercising before their heart rate has reached the maximum predicted based upon age. In these cases, the minute ventilation (the amount of air being breathed each minute) may be very large in comparison with the person's capacity or reserve. Remember that people with normal lungs seldom breathe more than 70% of their MVV, even during strenuous exercise. People with CF often use more than 80% of their MVV (in some cases, more than 100% of their "maximum" capacity is used!). Even as you can't expect a person with a normal heart to make the heart beat faster than its maximum, you can't expect *anyone*—with or without healthy lungs—to be able to use more than 100% of the lungs' capacity.

Most patients with CF maintain their blood levels of oxygen and carbon dioxide during exercise. In some patients, the blood oxygen level actually *increases* with exercise. However, in people with severe lung disease, the blood oxygen level may fall during exercise, and in some of these patients, the carbon dioxide level may increase. [This decrease in oxygen level does not occur in anyone whose forced expired volume (FEV_1) is greater than 50% of their forced vital capacity (FVC; see Chapter 3, *The Respiratory System*), and it doesn't occur even in most people whose FEV_1 is that low.] This means that for the amount of oxygen being used and the amount of carbon dioxide being produced by the exercising muscles, the person is not breathing enough. It is not known if this is harmful, but most CF physicians recommend that patients avoid this situation. That does not mean to avoid exercise altogether. Specific exercise guidelines are discussed later in this chapter.

Some people with CF also have asthma, particularly in response to exercise (*exercise-induced asthma*, or *EIA*). This is a common condition, and one that need not curtail your exercise program—about 10% of the United States Olympic team had *EIA*! I mention this not to guarantee you a spot on the Olympic team, but just to let you know that people with exercise-induced asthma may still be able to exercise and compete at a very high level. People with EIA will experience cough, wheeze, chest tightness, chest pain, or a combination of these symptoms when they exercise—typically, it's a few minutes *after* they exercise. The exercise that is most likely to bring on these symptoms is vigorous exercise—especially running—lasting 6 to 8 minutes, and especially in the cold air. The problem can be prevented in the majority of people with a couple of puffs from a bronchodilator (like albuterol) metered-dose inhaler about 15 minutes before exercise.

Many people with CF (whether or not they have asthma as well) cough during or after exercise. This may be distressing to someone who is watching, if they don't know about CF, and may be somewhat uncomfortable to the person coughing, but it is not dangerous. In fact, it is probably helpful in bringing mucus up out of the lungs.

Exercise in the Heat

Having CF should not prevent someone from exercising in the heat. People with CF have the same ability as people without CF to keep their body temperature down while exercising in hot weather. However, since they have the same mechanisms for doing this, including sweating, and since CF sweat is so much saltier than any other sweat, athletes with CF lose much more salt than their non-CF friends. They may lose so much that the blood levels of sodium and chloride drop. In most cases this does not cause a problem. Young people with CF also have an extremely accurate salt "thermostat" that enables them to know exactly how much salt they need to take to replace what they've lost. Replacing salt is something that can be done over a period of hours, and does not have to be done immediately after it's lost.

Replacing lost fluid is quite another matter, though, for anyone, with or without CF. It is very important for all people who exercise in the heat to drink plenty of fluid, but it is particularly important for children and adults with CF to drink while they exercise in hot weather, because while their salt "thermostat" works very well, their fluid "thermostat" is a little sluggish. All children tend to drink less fluid than they lose during exercise in the heat, but children with CF are especially neglectful of drinking as much as they need.

Exercise Tolerance

Many children and adults with CF who have good lung function are limited in their exercise capacity by the same factors that limit their classmates; namely, the heart reaches a limit to how much blood it can pump, and/or the muscles reach a limit to how much oxygen they can process. These factors will be especially limiting if someone has not exercised much and is out of shape. But those whose lungs are affected more extensively by their CF are likely to be limited by the lungs before the heart and muscles are pushed to their limits. This does not necessarily mean that their blood oxygen levels will fall, but rather that the work of breathing may just become too great and they will need to stop because of that discomfort. Even in most people whose oxygen level does fall, it is probably the discomfort of hard breathing and not the lowered oxygen level that forces them to stop running or pedaling. There are certainly a few people who benefit from using oxygen during exercise, and are able to do considerably more exercise if they use extra oxygen when they are active.

Although coughing may be severe, it seldom limits exercise.

Exercise Programs for People with Cystic Fibrosis

Exercise programs have the same benefit for people with CF that they have for people without CF, namely, increasing their fitness and sense of well-being, and probably improving their overall outlook on life. "Increased fitness" is defined as being able to do more physical work, and having a lower heart rate for the same workload. Some studies have shown better lung function after a CF exercise training program, and other studies have shown no change in lung function. A very important study showed that CF patients' fitness level corresponded more closely with their survival (how likely they were to be alive eight years later) than any other factor did. So, although it hasn't yet been proved that becoming more fit means you'll live longer, it's tempting to think so, and act as if that's so by working to get and stay in shape!

For people with normal lungs, strenuous aerobic exercise programs should raise the heart rate to 75% of its maximum, or about 150 beats per minute. Many people with CF will not be able to exercise this hard, because their breathing will stop them before their heart rate has risen that high. This does not mean that someone with CF cannot become more fit. In fact, it seems that CF patients can become more fit by exercising hard enough to raise their heart rates to 75% of their own maximum, and not the maximum that you'd predict on the basis of their age. Thus, if someone with CF has a maximum heart rate of 150 beats per minute (that is, the pulse goes up to 150 during the most strenuous exercise he or she can tolerate), that person will be able to benefit from regular exercise sessions with the heart beating around 115 beats a minute (roughly 75% of 150).

Fortunately, it's not necessary to measure the heart rate precisely during all exercise sessions to know if you're working hard enough to bring about improvements; instead, you can strive for a pleasantly tired feeling. If you're not at all tired, you are not working hard enough. On the other hand, if you're so tired that you don't feel at all good, you're pushing yourself harder than you need. That becomes important in planning a long-term exercise program because human nature is such that no one wants to do unpleasant things, and exercise is no exception: if your exercise sessions leave you exhausted and feeling bad, you will be much more likely to find excuses to skip them than if they are enjoyable. In the section after the next there will be an introduction to the nitty-gritty of carrying out an exercise program.

Heat Training in Cystic Fibrosis

Like everyone else, *people with CF can become adapted to exercise in the heat.* If you exercise in the heat every day for a week or more, at the end of that period, your heart rate and body temperature will be lower when you exercise than they were at the beginning.

When you have CF, you are likely to lose large amounts of sodium and chloride during each exercise session in the heat. If you allow yourself to eat and drink without restriction, you will find that you automatically select items that will completely replace the lost salt. This is very important because a major difference between the normal response to heat training and the CF response is that CF sweat glands cannot decrease the salt content of sweat. This means that even though you have greater tolerance for exercise and heat stress, you still lose much more salt than is normal. In addition, after you've trained for a while, you will begin to sweat earlier in the exercise session (this change occurs in *everyone* during heat training) and you will also be able to exercise for a longer period, thus losing even more salt after you've become adapted to the heat.

GUIDELINES FOR AN EXERCISE PROGRAM

General

Most CF physicians now feel that exercise is beneficial for all CF patients, and that an active lifestyle should begin early in childhood, well before a formal "program" is prescribed. In most cases, more activity is better than less, and parents should encourage activity from very early on. As with any child, parental *encouragement* is good; parental *aggressive pushing* is probably not. Parents can often help establish the exercise habit in their children by example: if they exercise, their children are likely to. And the family that exercises together is most likely to maintain the exercise longer than those who don't. As children get older, they may want to participate in sports, and this is fine. There are virtually no limits to what sports or activities they can engage in. Patients' bodies will usually tell them when they need to stop, so they need not be limited by parents or coaches. However, for patients with some degree of lung disease, their coaches must be aware of their condition, and must allow the patients to limit themselves: the patients should not be pushed beyond their comfort/tolerance. Teenagers and adults may want to have some guidelines for setting up their own exercise program. Read on.

Medical Advice

Check with your doctor before you start. If your lungs are severely affected by CF, your doctor may recommend an exercise test first to check your oxygen level. If your FEV_1 is less than 50% of your FVC (or 50% of the predicted normal level— that's about the same as 50% of FVC), it's a particularly good idea to see if your oxygen level falls during exercise, and if so, at what intensity: If your oxygen level is good until your heart rate reaches 150 beats per minute, it's relatively easy to keep your exercise program light enough that your heart rate stays below 145. Your doctor might even want to prescribe some oxygen for you to use while you exercise. For most people with CF, this will not be necessary.

Time Allotment

Set aside a time to exercise. This should amount to about 30 minutes a day, three to five times a week for the exercise itself, plus whatever time you need to shower and dress. You should guard this exercise time jealously and keep it for yourself. It doesn't matter what time of day you exercise. Some people prefer to exercise in the morning, whereas others prefer to wait until they've been awake and active for several hours. Of course, if your exercise is in gym class or with a team, you won't have much choice as to timing.

Type of Activity

Pick an activity that is a good aerobic conditioner. These activities are ones that are continuous, not stop-and-go; they are light enough that they can be carried out for many minutes at a time, without causing total exhaustion. Typical aerobic activities that are discussed below in greater detail include running, swimming, and biking. Others include rowing, skating, stair-stepping, cross-country skiing, indoor "skiing" on a NordicTrack® or similar equipment, and vigorous walking. Brisk walking (including race-walking) is excellent, and has recently become one of the most widely practiced forms of regular exercise.

Activities that are *an*aerobic include weight training, most racquet sports, and volleyball. These activities, are also beneficial, and many are fun; some may make you stronger and build your muscles, including the chest muscles that you use for breathing. Anaerobic activities will probably not help your endurance. For most CF patients, it's probably ideal to include a hefty dose of aerobic exercise, whether or not you also do anaerobic exercise.

Boxing is too dangerous even to be mentioned as an activity, except to condemn it.

Regular daily activities should not be overlooked in planning a more active lifestyle. If you usually walk the dog around a short block, try going around a long block instead; walk or ride a bike to the corner store when you run out of milk instead of getting a ride; take the stairs instead of the elevator whenever possible; and so on. Try cutting down on TV time in favor of exercising time. It does you a lot more good to walk or run around the block than to watch someone else doing it on TV.

PACING YOURSELF

Getting Going

Whatever activity you pick, remember not to overdo it, especially when you first begin to train. Listen carefully to what your body is telling you about how hard or fast or far you're going. It's much better to take a few days, weeks, or even months to work your way up to the desired amount of exercise than to get injured or discouraged by trying too much too soon. If you haven't been particularly active, limit your first exercise session to no more than 10 minutes. Continue to exercise for 10 minutes each day for the first week. With each successive week, try adding 2 minutes to each session. By the time several months have passed, you'll find that you're exercising for as long as 30 minutes.

Listen to Your Body

If you're getting winded, go slower until you've caught your breath, and then continue at an easier pace. If you feel as though you've hardly exerted yourself after 10 minutes, you can push a little harder for a little longer.

Injuries

Minor injuries can occur with most forms of exercise. Don't ignore them. While you can continue to exercise with some discomfort, real pain is a signal to stop. Let a few days pass without exercising, and if your pain persists, inform your doctor.

Medications, Food, and Drink

If you have asthma or if you take any inhaled bronchodilators, it's advisable to take an inhalation before you exercise. It is not wise to exercise after a heavy meal; in fact, waiting several hours after a meal before you run or swim will make your exercise more pleasant. If you're exercising in warm weather, you should drink while you exercise—probably even more than you think you need. You do not need to take salt pills.

RUNNING

Equipment

The only special equipment you need for running is a good pair of running shoes. Gym shoes or tennis shoes are not appropriate for regular running. A long-term running program involves a lot of pounding of your feet on the pavement. If you don't have the proper shoes, this pounding travels from your feet to your shins, knees, and hips and can cause an injury. It is advisable to buy your shoes in a store that specializes in runners' supplies. When shopping for running shoes, pick a shoe that feels good on your foot. Do not expect an uncomfortable shoe to "break in" after a while the way a leather shoe might (most running shoes are made of synthetic materials that do not change their shape with time and wear).

Clothes

You can run in clothes that you probably already have. For summer running, dress as lightly as possible. Nylon shorts and shirts are light and dry out quickly, but cotton is more absorbent. Some newer synthetic materials like "polypro" help wick sweat away from the skin for better evaporation and cooling. For running in colder weather, you are more likely to overdress than underdress. When the temperature is below freezing, cotton socks and sweat pants or stretch tights are the best. Cover your chest with several light layers rather than one heavy layer. On the coldest days, a T-shirt, cotton turtleneck, and hooded cotton sweat shirt should be enough. If it is very windy, a thin nylon shell suit over your running clothes will insulate you and keep the wind out. GoreTex® and similar high-tech fibers are expensive, but are impressive in their ability to keep you dry: they don't let rain or snow in, but they do let sweat out. Be sure to cover your head with a wool cap or the hood from your sweat shirt or jacket, because much of the body's heat is lost from the head. A scarf or mask over your nose and mouth may make breathing easier, particularly if you have exercise-induced asthma. Your feet are working hard, so they won't get very cold, but your hands will. To keep your hands warm, mittens or socks are better than gloves, since they let your fingers keep each other warm. Some petroleum jelly on your lips and cheeks will reduce the sting of the cold.

Starting to Run

Remember not to push yourself too hard, especially at first. You should be exercising to make yourself feel good; if you push so hard that you feel bad, you've missed the point. Start with a 10-minute run/walk session. Run slowly, and when you get tired, start walking. When you are ready, run again. Continue this for three or four sessions during your first week, trying to run for most of the 10 minutes. As the weeks go by, you should gradually add time to your run/walk sessions. Add 2 or 3 minutes each week, so that, after 7–10 weeks, you are running for most of each 30-minute session. If it takes longer to add the extra minutes, don't worry, there's no rush. It doesn't matter how far you go or how long it takes you to work up to 30 minutes of running.

Safety

You should be able to avoid injury to your muscles if you warm up properly before running, stretch and cool down afterward, and build up gradually to a regular exercise program. However, if you feel pain after running, be sure to have it checked. Other safety factors to consider include not running in traffic or other polluted areas, and not running in dark clothes at night. You can avoid these problems by running on an athletic field, golf course, track, or jogging trail rather than on the sidewalk or street.

If you start your running program in the spring, summer, or fall, you may become discouraged when the weather turns bad in the winter months. There is really no reason you shouldn't run in the winter, as long as you dress properly. Running on icy or slippery surfaces is dangerous, so be careful and sensible about running in the winter; a broken leg or sprained ankle will not promote your general conditioning. Running in cold weather may be hard for people with exercise-induced asthma. Two easy steps can make it much easier: take two puffs of albuterol or other bronchodilator before you go out, and wear a mask or scarf around your nose and mouth, so the air you breathe in will be warm and a bit moist.

SWIMMING

Where to Swim

You will need a pool, lake, river, or ocean. Unless you live in a part of the country where the weather is good and you can swim outside all year round, you will want to swim in a pool that is convenient to get to and affordable to use. A summer swimming program at a beach or lake won't give you any long-term benefit if you only swim for 2 or 3 months out of the year. Additionally, rivers and oceans have currents, waves, and tides that may interfere with a regular, sustained swimming program. If you don't have a pool or ocean in your backyard, there are a lot of places where you should be able to swim for free or at a moderate cost. Many high schools and colleges have pools that are open to the public during certain hours. Many people swim at municipal or community pools. Most YMCAs and many health clubs and hotels have swimming pools that can be joined for a reasonable fee.

Equipment

Once you have found a place to swim, the only equipment or special clothing you really need is a bathing suit. For a regular exercise program, a one-piece nylon or lycra tank suit is best. Both nylon and lycra suits wear well and dry out quickly. Goggles are useful if you are swimming in a pool or in salt water, since both chlorine and salt can be very irritating to the eyes. If you wear glasses or contact lenses you can purchase goggles with corrective lenses for very reasonable cost (ask your eye doctor or swim shop for details). If you have long hair, a bathing cap will keep your hair out of your face, as well as out of a pool's filter system. Caps also protect hair and scalps from the drying effects of chlorine.

Safety

NEVER SWIM ALONE! There should always be a lifeguard at the pool or beach. While you are probably less likely to drown in a swimming pool than in a lake, river, or ocean, always make sure that there is a lifeguard present. Failing that, use the "buddy system," swimming with a friend who can pull you out of the water or run for help if you need it. You should also learn some basic water safety techniques. The risk of pulling muscles or tendons while swimming is much less than while running or bicycling. If you are swimming smoothly, your muscles should get an even workout. Most injuries occur from diving into shallow water, swimming into the side of the pool, or sustaining cuts from rocks or trash on the bottom of a river or lake.

Learning to Swim

Swimming is most enjoyable when you have a smooth, comfortable stroke. If you do not know how to swim well or if you want to improve your stroke, swimming lessons will be helpful. This does not mean that you have to start training to make the Olympic team, but you should be able to execute the various strokes properly. As in running and bicycling, the goal is not speed, but rather sustained, even exercise over time. There are many places where you can learn to swim. The Red Cross and the YMCA are probably best known for their swimming programs, but any reputable class will do. Many places offer swimming lessons designed especially for adults.

Starting to Swim

As with running, don't push yourself too hard or too fast at first. A 10-minute session that alternates a strenuous stroke like the crawl (free-style) with a more restful stroke (breast stroke or side stroke) should get you off to a good start. Try to schedule your swimming sessions three or four times each week for the first few weeks. Gradually work up to longer sessions by adding a few minutes to each session after the first week or two. Your goal should be to swim for at least 30 minutes during each session. Again, remember that you can take as many weeks as you need to reach this goal. It doesn't matter how many laps you swim or how fast you swim them.

BICYCLING

Equipment

If you plan to cycle out-of-doors, a sturdy bike with 3 to 12 speeds is your basic piece of equipment. A cycling helmet is also essential to prevent head injuries if you fall or are thrown from your bike. If you plan to cycle indoors, there are many good models of stationary exercise bikes. However, before you buy one, remember that riding a stationary bike can be extremely boring. Some people set the bike up in front of the TV and pedal as they watch. Others listen to music or read while they ride. Most people who just cycle in a bare cellar don't stay with it very long.

Preparing Your Bicycle

Your bicycle should be in good condition each time you begin a ride. Make sure that the seat is properly adjusted, because this will increase the efficiency and comfort with which you ride. Raise or lower the saddle so that your leg is fully extended when your heel is placed on the pedal at the bottom of its cycle. This will cause your leg to be slightly bent while pedaling with the ball of your foot on the pedal. Before each ride, briefly inspect the tires, brakes, and wheels of your bike to make sure that they are in good order. If any part is not working properly, have it fixed. Proper maintenance of your bike will help to ensure safe riding.

Safety

Wear a bike helmet! Bike paths and lightly trafficked roads are recommended over city streets and highways. *Wear a bike helmet!* Familiarize yourself with the traffic laws regarding bicycling and obey them. *Wear a bike helmet!* If you plan to ride in the evenings, be sure that you have the proper lights and reflectors on your bike and wear light-colored clothes so that motorists and other riders can see you. There are wonderful little battery-powered blinking lights available to attach to your belt or bike seat that are visible from a long way aware. And, did I mention?: *Wear a bike helmet!*

Clothes

The clothes needed for bicycling are similar to those for running, except that you will build up less heat, and give off more heat on a bike than on foot, so you'll have to dress more warmly (and with more wind protection) on the bike. Be sure that your pants legs fit snugly so that they won't get caught in the gear sprockets or chain. Be sure that your shoe laces are tucked in so that they don't get caught in the sprockets or chain. And on your head? *Wear a bike helmet!*

Starting to Cycle

As with running and swimming, start out slowly and build up to longer periods of exercise. A 10- to 15-minute ride three or four times a week is a good way to start out, adding extra minutes to each session after the first week or two. Alternate slow, easy riding with fast, hard riding until you are riding for 30 minutes, three to five times a week. Strive toward a continuous, comfortable ride of increasing duration, rather than a ride that covers a certain distance.

SUMMARY

Patients with CF can and should exercise, at virtually every stage (and age) of life. They reap the same benefits from exercise programs and an active lifestyle that other people do (and perhaps even more): they can become more physically fit, and can do more exercise than if they are sedentary. Exercise helps CF patients keep their lungs clear of mucus. Exercise helps a lot of people emotionally, too, by reducing stress. Exercise may even enable CF patients to live longer.

11

Genetics

THE BASICS

1. CF is inherited. In order to be born with CF, you have to get two abnormal CF genes (one from each parent).
2. People with just one abnormal CF gene are called "carriers," and do not have CF.
3. Each time two carriers have a baby, the chances are 1 in four that that baby will have CF, even if the couple has already had one or more babies with CF.
4. It is possible to test during a pregnancy whether the baby will have CF.
5. It is possible to test to see if someone is a CF carrier, but the test will miss some carriers.
6. Gene therapy may some day be possible to cure CF.

INTRODUCTION

Cystic fibrosis (CF) is a genetic disorder, which means that it is determined by the genes a person has inherited. There are millions of genes located on the chromosomes within each cell in the body. The genes are made of DNA, the basic determinant of our body makeup. Genes come in pairs, with one gene having come from each parent. As a mother's eggs are formed, each egg has only one set of genes, rather than the double set that exists in all the other cells in her body. Similarly, each of the father's millions of sperm has only one gene for each characteristic. When the sperm and egg unite, the fetus they develop into will have one set of genes from the mother and one from the father. The genes determine all of our physical characteristics, from the shape of our ears to the color of our hair. What makes each of us unique physically is the combination of genes that make up our cells.

Different gene combinations work in different ways. In some cases, a gene is *dominant,* meaning that it is the gene that will be expressed, regardless of what the gene is that accompanies it. The dominant gene completely determines the outcome. An example of this (although it's a bit oversimplified) is the brown hair gene. If a baby gets one brown hair gene, he or she will have brown hair, no matter what the other hair-color gene is. In other cases, there is the *recessive* gene, which will not be noticed at all unless it is paired with an identical gene. At a first approximation, red hair is a recessive characteristic, so most redheads have received two red-hair genes—one from each parent. A baby with one red-hair gene and one brown-hair gene will usually have brown hair. Finally, there is the gene interaction where each gene contributes something so that the resulting characteristic is a combination of what each would have determined by itself. An example of this is skin color. When a very dark-skinned person and a very fair person have a baby, the baby's skin is often a color that is in between the parents' skin colors.

We all have two copies of the cystic fibrosis gene—the gene that determines whether or not we have CF—but for most people both copies are normal. Cystic fibrosis is a recessive disorder, which means that a baby who gets an altered (abnormal) CF gene from only one parent will not have CF, and will have no sign of CF. CF occurs *only* if a person has received an altered CF gene from each parent. For a parent to pass on an altered CF gene to a child, she or he obviously must have one of those genes. In almost every case, the parent carries one altered CF gene and one normal CF gene in each of his (her) cells. Yet there is no evidence at all that they carry the altered CF gene until they have a child with CF. People who have one altered CF gene and one normal CF gene are called *carriers* because they are not affected by the gene but carry it and can pass it along to their children. Whether their children will have CF depends on what gene the other parent contributes. In the unusual case where a parent has CF him- or herself, he (she) has two altered CF genes in each cell, and *must* pass on one of those to each child. As with carriers, whether their children will have CF depends on what gene the other parent contributes.

Figure 11.1 shows the possible combinations if two parents who are each carriers have children. For each of them, half of their eggs or sperm will have the altered CF gene, and half will have the normal CF gene. The chances of a sperm that carries the altered CF gene fertilizing an egg with the CF gene are exactly the same as its fertilizing a normal egg. This means that there are only four possible combinations of genes from these parents, and each is just as likely to occur as the others. *Each time this couple has a child,* the chances are 1 in 4 that the baby will get two altered CF genes, and will have CF; 2 in 4 (a "fifty-fifty" chance) that the baby will get one altered CF gene, and therefore will not have CF but will be a carrier; and 1 in 4 that the baby will not get any altered CF gene at all.

Chance and statistics can be confusing to understand at first. People may assume, mistakenly, that if their chances are 1 in 4 that a baby will have CF, and they've already had a baby with CF, then the next three children can't have CF.

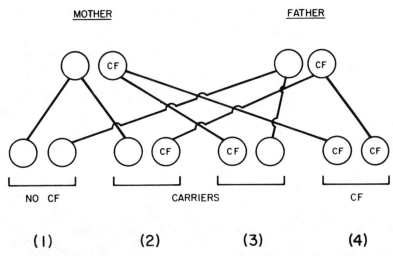

MOTHER   FATHER

NO CF   CARRIERS   CF

(1)   (2)   (3)   (4)

Figure 11.1. The inheritance of CF. Each parent of a child with CF has one abnormal CF gene (*circle labeled* "CF")1. The abnormal CF gene causes no problems if it is paired with a normal CF gene (*blank circle*). When two parents who each carry an abnormal CF gene have children, each parent passes on either the abnormal or the normal CF gene. The figure shows the possible combinations of genes which children of carriers can have: **(1)** A normal CF gene from both father and mother; **(2)** a normal CF gene from the mother and an abnormal gene from the father; **(3)** an abnormal CF gene from the mother and a normal gene from the father; and **(4)**; an abnormal CF gene from each parent. Each of these four combinations is just as likely to occur as the others, meaning that the chances of two carrier parents having a child with CF is one in four each time they have a child.

This is not so—*each* time they have a child, there is 1 chance in 4 that the child will have CF. There are families with three children, *all* of whom have CF, and others in which both parents are carriers, yet *none* of their children have CF. With statistical chance, the numbers work out over hundreds or thousands of cases, which doesn't much help the individual family.

Consider the example of a deck of cards. There are four suits: hearts, diamonds, spades, and clubs. If the cards are shuffled well and are not marked, and you try to pick a diamond, your chances will be 1 in 4. But you know very well that you might pick 10 cards one time before you get a diamond, and another time you might pick four diamonds in a row. If you picked cards all morning, by the time you'd picked 1,000 cards you'd have come pretty close to 250 diamonds, but those first few might have been almost any pattern.

Thus, while you can know the overall statistics, they won't necessarily be helpful in an individual case. So, in families trying to decide on their family's future, they can consider their statistical chances. If they have had a child with CF, that means the parents are both carriers, and the chances for each pregnancy resulting in a child with CF are 1 in 4. Some people consider 1 chance in 4 to be great odds, while others think they're dreadful. Great chances or dreadful, brothers and sisters of CF patients should all be sweat-tested to see if they have CF, even if they have been perfectly healthy, since each child born to the parents of someone

TABLE 11.1. *Risks for Individuals of North European Caucasian Background of Having a Child with Cystic Fibrosis*

One Parent	Other Parent	Risk with Each Pregnancy
No CF history	No CF history	1 in 2500
No CF history	First cousin has CF	1 in 400
No CF history	Aunt or uncle has CF	1 in 300
No CF history	Nephew or niece has CF	1 in 200
No CF history	Sibling has CF	1 in 150
No CF history	Has CF	1 in 50
Sibling has CF	Sibling has CF	1 in 9
Sibling has CF	Has CF	1 in 3
Sibling has CF	Known carrier	1 in 6
Known carrier	Known carrier	1 in 4
Known carrier	Has CF	1 in 2

Risks are actually slightly higher than listed because the list assumes that (excluding siblings of CF patients) someone who is a carrier has *one* parent who is also a carrier; it is actually possible that *both* of this person's parents are carriers, and that means that each of this person's siblings has greater than a 50–50 chance of being a carrier. Risks to other ethnic groups will generally be different (see Table 11.2).

with CF does have a 1-in-4 chance of having received the two altered CF genes, and many people with CF can be healthy for a long time before symptoms appear.

What about the chances of having a child with CF if there is CF in the family of one parent (or parent-to-be) or the other? What if you have a nephew, niece, brother, sister, or cousin with CF? Table 11.1 shows the chances in different situations, depending on the parents' family background.

HOW COMMON IS THE CYSTIC FIBROSIS GENE?

Sometimes it can seem to new parents of a child with CF that they were just unbelievably unlucky for two carriers of a disease-gene to get together. But carrying a harmful gene is very common: geneticists estimate that every healthy person carries between 3 and 5 different harmful genes. And the altered CF gene is not unusual. In fact, it is quite common, occurring in about 1 in every 25 white people in North America. It's less common in other ethnic groups (one in 17,000 African-American people in Washington, D.C.; one in 90,000 Asian-Americans in Hawaii), but has been reported in individuals on every continent (except, perhaps, Antarctica!), and from virtually every racial background. Table 11.2 shows how common CF is in different countries.

Not only is the CF gene common, it's also old: CF has been with us for somewhere between 3,000 and 53,000 years. People sometimes wonder how an altered gene that causes disease can persist for so long. Getting two copies of the altered gene clearly gives a person big disadvantages. Until very recently, no one with CF lived long enough to have children, so why should the gene still be around? For some other genes that cause recessive disorders (remember, those are prob-

Table 11.2. *Incidence of Cystic Fibrosis in Different Countries*

Country (or Group)	1 Baby With CF per Live Births*
Alberta (Canada) Hutterites	*313*
Afrikaners (Southwest Africa)	*622*
Ireland	*2,000*
Australia	*2,500*
United Kingdom (England)	*2,500*
North America	*2,500*
France	*3,000*
Netherlands	*3,500*
Germany	*4,000*
Denmark	*4,500*
Ashkenazi Jews in Israel	*5,000*
Sweden	*8,000*
Italy	*15,000*
Finland	*40,000*

*Numbers listed are CF patients per live births (so, for Ireland, of every 2,000 babies born alive, 1 has CF).

lems where you need to get one abnormal gene from each parent), there has been discovered a "carrier or heterozygote [see below] advantage," meaning that carriers of the gene have some benefit, some advantage, over those who do not carry the gene. A well-known example is sickle cell disease, a terrible problem that kills many young black people. Carriers of the sickle cell gene are said to have "sickle cell trait," and they have been known for some time to be less susceptible to malaria. Well, if malaria is killing off whole villages in Africa (as it has done throughout the ages), and you have something that keeps you alive when many others are dying from malaria, then you—and that gene that protects you—will survive.

Many different guesses have been made about what the "heterozygote advantage" might be for CF carriers. Things like increased fertility of the carriers, less asthma, or increased resistance to intestinal infections have all been suggested, but none has been proven. New work with the CF mouse (see below) has finally provided what seems to be a reasonable explanation (although one that is still a little controversial). It appears that mice with one altered CF gene and one normal CF gene (that is, carriers) are protected from the ravages of cholera. Cholera causes extremely severe watery diarrhea, with the loss of tremendous amounts of fluid, and many people infected with cholera die of dehydration. But the CF-carrier mice exposed to the cholera toxin that causes the diarrhea had much less watery diarrhea than mice who did not carry the altered CF gene. (This is discussed a little more in Chapter 1, *The Basic Defect*.) So, it may be that human CF carriers have been protected over the centuries from cholera or similar intestinal infections, and therefore their protective gene has stayed around, even though when it unites with a similar gene it causes CF.

Recent advances in molecular genetics enabled researchers to zero in on the CF gene, to determine that CF is caused by a single gene (and not a series of genes), and, in 1989, to discover and analyze the gene itself. That gene is located on the seventh of the 23 human chromosomes. The discovery of the gene has led to a virtual explosion in our knowledge about CF, has made possible the creation of a "CF mouse," has expanded our ability to identify CF carriers, and to diagnose CF in living patients, in unborn fetuses, and even sometimes in patients who have already died. The discovery of the gene has even enabled people to hope that the day may be approaching when CF will be *cured* with gene therapy.

To understand the importance of this discovery, let's take a little detour, to a crash course in basic genetics. Hold on to your hats!

WHAT IS A GENE?

A gene is a unit of DNA that directs the production of a protein. DNA is considered by scientists to be the basic blueprint of our body's structure and function. DNA in turn is made of pairs of chemicals called *nucleotides*. The chemicals or *bases* that make up these nucleotides are adenine, guanine, thymine, and cytosine (abbreviated A, G, T, and C). These nucleotides form long double chains, wound around each other in a "helix." The strands are held together by specific pairing of the nucleotides. Adenine always pairs with thymine, and cytosine with guanine. These chains of pairs of nucleotides ("base pairs") are the DNA. The incredible array of different information that is contained in these structures seems to be explained entirely by the order in which those four simple chemicals line up with one another.

The average gene is made up of about 30,000 nucleotides or base pairs. All of the human genetic information is stored on 23 paired *chromosomes*; each chromosome stores about 5,000 genes. This dizzying amount of material is all stored within each and every one of the millions of cells that make up our bodies! To get an idea of the dimensions we're dealing with here (Table 11.3), let's look at the genetic information in terms of *distance*: if one nucleotide were 1 inch long, a gene would be 700 yards long, a chromosome 1,900 miles, and all of the human genetic information (called the human *genome*) would stretch twice around the earth's equator! Instead of distance, what if genes were *time* (a kind of crazy idea)? Well, if a nucleotide were 1 second, a gene would be about 8½ hours, a chromosome nearly 4½ years, and the whole genome 1 century! And all this is packed into each of our body's cells, cells too tiny to see without a microscope.

The way genes dictate what our body's cells do is by directing ("coding") the production of proteins; it's the proteins that really do the work. These proteins are made of *amino acids,* and the various portions of the gene call for various amino acids, with 3 pairs of nucleotides per amino acid. All together, the particular amino acids and the order in which they are placed determine what the resulting protein looks like and does. It turns out that not all of the gene is involved in coding for

TABLE 11.3. *The Relative Dimensions of the Components of Human Genetic Material, Expressed as if They Were Time or Distance*

Unit	Time	Distance
Nucleotide	1 second	1 inch
Gene	8½hours	700 yards
Chromosome	4⅓years	1900 miles
Genome	1 century	2 equators

Thanks to Dr. John Mulvihill, University of Pittsburgh.

protein production; relatively short portions, called *exons*, do the directing of amino acid placement and protein production. These exons are separated along the length of the gene by long stretches of inactive DNA. The inactive stretches are called *introns*.

THE CYSTIC FIBROSIS GENE

The CF gene is very large, containing about 250,000 base pairs (about eight times as many as the average gene). The protein made under the direction of the CF gene contains 1,480 amino acids. (For those of you who've been following the complicated math here, you'll have noted that if it takes 3 base pairs for one amino acid, 250,000 base pairs could have resulted in over 80,000 amino acids, instead of a measly 1,480; this shows how much of the CF gene—like most genes—is made up of introns, that is, inactive DNA.) This 1480-amino acid protein has the unwieldy (but accurate) name *CFTR,* for **c**ystic **f**ibrosis **t**rans-membrane conductance **r**egulator protein. The main function of this protein is to direct traffic across cell membranes, especially traffic of salt (sodium and chloride). Abnormal movement of chloride and sodium (and water) across cells seems to explain virtually all of the problems seen in people with CF, and this cell defect is now felt to be the basic defect in CF. It is discussed at length in Chapter 1, *The Basic Defect.* Since the CF gene is responsible for producing the CFTR protein, the gene is sometimes referred to as the CFTR gene. To make things even more complicated, *everyone,* not just people with CF, has two CFTR genes, and makes CFTR protein. The difference between CF patients and people without CF is in the structure (and therefore also the function) of the CFTR protein. When the CFTR protein is normal, sodium, chloride, and water all act normally, secretions are not extra thick, and no disease results.

When the CF gene is abnormal, in any of a number of ways, the protein it produces will have a different amino acid composition, and therefore a different function, and, if both copies are abnormal, will cause the problems that make up CF. Far and away the most common alteration (*mutation*) in the gene that causes CF occurs in exon 10, and is the loss of 3 (out of a total of 250,000!) base pairs, leading to production of a protein that is missing one (of 1,480) amino acid. The missing amino acid is phenylalanine, and it is missing from position 508 of the protein structure. By a strange spelling agreement, geneticists abbreviate phenylalanine, "F." Together with the scientific notation "delta," written "Δ," meaning *deleted,* this gives the common CF mutation the name "delta F 508," or "ΔF508." About 70% of CF chromosomes (in North America) have the ΔF508 mutation. About 50% of North American CF patients have 2 copies of ΔF508 (one from each parent), while 20% have one ΔF508 gene and one of the other abnormal CF genes. (Someone with 2 copies of the same gene mutation is called *homozygous* for that mutation, from the Greek "homo," meaning "the same," and "zygote," for yoke, meaning two of the same genes are yoked or linked together. This contrasts with *hetero*zygous, meaning two *different* things linked together; "compound heterozygote" is the term used for someone who has two different mutations. A CF carrier, with one normal and one abnormal gene, is also sometimes called a CF heterozygote.)

TABLE 11.4. *Some of the More Common Cystic Fibrosis Gene Mutations and Their Characteristics*

Mutation	Geographic/Ethnic Incidence	Other
ΔF508	70–75% in North America	Pancreatic insufficiency
W1282X*	50–60% in Ashkenazi Jews; 2.1% worldwide	Pancreatic insufficiency
G542X*	3.4% worldwide	Pancreatic insufficiency; ?more meconium ileus
G551D*	2.4% worldwide	Pancreatic insufficiency
3905insT*	2.1% worldwide	Pancreatic insufficiency
N1303K*	1.8% worldwide	Pancreatic insufficiency
R553X*	1.3% worldwide	Pancreatic insufficiency
621+1G→T*	1.3% worldwide	Pancreatic insufficiency
1717-1G→A*	1.3% worldwide	Pancreatic insufficiency
A455E*	3–7% in Netherlands; 0–0.2% in North America	Pancreatic sufficiency;[†] mild lung disease
3849+10kb C→T*	1.4% worldwide; 4% in Israel	Pancreatic sufficiency,[†] normal sweat chloride; most males not sterile; lung disease varies from mild to severe
R117H*	0.8% worldwide	Pancreatic sufficiency[†]; slightly lower sweat chloride; older age at diagnosis
R334W*		Pancreatic sufficiency[†]; older age at diagnosis
R347P*		Pancreatic sufficiency[†]
P574H*		Pancreatic sufficiency[†]
Y563N*		Pancreatic sufficiency[†]

*"Compound heterozygotes," in most cases, meaning these patients had one copy of the particular mutation noted and one other CF mutation (usually ΔF508).
[†]Pancreatic sufficiency in most, but not all, cases.

After $\Delta F508$ was discovered, it was originally thought that there would probably be five or six other mutations that would account for the other 30% of CF chromosomes. By the time of the writing of this book, six years later, more than 500 different CF mutations have been identified! Most of these mutations are very rare, occurring in only a very few cases, some in only one case. There are a few mutations that are not so rare, and the frequency of different mutations varies, depending on a population's ethnic and geographic background. For example, "W1282X" is uncommon in non-Jewish people, but found in nearly 50% of all Jewish CF patients' chromosomes. "G551D" is relatively common in people of Celtic origin, occurring in 5–10% of abnormal CF genes in Ireland and England. See Table 11.4 for other examples. Taken all together, the known mutations explain about 90% of all CF chromosomes. In a few specific ethnic groups, a very few of the known mutations account for almost all of the CF patients (see Table 11.5).

DIFFERENT MUTATIONS: DIFFERENT DISEASES?

Whenever several different variations of a gene can cause problems, people wonder if the different variations of the gene cause different problems. Geneticists talk about the *genotype–phenotype relationship*. Genotype just means the type of gene one has. "Phenotype" comes from the Greek word that means appearance, and refers to what you see in a person: the outward evidence of various processes. In the case of CF, we know that some people seem to have a worse form of the disease, with severe lung disease and lots of hospital admissions, while others are pretty healthy, and some don't even need to take pancreatic enzymes. Whether someone needs to take enzymes, and how healthy his (or her) lungs are, make up his or her phenotype. So when people wonder about the genotype–phenotype relationship in CF, they wonder whether different CF mutations cause any of the variations we see in how CF affects different patients.

As with so many things, the answer seems to be "yes and no." The "yes" part has mostly to do with pancreatic function, and whether someone needs to take enzymes or not. Almost everybody with two copies (one from each parent) of the most common CF mutation, $\Delta F508$, needs to take enzymes (they have "pancre-

TABLE 11.5. *Ethnic Groups Where a Few Mutations Account for Most of the Cystic Fibrosis Chromosomes*

Group	Number of Mutations	% of CF Chromosomes
Alberta (Canada) Hutterites	2	100
Welsh	29	99.5
Brittany Celts	19	98
Ashkenazi Jews	5	97
Belgian	17	94.3

*Information from Dr. Gary Cutting.

atic insufficiency"). There have now been several different CF mutations discovered that are associated with pancreatic sufficiency (that is, you don't need to take enzymes), even if you have one of these genes and one ΔF508 gene. Table 11.4 lists some of these genes. Unfortunately, some geneticists have referred to the genes associated with pancreatic insufficiency as "severe," while those associated with pancreatic sufficiency are called "mild." The "mild" versus "severe" distinction holds true only for how the pancreas is affected (the need to take enzymes or not). This is confusing, since the pancreas has relatively little to do with the overall health of CF patients and how long they live.

The more important question is harder to answer: are variations in the amount of lung disease related to different CF mutations? With few exceptions, the answer seems to be "no." The differences in the severity of lung disease among people with two copies of ΔF508 seem to be much greater than differences between those with different genes. That is, factors other than the particular brand of abnormal CF gene are most important in determining how bad someone's lungs are. These factors could be environmental or genetic.

Factors that are known to influence lung health in CF patients more than their particular CF mutation include things in the environment, including exposure to cigarette smoke and viruses, and the aggressiveness of treatment. In a way, this is good news, since things over which patients and families have no control (what gene they happen to have) may end up being less important to their survival than some things over which they do have control (treatments, avoiding cigarette smoke).

It is possible that there are genetic factors other than the CF mutation itself that influence someone's CF phenotype. As one example, let's consider a gene that controls the amount of a protein called alpha-1 antitrypsin. This protein helps protect the lungs against some destructive chemicals that can be released by bacteria and by white blood cells sent to fight those bacteria. If you don't have enough of this alpha-1 antitrypsin protein, your lungs can be damaged (in fact, extreme deficiencies of this protein can cause emphysema in young nonsmokers similar to the emphysema seen in older people after a lifetime of smoking cigarettes). One small study from Denmark hinted that CF patients with the gene for lower levels of the protective protein have worse problems with infection in their lungs than those with normal alpha-1 levels. If someone with CF has another lung-damaging gene, the lungs will likely be worse. Similarly, inherited susceptibility to infection should make CF lung disease worse, since so much of CF lung disease has to do with infection. In real life, there have not yet been other specific genes discovered that have explained differences in the health (or "phenotype") of groups of people with CF.

THE CYSTIC FIBROSIS MOUSE

Until very recently, no animal had CF. Now, with genetic engineering, scientists have been able to alter the genes of a developing mouse embryo, resulting in mice with two abnormal copies of the CF gene. In some important ways, these mice can be considered to have a mouse form of CF. This is enabling researchers to examine the effects of different forms of the CF gene on the functioning of different cells and organs. Scientists hope that this will increase our understanding of CF, and will allow for the speedier testing of new CF treatments. It is important to remember that, some certain Disney characters aside, mice are not people, and it may be difficult to translate some of the findings in the "CF mice" into humans. For two examples: the earliest versions of the CF mouse had no lung problems, but did have severe intestinal blockage, which killed most of the animals within the first 40 days of life. This intestinal blockage may be something like human meconium ileus (see Chapter 4, *The Gastrointestinal Tract*), but it's clearly not identical to what happens in most people with CF. The second example is that the very structure of mouse lungs is quite different from human lungs; mice don't have some of the important mucus-secreting glands that humans have, and these glands are thought to be a source of much of the lung trouble in people with CF.

PRENATAL TESTING

For nearly every couple who already has a child with CF, it is now possible to tell reasonably early in pregnancy (16–18 weeks) if an expected child will have CF. To do this testing, a sample of the amniotic fluid (the fluid that surrounds the fetus inside the uterus) must be taken by putting a needle directly through the mother's abdominal wall into the uterus (amniocentesis). This procedure has some risks, but has been used safely for many years for a range of prenatal tests, the best known of which is the test for Down syndrome (performed mainly for women older than 35 years). The fluid includes cells from the fetus, and these cells can be analyzed to see if they contain the altered CF genes already known to be in this family. If they do, then the fetus would be born with CF. If they have only one abnormal CF gene, the fetus would be a carrier, and if the cells have none of the CF mutations, the fetus would neither have CF nor be a carrier.

Another method of obtaining cells from a fetus to test for CF can be carried out even earlier in pregnancy (at 10–13 weeks). This method is called chorionic villus sampling (CVS). In this procedure, a small tube is inserted through the vagina and cervix into the mother's uterus. Once the tube is in the uterus, suction is applied, and a small sample of cells from the placenta is taken for analysis. The analysis and significance of the results are the same as for amniocentesis. Both amniocentesis and chorionic villus sampling have risks to the fetus and to the mother, but the risks are usually quite small. Both tests have been in use for a long time, and—in experienced hands—are quite safe.

Many families have used these new methods to decide to continue a pregnancy if the fetus is shown not to have CF, or to stop the pregnancy (with an abortion) if the fetus has CF. For people who would not consider having an abortion, these tests are less useful. In unusual cases, the family might be opposed to abortion, but might feel so strongly that they wanted to know ahead of time (for their peace of mind if it turns out that the new baby will not have CF, and for planning their lives if the new baby will have CF) what the baby would have, that the small risks to the fetus and mother could be justified.

The main use of these tests is for couples with a CF child. But there are a few other instances where they might be used. For instance, if the cousin of a patient with CF wants to get pregnant, and she and her husband are found to be carriers, they would be able to use the prenatal testing. In fact, in any couple where both partners are carriers, testing could be done to see if their baby would be born with CF. Of course, if carrier testing (see below) shows that one spouse is *not* a carrier, then no further testing would be required, since both parents must be carriers for a child to be born with CF.

CARRIERS

If a brother or sister of someone with CF does not have CF, there are two chances in three that this sibling is a carrier. Here's why: as illustrated in Figure 11.1, if both parents are carriers, there are only four possible combinations of CF and non-CF genes that their children could have. One combination gives CF (two CF genes); two combinations result in carriers; and one combination has no CF gene. Once you know that a brother or sister does not have CF (and you'll know that after a properly performed sweat test), there are only three possible combinations, two of which result in carriers. Table 11.6 shows the chances of various people being CF carriers. Until very recently there was no carrier test for CF. The only way you knew if someone was a carrier was if he or she had a child with CF. With recent advances in molecular genetics, a genetic test can now tell if a relative of a CF patient is a carrier. The test can even be used in some cases where there is no family member with CF.

The way the test is done is to send some of the person's cells to one of the genetic diagnostic laboratories for analysis. The cells can be obtained from a routine small blood sample or by gently swirling a cotton swab inside the person's

TABLE 11.6. *Risks of Being a Cystic Fibrosis Carrier*

Relationship to CF Patient	Risk of Being a Carrier
Parent of a CF patient	1 in 1 (100%)
Unaffected sibling of a CF patient	2 in 3
Aunt or uncle of a CF patient	1 in 2
Nephew or niece of a CF patient	1 in 3
Cousin of a CF patient	1 in 4
None known (northern European)	1 in 25

Risks are actually slightly higher than listed, because the list assumes that (excluding siblings of CF patients) someone who is a carrier has *one* parent who is also a carrier; it is actually possible that *both* of this person's parents are carriers, and that means that each of this person's siblings has greater than a 50–50 chance of being a carrier.

cheek. The laboratory technologist will then look at the cells' DNA for anywhere between 1 and 3 dozen of the most common CF mutations. In the case of a close relative of a CF patient, the important mutations are the ones that the patient has. If a brother or sister of the CF patient does not have one of the same CF mutations that the patient has, he or she is not a carrier. Period. If cousins, aunts, or uncles are being tested, and they don't have one of their relative's known CF mutations, they probably are not carriers either. For someone with no family history of CF, or where the CF relative's mutation was not known, the laboratory technologist will look for all of the most common mutations. Finding one of these mutations confirms that the person is a carrier. Not finding a CF gene makes it less likely that the person is a carrier, but in most populations does not rule it out completely. Just how much less likely you are to be a carrier with a negative carrier test depends a bit on your ethnic background. As Table 11.5 shows, in a few ethnic groups just a few mutations account for virtually all cases of CF, whereas the 2-to-3 dozen most common mutations account for about 85–90% of CF chromosomes.

GENETIC DIAGNOSIS OF CYSTIC FIBROSIS

In some cases, gene testing can be used to help make the diagnosis of CF itself. This issue is discussed at greater length in the *Introduction,* in the section called "Making the Diagnosis." The procedure for obtaining cells for testing is the same as for carriers: either a blood sample or a gentle brushing from the inside of the cheek can be used. If two of the known CF gene mutations are found, then almost certainly the person has CF. If one or none is found, it is less likely, but not impossible, that the person has CF.

Even though DNA analysis has a gee-whiz, high-tech gloss to it, in most cases, the sweat test remains the "gold standard" for diagnosing CF. This is true in part because there have been rare cases where the genetic testing appeared to confirm two abnormal CF genes, and yet the person did not have CF. This may be particularly true for men who are healthy and are discovered to have two apparent abnormal CF genes as they are being evaluated for infertility: you'll recall from Chapter 5, *Other Systems,* that most men with CF are sterile because they have a complete blockage, or even absence, of both the right and left *vas deferens,* the tubes that normally carry sperm from the testicles to the penis. There is an uncommon form of male infertility not associated with any other evidence of CF, called congenital bilateral absence of the *vas deferens,* usually abbreviated CBAVD (congenital: you're born with it; bilateral: both sides). It turns out that a lot of these men have one abnormal CF gene. Some have two unusual CF genes. One abnormal CF gene that has been associated with this form of infertility is D1270N, and another is R117H-7T. Men with CBAVD and two copies of R117H-7T, or one D1270N together with one ΔF508, but no other evidence of CF, should not be considered to have CF. In this case, finding two abnormal CF genes does not make the diagnosis of CF.

Three particular cases stand out where gene testing may be very useful in making the diagnosis of CF. The first and most common is in someone who has signs, symptoms, and perhaps even family history that suggest CF, yet the sweat test does not give a definitive answer. This is quite unusual, but the occasional baby does not produce enough sweat to analyze, and the occasional baby or older person has a sweat test result in the "gray zone": not definitely positive, not definitely negative. Finding two CF genes in someone like this will make the diagnosis of CF much more likely.

The second situation in which DNA analysis for the CF gene may be useful in diagnosing someone with CF (or helping to rule it out) is the very unusual one where there is not an accredited CF center for performing the sweat test. If someone lives 'way out in the boonies, and travel to a laboratory skilled and experienced in performing sweat tests is temporarily impossible, a blood sample could be sent by express mail to a diagnostic laboratory, with results back within a week. The cost of the DNA testing is comparable to that of a sweat test (even cheaper in some labs!).

The final situation where DNA testing can help make or confirm the diagnosis of CF is in someone who has died. This situation arises more often than you might think: a baby gets very sick and dies before testing can be done (or before CF is considered), or someone has a relative who died a long time ago, and only now has the possibility of CF been considered. If blood or a small piece of tissue is obtained within a few hours after death, the cells will still be enough for testing. Amazingly, if an autopsy was done (even *years* before), it may be possible to do DNA analysis on any remaining autopsy microscope slides or tiny blocks of tissue that have been preserved embedded in paraffin. Obviously, in these cases, making the diagnosis cannot help the patient who has died, but it can be tremendously helpful for the patient's family.

GENE THERAPY

Gene therapy is discussed at greater length in Chapter 16, *Research and Future Treatment*. Gene therapy is placing a healthy gene into cells affected by an abnormal gene, and having that healthy gene take over the function of those cells. In CF, this would be getting a healthy CFTR gene into cells in order to correct the abnormalities in salt (sodium and chloride) and water traffic across the cell membranes. This would be most important in the lungs. Big strides have been made toward developing successful (safe and effective) gene therapy since the discovery of the CF gene in 1989: gene therapy *has* worked in the test tube, in individual CF cells, and it seems to have worked in CF mice. But it is a long way from here to having it work in human beings. Nonetheless, work continues, and most CF researchers think the day may come when gene therapy will provide a cure for CF.

12

The Family

THE BASICS

1. Hearing that a child has CF is very stressful for parents.
2. As parents learn more about CF, and see their children doing better, the stress lessens.
3. CF center staff expect you to have a lot of questions, and want you to ask them. They know that it takes a long time (years) to learn all there is to know about CF.
4. Children with CF should be treated normally: they need to do homework and chores, and should be allowed to participate in all normal childhood activities. Children treated this way grow up healthier emotionally and physically.

As a chronic disease that requires a vigorous schedule of daily treatments, cystic fibrosis (CF) imposes significant stress on the affected child, the parents, and any brothers and sisters (whether or not they also have CF). Understanding the reactions to this stress and learning about effective methods to cope with them are important to the care of the child with CF and to the functioning of the family.

This chapter discusses the variety of reactions that parents have to the diagnosis and management of CF, the methods for dealing with the daily stresses, and suggestions for how the family and the medical team can work together most effectively.

YOUR CHILD HAS CYSTIC FIBROSIS

Parents and other family members experience a variety of emotions when told a child has CF. Family members may say to themselves, "I can't believe this. This can't be happening to *my* child and *my* family. I don't know what to do. What does the future hold? Is there anything I can do for my child? Could I have prevented this?" All of these reactions—anger, denial, shock, grief, helplessness, confusion, despair, sadness, and fear—are very normal responses. These emotions are part of a *grieving* response. Just as a person experiences many of these feelings when a loved one dies, parents feel many of the same emotions when they learn that a child has a serious health problem. The parents "mourn" the loss of the perfect, healthy child that they had expected. Another very common response upon learning the diagnosis of CF is one of relief—if a family has taken their child to many doctors over a long period of time, they may be *relieved* finally to have been given a reason for their child's health problems. This sensation of relief may be very puzzling, and the parent may even feel guilty about it.

No matter what the reaction, it's important that each family member has someone to confide in—a trusted, understanding friend or health professional with whom he or she can share feelings. It may be difficult for the parents to talk about CF with one another, especially immediately after the diagnosis is made. Strong emotions may make it too hard to listen and understand another person's pain, grief, or anger—even if it is a spouse. A husband and wife may find that they react very differently to the diagnosis ("how could he feel *that* way?"), making discussion even more difficult. Since they are two individual people, they may experience varying reactions at different times. And it is hard to *give* support and understanding to anyone—even your spouse—when *you* may be hurting badly yourself. This can put a strain on the relationship unless both husband and wife try to remember that it is normal and that the spouse's reaction does not reflect a lack of caring. It is important to try to be open and nonjudgmental about each other's reactions. A third person may be able to help a couple get through this difficult time.

At the time of diagnosis, the family will be given extensive information about CF and its management. The flood of emotions may make it hard to concentrate on what the doctor is saying and to remember this information. Despite an initial lengthy discussion with the doctor, it is not uncommon for parents to retain very little of what they have been told; they may feel that they have a poor understanding of CF and have many unanswered questions.

The team at the CF center is aware that it is difficult to comprehend all this information at such a stressful time. They know that it is important to review the information many times and they plan to spend ample time with the family for this purpose. Learning about CF is a continuous process that goes on over many months and years. The CF center staff *expect* this, view education as a very important part of their jobs, and *want* you to ask your questions, great or small.

Many parents find it helpful to write down their questions and discuss them with the doctor, nurse, or social worker, in person or by phone. Typical questions that many parents ask are the following:

- Will CF affect my child's brain function?
- Will my child look any different from other children?

- How will CF affect my child's daily life?
- How long will my child live?
- Is there something I did during the pregnancy to cause my child to have CF?
- Could I have prevented this?
- Should I limit my child's activity?
- Can my child go to daycare and school?
- Do my other children have CF?

Some families are reluctant to ask these questions out of fear of what the answers might be, or fear that they may appear insignificant or too simple. Your physician and the team members at the CF center understand and encourage the families to ask *all* their questions—no question is too insignificant to be considered, and even answers that are hard to hear are seldom as horrible as people's imaginations.

Because manifestations of CF are so different in each child, it is often difficult for the doctor to be specific in answering many of the parents' questions. No one can predict the exact effect of cystic fibrosis on a child's lung function, growth, activity, or life span. The uncertainty is very frustrating and frightening, for it means that the family must live with the unknown from day to day. Even though the doctor cannot make any predictions for a specific child, he or she can explain to the parents the range of disease in CF and perhaps where the child falls in this range. On the whole, most children with CF should be expected to attend school regularly, to be able to participate in sports, and to play with other children without restriction, that is, in general to carry out the work and play of normal children.

BEGINNING HOME CARE

In addition to obtaining *information* about CF, it is important that parents learn *techniques* in caring for their child with CF—particularly the methods for respiratory treatments and enzyme administration. Many physicians recommend that the newly diagnosed infant or child be admitted to the hospital for thorough evaluation of respiratory function and growth and for education of the parents. While this idea may be frightening to the family (and disapproved by short-sighted "bottom-line" oriented insurance clerks), it often helps if they realize that an admission to the hospital provides the valuable opportunity for the parents to have daily contact with the CF team, and lays the groundwork for a lifetime of successful health care—perhaps preventing or minimizing the need for future hospitalizations. The doctors, nurses, social worker, respiratory therapists, and dieticians use this time to teach the family about home management of CF and begin to develop an important working relationship with the family.

No matter how thorough the instructions and how skillful the parents, most families are nervous about beginning therapy at home. At the same time they are beginning enzyme administration and respiratory treatments, they may be facing an already busy child-care schedule, work schedule, or both. With the help of a nurse or social worker, the parents may benefit from sketching out a daily schedule, which takes into consideration *their* family's needs. The doctor, nurse, or social worker may be able to arrange for a meeting with a family more experienced with CF who can serve as an important source of information and support.

In addition to the confusion of a new schedule and nervousness about new treatments, parents may find themselves faced with a cranky baby who is hard to comfort. Some babies with CF are fussy eaters, and before diagnosis have been irritable because of lung infection, hunger or chronic abdominal discomfort, and diarrhea. Because they have been hard to feed, hard to soothe, and haven't grown well, their parents may feel helpless and incapable.

Many parents say that they find it difficult to *like* their infant because he or she is so irritable and is frustrating to care for—and they feel guilty about resenting their own child. It may be hard for the parents to talk about these feelings or even for parents to admit them to themselves. These feelings, while very troublesome to the mother and father, are very common, normal reactions.

Gradually, as babies become accustomed to their new medications and treatments, the chronic digestive symptoms will be relieved and they will begin to gain weight. As babies feel better, they become more contented, and their parents can draw much satisfaction from their daily efforts and the successful "settling in" at home.

EXPLAINING CYSTIC FIBROSIS TO OTHERS

Once they are at home, the parents must begin to explain CF to grandparents, other family members, and friends. This may be difficult to do. However, an honest, simple explanation is essential—it will set the tone for how others react to their child for many years to come. Although CF is a chronic progressive disease that may result in shortened life span, many patients live to middle age. As the prognosis for CF improves, it is important that children and teenagers be raised with the idea that they should look forward to being active, productive adults. In order to promote independence and goals for the child with CF, the parents and others with whom the child lives and works must share an outlook of hope and encouragement for the child. Many questions are difficult to answer, but each successful encounter makes the next one easier to handle.

Following are some of the important points that parents may want to share with others:

- CF does not affect the brain or intelligence.
- No part of CF, including the cough and loose stools, is contagious.
- CF is a genetic disease caused by inheriting a gene from *each* parent; it could not have been prevented and it is no one's *fault* (some grandparents have difficulty accepting the idea that an abnormal gene came from *their* side of the family).

- CF is not curable, but it is treatable.
- The treatment for CF must be carried out each day and consists primarily of respiratory care and enzyme administration, both of which must be made non-negotiable and normal parts of *every* day.

YOU AND YOUR CHILD

One of the most valuable gifts you can give your child with CF (and yourself) is to treat him or her as a *normal* child *who happens to have CF,* and *not* as a *case of CF,* nor as a poor, sickly weakling who should not be expected to do normal things. First of all, the large majority of children and adolescents with CF *are not limited* in their physical or mental capacities by their disease. Many play sports, some even excel at sports; many excel in school. But as surely as day turns into night, children whose parents *expect* them to fail and to be unable to take care of themselves *will* fail, and will grow up thinking poorly of themselves. Children should know that they have CF, and that having CF means certain things are different from other kids (need to do chest treatments, need to take enzymes with meals). Many children who feel unfairly singled out because of having to do special things because of their CF take some comfort in knowing that *many* kids have to do different things: some children may have diet restrictions that the CF child doesn't; some may need a wheelchair, as the child with CF doesn't; some may need braces, etc.

But they should also know that they have the same rights, privileges, and responsibilities as anyone else in the family or school. They go to school, have friends over, play sports, and so on. They need to do homework, help with the dishes, and so on. Treated normally, they will think of themselves as normal, and will *be* normal. In reviewing this book, several teenagers and young adults with CF urged me to stress that children with CF should never be allowed to use CF as an excuse for getting out of unappealing chores or responsibilities.

In fact, most parents and children with CF are able to adopt this very positive outlook, which in turn not only makes the children wonderful to be around, but also has a very positive influence on their health.

YOU AND YOUR OTHER CHILDREN

In many ways, having two children is more than twice as hard as having one. Although the bond between siblings in most cases ends up being among the strongest on earth, sibling rivalries and jealousies exist at one level or another in most families. Most parents are able to keep these rivalries and jealousies from erupting into outright armed conflict, but at times the peacekeeping role can be challenging. If one child has CF, this can add a dimension to the challenge. The child with CF may resent the other child for *not* having it ("Why me? It's not fair!"), while the child without CF may resent the extra attention the child with

CF gets (treatments, trips to the clinic, perhaps even visits and gifts in the hospital). It's a balancing act—that most parents end up doing very well—to make absolutely certain that the child or children with CF get all the needed treatments, while the other child or children realize that they too are cherished.

YOU AND YOUR SPOUSE

In conjunction with the treatment of CF, parents find themselves faced with new stresses on their marriage: care of the child takes up more time—how should they divide the responsibilities? Medicines and doctor visits are expensive—how can their budget accommodate this? There is a risk of subsequent children having CF—how can they work out their sexual relationship and family planning? The child with CF needs discipline as any other child—how should they handle discipline for a "sick" child? The other children need attention or one parent's job may be in jeopardy—how can they cope with preexisting family problems in the midst of this new stress?

An important starting point for handling each of these stresses is for the couple to be open and honest in sharing their feelings with one another. Good communication will help to define the problems from each partner's perspective, starting them on the path to developing mutually acceptable solutions. As the husband and wife work *together* to resolve conflict, many couples report that their relationship is strengthened and they are better prepared to face future challenges together.

If one spouse is employed outside the home and the other is responsible for child care, the employed spouse will probably have a limited amount of time to administer treatment. However, it is important that parents share responsibility for the child's care, even if it can only be to a limited extent. This shared responsibility demonstrates to children that their parents are unified in their approach to their care; it also may help to avoid resentment that can arise when one spouse is solely responsible for treatments.

Financial worries can cause much strain within a family. Insurance coverage may be inadequate or nonexistent. State-aid programs may be helpful in some situations. Many clinics have a "patient representative" or a social worker who can put parents in contact with appropriate financial resources.

As the husband and wife cope differently with their reactions to the diagnosis of CF, their desire for sexual intimacy may be altered. These differing needs may serve to create further conflict and misunderstanding. Overshadowing these differences may be fear of another pregnancy and the birth of another child with CF. An atmosphere of open, honest communication is essential for the resolution of these differences.

Sometimes the stresses associated with a diagnosis of CF are too much for a couple to handle without outside help and guidance. The cystic fibrosis center team can be a valuable resource in assisting the family; they may recommend further assistance from a psychologist, counselor, or clergy. The family's pediatrician or family doctor may also be of great assistance. Although these professionals are not CF experts, they may have known the family for a long time and often are very willing to provide support. It is essential that a family seek help promptly if difficulties arise in coping with the diagnosis of CF or with related issues. Such problems do not "just go away" and must be handled directly and aggressively. Unless properly managed, problems with stress and communication within the family may persist, having an impact on CF management and adversely affecting the child's health.

GOING TO THE CYSTIC FIBROSIS CLINIC

Most CF patients will have clinic visits scheduled for between four and eight times a year, more just after diagnosis and when someone is sick. These visits are very important to maintaining the patients' good health, but for many people they are not easy. Depending on the distance you live from the center, the number of tests to be done, and how busy or organized the clinic happens to be that day, a variable amount of time (often a whole day) is lost to other activities. This may mean losing a day's work (and wages), spoiling a perfect school attendance record, missing a team or chorus practice, and so on. It may be expensive to drive and park.

Beyond the financial and logistical nuisance of clinic visits, they may be difficult emotionally, too. For some young patients, there is the fear of shots (despite experience and assurances that there are unlikely to *be* shots, except for a yearly "flu" shot) or the fear of hospital admission. For some patients and families, it may be less focused, but scarier than that: going to CF clinic is a rude reminder that the child *has CF.* Many families—including many who do absolutely every treatment, every day—are able to put CF aside and not think of it or its long-term implications most of the time. But a clinic appointment brings CF back into the center of the family's existence for a brief time.

There are some things that may help ease the emotional burden of a trip to clinic. The first is the realization that most clinic visits are actually quite pleasant, with a number of people who are truly glad to see you and your child, and with a minimum of unpleasant tests or treatments. At most visits, there's a positive report from the physician, or an optimistic and realistic plan arrived at to attack a problem you knew about before you came: it's relatively unusual for a bad problem to be discovered at the clinic visit that is a big surprise. Parents can help nervous children prepare by stressing the positives: "You'll get to see_____" (fill in the blank with a favorite nurse or doctor or waiting room toy), and we'll go out to eat afterward (or to the museum, zoo, mall, etc.). It is *not* helpful to say over and over to a frightened toddler, "They're not going to *HURT* you; I won't let them *HURT* you," as that can even plant the idea of hurting in the child's mind.

GOING TO THE HOSPITAL

Occasionally, hospitalization may be necessary. Admission to the hospital upsets the daily routine of a family, and, in effect, creates a crisis. This topic is dealt with at length in Chapter 7.

SUMMARY

Having a child with CF adds stress to a family, particularly when the diagnosis is made. With time and education, if parents make an effort to work together, the stress eases, and the family can even be made stronger by this stress. Parents can work together with CF center staff to learn about CF. CF center staff expect (and want) parents to ask many questions, since learning about CF is very important, and takes years. Children with CF should be brought up normally, with the same plans, expectations, and responsibilities as other children. The large majority of children with CF grow up with healthy positive attitudes they've gotten from their parents, and this positive outlook helps their physical health as well.

13

The Teenage Years

THE BASICS

1. The teenage years can be wonderful and healthy for people with CF.
2. The teen years are a crucial time for CF patients' health. If the lungs are neglected, they can easily be damaged irreparably; with good care, they can often remain very healthy.
3. Teens with CF can do virtually everything that their friends with CF do: school, college, date, plan careers, etc.

HOW DO TEENAGERS RATE THEIR OWN CHAPTER?

If you read the *Preface* to this book, you saw that teenagers with CF are one of the main reasons for this book's having been written. There are a few reasons for that, and a few why you deserve your own special chapter. Teenagers are caught between two extremes: adults—out on their own, totally *independent,* and with their own chapter in this book—and children—totally *dependent* on parents for everything, and with a lot of the rest of the book focused on their needs. There are special questions of concern to teenagers more than other people (education, deciding on a career direction, establishing relationships—including intimate relationships with people of the other sex, and even deciding who you are and who you are going to be). And, there are a lot of you: in 1994, there were 19,517 CF patients aged 0 to 70 years (that's right, 70!) seen in CF centers in the United States, and 4,283 of them were aged 13–19 years. That means about 22% of all CF patients are teenagers. Finally, perhaps more than any other 7-year period, the teenage years determine what will happen to your health for the rest of your life, based in large part on what you yourself decide to do about it. Unfortunately, many teens with CF have made what they later realize have been *bad* decisions about their health, and have paid a big price for those decisions, for the rest of their lives. I want to help convince you to make *good* decisions, and be able to reap the benefits of them, for the rest of your longer, healthier lives. In addition to the problems that everyone always talks about with the teen years, these years can be wonderful, and your CF does not need to change that.

You will find some of the information in this chapter other places in the book, as well, particularly Chapter 14, *Cystic Fibrosis and Adulthood.*

MEDICAL ISSUES

In this section, I'll address the various organ systems of the body that are affected by CF, and how either the effects or the treatment might be different for teenagers. You'll find more details about each organ system in its own chapter (for example, lungs are discussed at great length in Chapter 3, *The Respiratory System*). You probably know a lot of this stuff already, since you've had CF all your life, but most likely you haven't had the opportunity just to sit down and learn about CF; rather—if you're like 99% of teenagers with CF, it's been a matter of picking up a bit here and a bit there as you go to clinic, get your treatments, have arguments with your parents, etc.

Lungs

Far more than any other part of the body, it's the lungs that determine the health of people with CF, and how long they live. The lungs account for 95% of the deaths from CF. Fortunately, there's a lot you can do to influence the health of your lungs.

First, you need to know what happens in the lungs of people with CF. For the full story, you can go back to Chapter 3, *The Respiratory System*, but for the brief version, here we go: Thick mucus blocks the bronchi (air tubes, sometimes called *airways*) of people with CF. It doesn't *totally* block them, but it blocks them enough that infection and inflammation can take hold. Infection you understand: germs (mostly bacteria, but also viruses, and occasionally *funguses* [or *fungi*]) can grow in the bronchi and cause damage. *Inflammation* is what happens when the body responds to these invading germs: white blood cells are sent to fight the infection, and—in a kind of chemical warfare—they release toxic chemicals that attack the bacteria. Unfortunately, these chemicals can also damage the cells that line the airways, causing swelling and cell damage. Some of the bacteria themselves release the same kinds of chemicals and cause the same kind of damage. If the infection and inflammation go on too long or too often (and nobody knows exactly how long "too long" is, or how often "too often" is), airway cells are killed, and scar tissue is formed. For each little infection, it's probably only a little bit of scar tissue that's formed, but once scar tissue forms, it can never become normal, and over months and years that "little bit" of scar tissue for each little infection adds up, so that eventually virtually the whole lung becomes a mass of infected *cysts* (fluid-filled sacs) and scar tissue. In fact, since scar tissue is called *fibrosis,* you can see where the name *cystic fibrosis* comes from.

So, the idea in treating the lungs of someone with CF is to prevent this progression of airway blockage, infection, inflammation, and scar tissue formation. Since there are three ingredients in the recipe for scar formation, there are three targets for treatment, namely, (1) reducing or preventing airway obstruction, (2) treating or preventing infection, and (3) treating or preventing inflammation.

Minimizing Bronchial Blockage

Airway clearance techniques are used to minimize bronchial blockage. These techniques include chest PT (for *chest physical therapy*), also called PDs (*postural drainage*), the Flutter, percussion vests, *huffing, autogenic drainage*, and several others. You've probably heard of one or more of these, and have probably had countless treatments with at least one of these techniques. You *may* even have realized how effective they can be in keeping your airways unblocked, and you never miss a one. But, there's a reasonable chance that you've thought they don't make any difference, or perhaps part of you realizes they help, but you skip a lot of treatments because they're a bother.

The thing is, they *do work.* Studies have shown a significant deterioration in lung function after 3 weeks of missed treatments, even in people whose lungs are in pretty good shape. But a big catch is that if your lungs are in pretty good shape, you will probably not *feel* a difference after getting (or missing) an individual treatment. Our lungs—all of us, CF or no—are notoriously insensitive. By that I mean that we cannot tell when our bronchi are blocked. In a famous experiment, people breathe through a small plastic tube, with their eyes closed. Then the doctor conducting the experiment gradually blocks the end of the tube until the person doing the breathing feels a blockage. Most people can't tell those tubes are blocked until they're more than 50% blocked! The same is true if the breathing tube is your own airways, and not a plastic tube you hold in your lips. So, you can't go only on the basis of how you feel: "my breathing feels good, so there must not be any blockage." There can be substantial blockage before you feel it. This is true if the blockage happens quickly (as you just saw, with that tube-blocking experiment); it's 10 times truer if the blockage develops slowly. As with so many other things, gradual changes are very hard to notice: you don't see a kid brother or sister (or the grass) grow taller from day to day, but let a few months go by and they don't fit their jeans anymore (and the grass now looks like a wild field). The difference between those examples and the lungs is that it's never too late to buy a new pair of jeans for your kid sister; and the lawn can be mowed when it's tall—it'll be harder, but it can be done. If the lungs are let go for too long, it may be impossible to get them back in shape again. You may be able to gain some control over infection and inflammation, but the parts that have been replaced by scar tissue can never be made into healthy lung tissue again.

One big problem with the older (and still useful) ways of clearing mucus from the lungs, like chest PT, was (and is) that for these to be done well, you had to have someone else do them to you. That "someone else" was almost always a parent. That's fine when you're a baby or young child, but gets harder when you and your folks may not see eye-to-eye on everything, including exactly *when* something is supposed to be done. You have your own schedule of activities, friends, and so on, and your parents have their own schedule, and the two might not coincide. This can be an area of conflict between teenagers and parents (ever notice how a *lot* of things can be an area of conflict between teenagers and parents?). If this has been a problem for you, there's very good news. There are some treatments that are as effective as (maybe even *more* effective than) the old chest PT. You can read more about these in Chapter 3, *The Respiratory System,* and in Appendix C: *Airway Clearance Techniques.* Here's exactly what Chapter 3 says about one of these techniques, namely, the *Flutter* valve.

> This is a hand-held device, small enough to carry around in your pocket, that looks a little like a kazoo. It has a stainless steel ball in it that vibrates up and down (flutters, you might say) as you blow into the tube. The vibrations are transmitted backward down through the patient's mouth into the trachea and bronchi, where they shake mucus free from the bronchial walls. Many teenagers and adults who had done traditional PDs for years have become "Flutter converts," saying that the Flutter is more effective in helping them bring up mucus, letting them feel when there's excess mucus there, and to know when they've cleared their airways. The Flutter has the advantage of enabling patients to work on airway clearance without help.

Airway Clearance Techniques

Autogenic drainage, the *PEP mask,* and the *active cycle of breathing* are all airway clearance techniques that also can be done independently. These last three techniques are used more in Europe than they are in the United States and Canada. They seem to work well, but you need to be taught how to do them by someone with a lot of experience in using them.

Exercise

Exercise is another thing that also helps to clear mucus. Many of you have no doubt noticed that you cough and bring up mucus when you exercise hard. Right now, most CF doctors recommend that exercise be used *in addition* to one of the other airway clearance techniques (and not instead of them) but it is clearly helpful.

Mucus-Thinning Drugs

CF mucus is hard to clear because it's so thick and sticky. Thinner mucus should be easier to move up out of the lungs. There are a few drugs available (and several others that will probably be available before too long) that make CF mucus thinner. These drugs work extremely well, in a test tube. It's hard to know ahead of time which actual patients these drugs will help, but for *some* people they *do seem* to be very good. The main drug in this family is DNase (Pulmozyme®). DNase is breathed in once a day, in an aerosol. One study with 900 patients (!) showed an overall small improvement in lung function in CF patients who took DNase once a day for 6 months, compared with no change in lung function in those who took a *placebo* (a drug that looked and tasted like DNase, but had no effect). Some patients definitely feel better when they take DNase, and some say they breathe easier. Almost no one is hurt by the drug (except financially, since it costs about $12,000 a year). A very few patients who have more severe lung problems and lots of thick mucus stuck in their lungs have had trouble when the DNase has freed huge amounts of newly thinned mucus all at once. For these few patients, it's been too much fluid in their airways for them to handle comfortably. Most patients do not feel any different, nor can differences be measured in most patients' PFTs.

Mucomyst® is an older drug that does the same thing as DNase: it breaks down mucus, and makes it thinner, in the test tube. Some patients have benefited from Mucomyst®, but many have had worsened inflammation within their airways, or even had asthma attacks after taking Mucomyst®.

Treating Bronchial Infection

Antibiotics are the main tool for fighting infections, including bronchial infections that people with CF get. (We often call these times of bronchial infections *pulmonary exacerbations,* which just means times when the lungs are worse than usual.) Antibiotics kill bacteria. They don't kill viruses, but they are often prescribed when someone with CF has a viral infection (like a cold), too, because the viruses can throw off the lung defenses enough that bacteria can take hold there more easily. Antibiotics come in different preparations, including oral, aerosol, and IV. Usually, with a new infection, oral antibiotics are used. Antibiotics are prescribed to go in your aerosol if the oral antibiotics aren't working well enough, and if the aerosol and oral antibiotics aren't controlling the infection, then IVs may be needed. IV antibiotics are usually given in the hospital, for at least 2 weeks, and sometimes as long as 3 or 4 weeks, depending on how long it takes to get you back to normal (back to your "baseline" is what we often say, meaning back to where you were before this particular *exacerbation* started).

The steps here are pretty easy to understand. It's *not* always easy to know when to start treatment at any of the steps, when to move on to the next step, or even when you've gotten back to your baseline. The reasons for this are a bit like what we just said about bronchial obstruction: you can't always tell when you've got worsened infection in your lungs, or when it's gotten as much better as it can get. Physicians can't always tell that easily, either.

How to Tell If You Need More Treatment

The amount of cough you have is the main clue for most pulmonary exacerbations. Someone who usually has no cough may start with a morning cough, while someone who usually does have some cough may have more cough. Your parents or brother or sister may tell you that they heard you coughing during the night (or the cough may actually awaken you during the night). Your mucus is the next clue. Someone who doesn't usually feel like there's extra mucus inside the chest might start to feel some, or start to bring it up. People who are used to bringing up mucus may have more, or it may be darker, thicker, or harder to bring up. Some people may have some trouble catching their breath (they are *short of breath*), either when they go up stairs or run, or even just sitting there. There are some signs that aren't obviously connected to your lungs that often go along with a pulmonary exacerbation, including being tired, losing weight, and having a crummy appetite. All of these changes can signal worsened lung infection (and inflammation). But it may be hard for you to detect any small changes from your baseline, particularly if the changes have developed gradually.

That's where your doctor can help. He or she may be able to tell some things by examining you. Listening with a stethoscope can help. If your lungs are usually clear, but now have *crackles* (some physicians call these lung sounds *rales*) when your doctor listens, or perhaps more crackles than usual, that suggests extra mucus and infection. (If you're wondering what crackles sound like to the physician, reach up to next to your ear, take a few strands of your hair and roll them back and forth between your fingers. The sound the hairs make rolling over each other is what crackles sound like: now you're a doctor! Well, maybe not, but now you know what we hear when we say we hear crackles.) But if you have no crackles, or only in the same places you always have them, the listening might not have told the whole story. Your weight will be important: if it's down, without another explanation, the most likely cause is your lungs (lung infections make you lose weight several ways: if you're breathing harder, your breathing muscles use up energy and calories, just as any other prolonged muscular exercise can do; your body also uses calories to fight infection; and finally, having a lung infection can often make you lose your appetite, so you won't feel like eating as much as usual).

Finally, PFTs (pulmonary function tests, breathing tests) can be a big help. You've probably had these a bunch of times: you blow into a tube, and a machine records numbers. These numbers mostly tell how quickly you've been able to blow air out of your lungs, and that tells how much blockage there is: the more blockage, the slower the air comes out. If the larger bronchi are blocked, that will affect the first part of the breath, and if the small bronchi (the ones further out in your lungs) are blocked, that will have more of an effect on the last part of the breath. The PFTs are much more sensitive tools than your doctor's stethoscope, or your ability to feel how hard it is to exhale, for telling just exactly how much obstruction you have in your lungs.

Since the physician (with or without the PFTs) can often detect changes that you hadn't been aware of, it's usual for regular checkups to be scheduled somewhere around 4 times a year. If an unexpected problem shows up at one of the regularly scheduled clinic visits, it's usually possible to start effective treatment before irreversible lung damage has set in. If you waited a year between appointments, it is certainly possible to have some lung damage that's gone beyond the stage of recoverability, *even if you feel pretty good*. That's why it's important to keep those clinic appointments.

Fighting Inflammation

The main way to fight inflammation is to fight infection. For most people, controlling infection with antibiotics will also control inflammation. But some people with CF (and lots of people with asthma) do better if they also get specific *anti-inflammatory* treatment. There are a couple of different kinds of anti-inflammatory medications. *Steroids* are the first kind, and *prednisone* is the most common form of steroids used for people with CF. These drugs are very powerful, and control inflammation very well: there are many people whose breathing is a lot more comfortable when they take prednisone. Unfortunately, prednisone (and all the other steroids, too) has some side effects that are unpleasant or even dangerous. The two side effects that probably bother teenagers the most are that they can cause acne, and they can cause some puffiness, particularly of the face ("chipmunk cheeks"). Another anti-inflammatory medication that's being used a lot recently is *ibuprofen*. You've probably used ibuprofen on occasion for headache or other minor ache or pain. A study has shown that ibuprofen taken in fairly high doses over a 4-year period seemed to slow the deterioration in CF patients' lung function. You'll note I didn't say that it *improved* lung function, but it *slowed* how quickly lung function got worse. So, this is not a medicine that is going to make you feel better after you've been on it for a day or so. Even if helps, you won't be able to tell. There are some other problems with the drug, too. Ibuprofen can cause kidney problems and can cause stomach ulcers. It's possible that your CF doctor will want you take this drug, and it might be good for you, but be sure you understand the possible side effects, and also understand that—even if it's helping—you probably won't *feel* any better on it.

There are a couple of anti-inflammatory inhalers that are very effective for people with asthma, and might be prescribed for you (even though we don't know yet if they are helpful for people with CF who don't have asthma). One family of these drugs is inhaled steroids (Vanceril®, Beclovent®, Azmacort®, etc.). One of the differences between these steroids and prednisone is that these are not absorbed into the bloodstream, so they don't cause side effects (no acne, no chipmunk cheeks). Another difference is that they are not as powerful, and don't do very much to make you feel better *right away* (even in people with asthma for whom they work extremely well, they work to *prevent* problems, and not to cure those problems once they've started). Another inflammation-preventing inhaler is cromolyn (Intal®), and its brother, nedocromil (Tilade®). Like the steroid inhalers, these are effective for people with asthma, have no side effects, and will not make you feel better, but *might* prevent you from developing more inflammation in your bronchi.

Complications of Lung Disease

Problems that are the indirect result of CF include *pneumothorax* and *hemoptysis*, and both are discussed in Chapter 3, and in Chapter 14, *Cystic Fibrosis and Adulthood*. Very briefly, *pneumothorax* is a collapsed lung, and can be serious, but is quite uncommon. Anyone who develops a very sudden sharp pain on one side of the chest, along with being short of breath, should call the CF center because this might be a pneumothorax and need quick treatment. At the other end of the spectrum of how quickly treatment is needed is *hemoptysis,* or coughing up blood. It's not uncommon to have some blood streaks in the mucus, and a few people have pure blood. This is very scary, but usually not nearly as dangerous as it might first appear. See Chapter 3 for more details.

Gastrointestinal System

There's not very much different for teenagers in the gastrointestinal (digestive) system. The main things are the need for enzymes with all meals and most snacks (all the ones with fat or protein in them; see Chapter 6, *Nutrition,* for details). About 90% of all patients with CF need to take enzymes for full digestion of their food. You're probably already familiar with what happens if you miss your enzymes, or don't take enough: abdominal pain, loose, greasy, smelly stools, and maybe more gas. Surprisingly, some teenagers may need slightly fewer enzymes than they needed as children. Intestinal blockage, called DIOS (distal intestinal obstruction syndrome), is more common in teenagers than in children, and can be extremely uncomfortable (abdominal pain, no stools). Treatment can sometimes be accomplished by drinking a very large amount of a special fluid (GoLytely®, or other similar products) your doctor will prescribe, but may need a special enema (in the x-ray department of the hospital), or even surgery. If the problem is caught and treated early, it's easier to avoid the more invasive treatments. So, if you're having "stomachaches" and fewer bowel movements than normal, let someone know.

Diabetes

About 10–15% of teenagers will develop diabetes, a condition where the pancreas does not make enough *insulin,* and therefore the amount of *glucose* (sugar) in the bloodstream increases, and some glucose is lost in the urine. Losing sugar in the urine means several things: you lose calories, so you might well lose weight and energy (before diabetes is diagnosed and treated, people often feel drained and dragged out without knowing why). Also, sugar in the urine makes you lose a lot of urine, and you're likely to notice that you're getting up in the middle of the night to pee, and you're thirsty all the time. If you have these symptoms, you should be checked for diabetes. Diabetes in people with CF seems to be less severe for some reason than diabetes in young people without CF. Diabetes is usually treated with a special diet (mostly cutting down on soda pop, candy, and other "concentrated sweets." Most people with CF diabetes end up getting insulin shots 1–3 times a day. These shots are surprisingly easy to get used to, and make an amazing difference in how good someone feels.

Some patients also have liver problems, and these are discussed more in Chapter 4, *The Gastrointestinal Tract).*

Other Systems

Sweat Glands

You probably know that people with CF have extra-salty sweat. That's what makes the sweat test such a good test for CF (analyze sweat, and if there's a lot of salt in it, that means the person has CF). It also means that people with CF lose more salt than normal when they sweat, and will have to take in more salt in their diet than others, especially during hot weather, and particularly if they're exercising a lot. This is something that your taste buds are pretty good at telling you: in most cases if you *need* more salt, you'll *want* more, and you'll find yourself heading for the chips or pretzels or pickles, or just using the salt shaker more at meals. It's not necessary or useful to take salt pills.

Reproductive System

General

Both boys and girls with CF may be delayed in going through puberty (growing and developing). This can be a big worry for young teenagers when their friends (or not-friends) are bigger and look more mature. Locker rooms make the differences and delays in development embarrassingly obvious. It's good to keep in mind that almost everybody with CF will catch up, even if it's a year or so later.

Males

Everything about the reproductive system in men with CF is normal, except one little tube. That tube, the *vas deferens,* is the tube that takes sperm from where they're made (the testicles) to the penis, and in 98% of men with CF it's blocked or even absent. That means that men with CF can and do have a completely normal sex life, but there are no sperm in the semen when they ejaculate. In almost every case this means that men with CF are *sterile,* that is, they cannot get a woman pregnant. You can have your semen analyzed to see if there are sperm present (as there will be in 2% of patients).

Females

Everything about the reproductive system in women with CF is normal, except for thick mucus in the cervix (the opening to the uterus). This makes it harder for women with CF to get pregnant, but yet hundreds of women with CF have gotten pregnant. Some women with CF have irregular menstrual periods. These can be regulated with birth control pills. A lot of young women have vaginal yeast infections (with itching and burning, especially during urination), and it seems that women with CF may be somewhat more likely to develop these infections than women without CF, probably because taking antibiotics makes it easier for the yeast to take hold. These infections can be treated successfully, but only if your doctor knows, and gives you a prescription.

YOUR MEDICAL CARE: WHO'S IN CHARGE?

Your medical care is like so many other aspects of your life where you're between childhood (where your parents take care of everything for you) and adulthood (where you take care of everything yourself). Ideally, during the teenage years (actually, *early* in the teen years), you should be starting to take charge. That means knowing your medications (names, doses, times, side effects you've had, and so on), being able to report your symptoms correctly (being honest with your doctor and—a necessary first step—yourself about new or worsened symptoms). That means making a call (yourself) to your doctor to report new symptoms, and get a new prescription, or arrange for a new appointment. It's extremely common for a teenager to tell the doctor, "I'm fine," leaving it to the parents to point out that the teenager has been coughing a lot more in the past week or two, and needing a nap in the afternoon. This inaccuracy on the part of the teenaged patient is almost never *lying,* but rather a kind of *optimism* that sometimes is called *"denial"* by physicians. The kind of optimism and positive outlook on life that so many people with CF have is very important and healthy, *if it doesn't blind them to symptoms that need attention.* We'll talk a little more about denial and optimism later in the chapter.

Your medical care team is going to include you, your parents, and your physician (as well as other folks at the CF center), and needs to be a cooperative venture. You may not always know when you need more care, more antibiotics, or a clinic visit. Your parents won't always know for sure, and in fact, your doctor can't know either, without good information from you. It's very common for parents to have a hard time giving up their control over their child's medical care. And it's not uncommon for their teenagers to resent this refusal to turn over responsibility. If the resentment is great (as it often is), there are two different ways teenagers express it: one is just to tune out, be sulky, and *let their parents and doctors get away with doing all the talking and making all the decisions for them.* The other is to refuse to have anything to do with treatments, medications, etc. By refusing to do treatments, some patients feel that they are taking over control of a part of their lives ("They can't make me do this!"). But it's an unfortunate mistake that ends up almost being: "I'll show you, I'll get sick!" And this approach actually hands control over to *the disease.* A way a patient can really take control of this important part of his or her life is to learn about CF, and say, *"I'll do the front-line monitoring of how I'm doing; I'll call when I'm doing worse; I'll make sure I get more treatments to keep myself healthy."* You can't get rid of CF, and it's no one's fault you got it, but there's lots you can do with your life, including getting as good control as possible of your CF.

PSYCHOLOGICAL AND FAMILY ISSUES

You and Your Parents and Cystic Fibrosis

Although most parents and teenagers get along reasonably well, some are constantly at each other's throats. Even the families that get on well together have times when they get on each other's nerves. The teenagers are embarrassed by and feel nagged and harassed by their parents, while the parents feel exasperated that the teenagers don't listen, and don't have a sense of responsibility. These occasional or constant irritations and disagreements can affect CF care. Some teenagers feel that their parents restrict their activities because of CF, and are always "on their case" about their diet or doing their treatments.

It's worth keeping in mind that parents who don't care about their children don't nag them about medications or treatments. So, most nagging parents nag because they care (not that that's the best way to show it, and not that nagging is easy to put up with, but it's worth checking back in with that fact now and then). One way a lot of teens with CF have found to get their parents off their case about treatments is to grab control of treatments and CF in general away from their parents: show that you can be more compulsive and reliable about your treatments than they ever were. Show that there is no need or point to nagging you, and you've won! They leave you alone, you've gotten control, and your health improves, all in one.

Your Parents, Prenatal Testing for Cystic Fibrosis, and Abortion

A very few teenagers will have the experience that their mother has gotten pregnant, had prenatal testing for CF, and decided to have an abortion because the test showed that the baby would have been born with CF. Others will have heard their parents discuss this question. Sometimes when this happens, the person who's already alive with CF gets the feeling, "Do they wish *I'd* never been born? Do they hate me *that* much?" Of course, this is seldom the case. Almost always when parents make the decision not to have another child with CF (either by not taking the chance and deciding not to have *any* more kids at all, or by using prenatal testing, and having an abortion if the prenatal tests show positive for CF), it's not because they regret having had the child or children they already have, but because they want to spare future children the hardships (and there are some, as you know) that come along with having CF.

You and Your Siblings and Cystic Fibrosis

Sometimes CF can seem to cause tension between siblings. Every single person on earth occasionally gets into a "poor me" mood. People with CF are no exception, and you may on occasion think of the unfairness of CF: why did you get it, and not someone else? If you have a healthy brother or sister, they are obvious examples of the "someone else" who could have gotten CF instead of you. Try to keep in mind that just as it wasn't *your* fault that you ended up with CF, it wasn't *their* fault that you did either, or that they didn't. Many brothers and sisters of CF patients also feel (particularly when they're in their own "poor me" moods) that they've been dealt an unfair hand too. It may seem to them that you get all your parents' love and attention, since your parents spend a lot of time giving you treatments, going to the doctor's with you, and perhaps visiting you in the hospital. If you've been in the hospital, you may have gotten gifts from friends and relatives, too, that siblings didn't get. All this might seem to confirm that you're luckier or more loved than they are. You can reduce these feelings by trying to include them in your life and making it clear to them that they are important to you. Of course, this isn't always easy, because younger siblings *can* be a royal pain sometimes.

You and Your Own Attitude Toward Cystic Fibrosis

There are almost as many different approaches to one's own CF as there are people who have CF. Most people have a very strong healthy positive outlook that serves them well. Psychologists who have studied groups of patients with CF are always impressed with what an emotionally healthy group of people they are. In practically all areas of life, a positive outlook brings positive results. You might have heard of "self-fulfilling prophecies." This means that if someone is convinced they'll succeed at something, it makes their success that much more likely (certainly the reverse is true: if you go into something convinced you'll fail, you will). So, someone with CF who approaches life with optimism and determination (as the majority of people do) ends up doing better, and being happier than those who have a more pessimistic approach. (If you find that you just can't seem to get that optimistic attitude, and are sad or depressed a lot of the time, you should let your doctor know, because you can be helped, by talking with someone—social worker or psychologist or psychiatrist, or by some very effective medications.)

Most teenagers with CF are able to go on about their lives without paying undue attention to CF. In fact, when CF rears its ugly head, for example, with an article in the newspaper about CF being a "fatal disease," or with a friend dying, or even with a parent nagging you about taking your aerosols, most people are able to push aside the darker thoughts about dying, and go on with their lives. By thinking, "this person who died isn't me," you are able to go on about your business. Some professionals call this "denial," meaning that somebody is denying that they have a disease, or refusing to face reality. Actually, though, I prefer to think of this approach as "optimism," and I find it a very healthy, positive way to live your life, with one qualification (see below). People who don't push away negative thoughts, and dwell only on the depressing parts of life (CF or other), get stuck in a quagmire, and will not have a very rewarding life.

The only qualification about this approach is that you can't be so unrealistically optimistic about life that you ignore (or deny the importance of) signs that you might need more treatment to maintain or improve your health. Don't dwell on them; don't let them run your life, but face them, deal with them, and move on. If you've got more cough, don't pretend you don't, but increase your treatments, contact your doctor for an antibiotic, and get on top of the problem. If your parents nag you about treatments, don't react to the nagging by skipping health-maintaining treatment.

Your Body Image

Body image means how you feel about your body. This is a problem for some teenagers with CF, which shouldn't be terribly surprising because it's a problem for lots of teenagers, period. Many people think they're too short or fat or whatever. In addition to the doubts about their bodies that many, many teenagers have, the teenager with CF may have some specifics to focus on: finger clubbing that might seem grotesque to him or her (and likely not very much noticed by others), big chest because of overinflated lungs, skinny, or perhaps puffy chipmunk cheeks from prednisone. For many of these things, nothing can be done other than to try your best to accept them as part of who you are and what you look like, remembering the dedication at the front of this book ("it's not just what you're given, but what you do with what you've got"). For some things, you may be in a position to do something (for example, a number of teenagers with CF were upset enough about being short and skinny that they agreed to have a gas-trostomy tube placed [see Chapter 6, *Nutrition*] for overnight feeds). Many of these people have liked the results of their taking some control over their bodies.

Friends

Friends Who Do Not Have Cystic Fibrosis

Most of your friends don't have CF (even though CF is among the commonest diseases, lots more people don't have it than do: of every 2,500 babies born, only one has CF). You should be able to do everything with your friends that they do with people who don't have CF. There are just a few qualifications to that last state-ment: if your friends are smoking and drinking, you shouldn't. It's not a great idea for *anyone* to smoke at all or drink heavily, but these can be more trouble for peo-ple with CF than for people without CF. Cigarette smoke is clearly very harmful to the lungs of people with CF, whether they are holding and sucking on the cigarette themselves or whether they're breathing in the *sidestream* or *second-hand* smoke from someone else's cigarettes (*sidestream* smoke is the smoke that comes from the lighted end of a cigarette that's just sitting there; *second-hand* smoke is what's exhaled from a smoker's lungs). And too much alcohol can depress your breathing; even a small amount of alcohol can react badly with certain antibiotics, and make you feel very sick. If you're old enough to drink, and plan to have a glass of wine or a beer, ask your doctor if that will be a problem with any of your medications.

Late nights, meals out, even trips away, shouldn't be a problem *if you contin-ue to take your enzymes, antibiotics, and other medications, and get in your air-way clearance treatments.*

Whom Should You Tell That You Have Cystic Fibrosis?

This is a hard question that everyone with CF has to decide for him- or her-self. People worry that if others know they have CF, they'll be treated as "a case of CF," or a freak, and not be treated for who they really are. And there certainly are horror stories of kids asking, "Why aren't you dead if you have CF?" or teachers announcing on a schoolwide PA system that someone has CF, and ask-ing the whole school to pray for them (these are true stories). Most CF physi-cians and social workers and psychologists feel that if you are just open and matter-of-fact about your CF, you will do much better overall, including deal-ing with the occasional jerk who does or says something hurtful. This is prob-ably the same jerk who might say, "all blondes are stupid," tall thin people look like Ichabod Crane, call overweight people "fatso," and so on. Just as the blonde doesn't go around trying to pretend she or he isn't blonde, it's a lot easier just to go about living your life, and not carrying around a deep dark secret. Keep-ing a secret is very difficult, anyway. If you tell *some* people, like your very best friends (and you *should*), it'll be hard for you to know who knows and who doesn't. Instead of going around scared that someone who knows might spill the beans around someone who's not supposed to know, if everyone knows (or at least if you don't care if they know), your life is a lot easier. This doesn't mean defining yourself as *a case of CF,* (you're *not;* you're a person who happens to have CF). And it doesn't mean going up to strangers on the street and saying, "Hi, I'm Arthur (or Anna); I have cystic fibrosis." It just means not hiding the fact, and being comfortable with discussing it. For example, you might meet somebody who complains about needing to take an inhaler for asthma. You can say, "Yeah, I know what you mean. I have cystic fibrosis, and I have to take inhalers too."

Friends with Cystic Fibrosis

Often people with a lot in common can support each other. We tend to seek out people with similar interests and experiences. CF is no exception, and many people with CF get comfort from knowing others with CF—people who can understand what it's like to have a hard coughing spell in the middle of class, or what it's like to have to swallow capsules with a pizza, and so on. (Some people choose *not* to associate with a lot of people with CF, because they don't want to define themselves too much as Someone With CF, and that's OK, too.) A recent change has occurred to make this a little more difficult for people with CF: physicians and families worry that CF patients can give each other possibly dangerous bacteria (the most notorious of which is *Burkholderia cepacia*, or just *cepacia;* see Chapter 3). Because of this concern, there is less opportunity to meet and mingle closely with other people with CF. This limited contact is a bother (and the reason for it can feel scary), but it has probably saved some people from getting sicker. Limiting contact does not mean eliminating it completely, so you still should be able to have friends, perhaps electronic correspondents, with CF.

Seeing Other Cystic Fibrosis Patients Get Sicker

This can certainly be hard. Some of your friends with CF will undoubtedly be sicker than you, and you might see some get sicker who you know didn't need to because they didn't take care of themselves. Some others might do every single treatment and still get sicker. Your job is to be as supportive as you can, and to keep in mind for yourself that CF affects different people very differently. Let your friends talk to you if they want, about anything, including their fears and wishes. Sometimes people who are worried about their health—perhaps even worried that they might die—have trouble finding people to talk to about their fears. It might be hard for their parents, who might tell them, "nonsense, you're fine, don't even think about it," and their friends can do them a big service by letting them talk, and being supportive and understanding. It can be sad for you to see someone you care about get sicker, and especially sad if they die. You may find a lot of different feelings arising, including sympathy, guilt that you're healthier than your friend, fear that you might get sicker, etc. You yourself may need someone to talk to about the feelings their sickness brings up for you. Parents sometimes *are* good people to talk with about this. Other friends may be able to help by listening to you. Your physician or CF social worker has a lot of experience with people going through exactly what you're going through, and they may be able to help.

Seeing Yourself Get Sicker Than Your Friends

This too can be hard and sad, and can raise the "it's not fair" feelings that we talked about a little bit ago. It is almost never too late for increased attention to your health to make some difference, so if you've not been taking good care of yourself and you realize that you're sicker, start taking care of yourself now. You won't be able to heal scar tissue, but you can slow your deterioration, and you will probably be able to make yourself feel better. There is an excellent chance that you'll be able to feel better *about* yourself if you've adopted a positive "I'm going to take control now" attitude.

DATING, MARRIAGE, FAMILY

Some of these topics are also discussed in Chapter 14, *Cystic Fibrosis and Adulthood.* When we said that CF should not keep you from having friends, that included boyfriends or girlfriends. People with CF have the same wishes as everyone else, and dating and forming intimate relationships with others are important parts of life for many people. There is nothing about CF to prevent this, although there are a few little points to keep in mind.

If You're Dating, Should You Tell Him (Her) That You Have Cystic Fibrosis?

As you have seen, most people think it's a whole lot easier if you are open about having CF. Certainly if you are close to someone, they need to know. If they are close to you and care about you, they will *want* to know. Their knowing about CF will help avoid a lot of otherwise awkward times and explanations: why you might have to excuse yourself more often to go to the bathroom; why you take those pills with your meals; what was that embarrassing explosive coughing spell just as you were getting ready for (or worse, in the middle of) a good-night kiss?

Sex

Most of the same things that are true about sex for all teenagers are true for teenagers with CF. In addition, there are a few special considerations. Some of the things that apply to *anybody* include being sure not to get pressured into having sex. Being physically close to someone else can be very special, and many teenagers feel, correctly, that that closeness (whether it's actual sexual intercourse) or holding, hugging, and kissing, shouldn't be entered into lightly, and certainly not done without a full understanding of the possible consequences. In addition to the tremendous emotional commitment that having sex with someone entails, there are definite medical consequences as well. The risk of pregnancy is the first that should be considered. You've already learned that *most* young men with CF cannot get someone pregnant, although they can have sex just the same as any other man, and that women with CF are less likely than other women to get pregnant. You absolutely must be clear that some men with CF *can and have* gotten women pregnant, and many women with CF have become pregnant. *Having CF is not adequate birth control.* For young women with CF, it also is essential to keep in mind that there are reasons not to get pregnant in addition to the huge responsibility that *anyone* would have if they got pregnant. Those additional reasons include the fact that pregnancy can in some cases be very harmful to a young woman's health. (Don't despair; if your lungs are in good shape, you may well be able to have a baby later, when your living situation is stable and you're able to take care of one; this is discussed in the next chapter.) Men can have a semen analysis done to see if they have sperm. If they do not have sperm, they might not need other birth control, **BUT** anyone having sex should be practicing safe sex. Using a condom can protect against STDs (sexually transmitted diseases), including AIDS, as well as protecting against pregnancy.

EDUCATION

Many young people with CF decide to further their education after high school. Many have gone away to college, and lots have even earned graduate degrees. Your CF certainly doesn't interfere with your ability to think, and many CF patients are outstanding academic successes. Plan your education so that it fits your lifestyle, and so that your health doesn't suffer.

Home or Away?

The decision to go away to college is a big one, especially for someone with CF. For many people—with or without CF—it's not something they want to do, and it certainly is not something that *needs* to be done. But if you want to attend college away from home, it can be a wonderful experience: an opportunity to establish your independence, in certain ways even to define anew who you are. If you decide to take the plunge, you must be certain that your CF care doesn't suffer. You will be in a place where your parents won't be reminding you to eat properly (and providing the food), to take your enzymes, to do your treatments, to insist that you go to (or call) the doctor if you have new symptoms. They won't be there to do your chest PT. All of these things must be done, though. One of the saddest things any CF doctor sees is his or her favorite patients going off to school full of enthusiasm and coming back with irreversible lung damage because they neglected their health while they were away. One of the *nicest* things we see is our patients going off, full of enthusiasm, and coming back grown up *and healthy,* because they took care of their health as well as their education! It can be done.

CAREER DIRECTION

Cystic fibrosis does not need to dictate your career choice. People with CF have successfully held a broad range of jobs: doctors, lawyers, businessmen and -women, secretaries, school teachers, coaches, construction workers, grave diggers, housewives and husbands, computer repair technicians, and so on. So if you really want a particular career, you can probably have it. It is worth keeping a few things in mind. It's not a great idea to have a job with heavy exposure to airborne pollution, smoke, dust, chemical fumes, etc... You should also keep in mind that very heavy physical labor might be difficult to sustain over a period of many years. There are people available who can help you make career decisions. Some of these people include CF social workers, and people connected with your state's Office (or Bureau) of Vocational Rehabilitation. (There's a lot more about careers and employment in the next chapter.)

SUMMARY

The teenage years are full of challenge for people with CF, just as for people without CF. However, for those with CF, the stakes are higher, in that if they neglect their health during these important years, they might never regain it. If teenagers with CF take good care of themselves, these years can be wonderfully happy, healthy, productive, and fun.

14

Cystic Fibrosis and Adulthood

THE BASICS

1. Most patients with CF live well into adulthood.
2. Most adults with CF are able to study, work, marry, and do most of the other things that adults do.
3. Adults may have more health problems than younger CF patients.
4. Adults have to deal with some difficult questions, including what kind of work they can do, whether they can or should have children, and how long they will live.

Until fairly recently, adults didn't have cystic fibrosis (CF); children had it, and they died. Today, most patients with CF can plan to live well into adulthood, with the pleasures and responsibilities that come with adulthood. In fact, fully one-third of all CF patients today are 18 years or older, compared with only 8% in 1969. In 1994, there were 6,614 CF patients 18 years or older, compared with only 624 in 1969. Patients now live to an average age of about 30 years, and some experts have predicted that survival will increase to 40 years for someone born today (even without any of the many new treatments that are on the verge of becoming available).

Adults with CF are living fulfilling lives. In 1994, 60% of CF patients 21 years and older had graduated from high school; this compares with the national rate of 32%! Many of those CF high-school graduates went on to college, and some to graduate school. Only 20% of CF patients over 18 years old listed themselves as unemployed, while 18% were students, 33% were working full-time, and 17% working part-time; 27% of these adults were married, and 5% were living with a partner.

Upon reaching adulthood, people with CF must contend with some special issues, in addition to those faced by all people as they approach adulthood, and in addition to the CF issues facing younger patients and their families. Since the lung problems with CF are progressive (that is, they tend to get worse, slowly, as time goes by), many adults with CF have more symptoms and limitations than they had as children and teenagers. What is true of the lungs is also true to some degree for the other body systems affected by CF: more CF-related problems happen in adults than in children. For this reason, we will have a brief discussion in this chapter of the different organ systems and how they may be affected differently for adults than for younger CF patients.

Newspapers, TV, and "the public" (whoever *they* are) often refer to CF as "a fatal disease," which forces even healthy adults to consider the issue of death and dying, which we will address with a brief discussion of death and the adult with CF. Fuller discussions of each of these topics can also be found in other chapters. We'll also discuss some other issues, including medical care, health insurance, employment, marriage and family, disability, and psychological issues.

Patients' attitudes and outlook on life have a tremendous influence on what they are able to do, and indeed on how long they live. Patients with CF typically have a strong, positive outlook, and therefore are able to accomplish many of the normal tasks and enjoy many of the normal pleasures of adulthood, despite having to contend with some difficulties.

DIFFERENT ORGAN SYSTEMS

Respiratory System

Upper Airway: Nose and Sinuses

There is little different about the involvement of the nose and sinuses in adults with CF compared with CF children and adolescents. In all ages, the sinuses will look abnormal on x-rays, and patients may develop nasal polyps, which may or may not respond to nasal sprays, and which may need to be removed surgically. The sinus abnormality is more apt to bother an adult with CF than a child with CF, and some adults will have problems with chronic (long-lasting) sinusitis. Headache, constantly stuffed nose, and even increased cough may signal infection of the sinuses, which will usually improve with antibiotic treatment. If sinus problems persist despite antibiotics, sinus surgery (to open up the sinuses and make it easier for them to drain) may be helpful in some cases.

Lower Airways: Lungs and Bronchial Tubes

The lungs, of course, especially the bronchial tubes, are the main source of problems for anyone with CF, with buildup of secretions, infection, and inflammation that if unchecked can lead to permanent replacement of healthy lung with scar tissue. The lung problems are more likely to occur, and be more difficult to manage, in adults. By age 15 years, about one-half of all CF patients cough up mucus each day, and 85% bring up mucus from their lungs occasionally. Adults have more episodes of infection for which they need to be treated with IV antibiotics, either in the hospital or at home. While pulmonary function tests do not tell the whole story, they can help give a general picture of this situation: You may recall from Chapter 3, *The Respiratory System,* that the FEV_1 is the amount of air that can be blown out of the lungs in 1 second, and is a measure of how much bronchial blockage there is (the higher the FEV_1, the higher the airflow, and the less blockage there is). The average FEV_1 for 7-year-olds with CF is 95% of normal (meaning that the average 7-year-old with CF can blow out 95% as much air in 1 second as a normal healthy 7-year-old), the average for 18-year-olds is 69% of normal, and for 30-year-olds is 50% of normal. What this shows is that adult patients are more likely to have considerable bronchial blockage and generally serious lung disease than younger patients. Adults are more likely than children to have difficulty exercising. Adults are more likely than children to need to use oxygen (although most will not). Adults are more likely than children to be referred to a lung transplant program for possible lung transplantation (see Chapter 8, *Transplantation*). But not everyone continues to get worse and worse after they reach adulthood. Some patients remain quite healthy, and even those who have gotten sicker as they have become adults may be relatively stable for a long time. Some adult patients tell us that they don't get sicker each year, but feel that they have to work harder to stay the same.

Of specific *complications* of lung disease (see Chapter 3, *The Respiratory System),* adults are more likely than youngsters to have hemoptysis (coughing up blood) and pneumothorax (collapsed lung caused by a hole in the lung). It is fairly common for an adult with CF to have blood-streaking of the mucus that they cough up and spit out, but bringing up a large amount (enough to require hospitalization, for example) is much less common: about 2.5% of patients older than 21 do so (this compares with less than 0.4% of children under 15 years old). Although pneumothorax is 3 times as common after the age of 15 years as before, only about 1% of older patients suffer this problem in a given year. So, even though both of these problems are more common in adults than children, neither one is a major problem for most adults with CF.

Gastrointestinal System

The symptoms and signs from the gastrointestinal system vary in their effects on adults. Most patients, young and old alike, need to take pancreatic enzymes for the digestion of their food. For some strange reason, it seems that many adults have less abdominal discomfort from their pancreatic problem (and may need fewer enzymes with meals) than children with CF. We don't know why this is so; it may be simply that by the time they are adults, patients have learned how to take their enzymes better, or they've learned to avoid problem foods. It may also be that with age there is a change in their pancreas, stomach, or intestines that we haven't identified. There may be another explanation, too: it may be that some patients are just *used to* the discomfort, so they notice it less.

DIOS

Intestinal blockage (DIOS, standing for **d**istal **i**ntestinal **o**bstruction **s**yndrome) occurs in as many as 20% of adults sometime during their adult lives. It's not known what causes DIOS, but one factor that has been blamed in many cases is not taking adequate enzymes. DIOS can cause symptoms ranging from mild cramping to severe abdominal pain—that seems a lot like appendicitis—and lack of bowel movements. It can be very serious, and occasionally may even require surgery. Because of the possible consequences, changes in bowel habits—especially having no bowel movements for a day—should make you call your CF physician right away. DIOS can usually be treated by drinking large amounts of special liquids (the best known is GoLytely®), or if that fails, by special enemas. Patients with CF should never undergo surgery for "appendicitis" without communicating with their CF physician, since DIOS can sometimes mimic appendicitis, but can be treated without surgery. Only very rarely is surgery necessary.

Gallstones

Gallstones appear in about 10% of patients with CF at some time in their lives. This is more likely to happen in adulthood. Gallstones can be completely innocent, or can cause pain, or block drainage of liver secretions. If they do cause pain, they are usually removed by surgery (taking out the whole gallbladder).

Diabetes

As you saw in Chapter 4, *The Gastrointestinal Tract,* diabetes is much more common in adults with CF than in children, with about 10% (or more) of CF patients developing diabetes each decade after age 10 years: Almost no one with CF gets diabetes before age 10; about 10% of patients between 10 and 20 years old develop it; by age 30 years, about 20% of patients have developed it. Diabetes is well-managed with diet and insulin injections (and in unusual cases, with diet alone). In some centers, oral medications are used to help control the blood sugar level. Other than the bother of watching the diet a little more carefully than before, and of taking extra oral medications or giving oneself injections, it is unclear what impact diabetes has on the CF patient's health. One report suggests that it has a negative impact, with diabetic CF patients dying earlier than nondiabetic patients, while most studies have found no effect on how long someone will live.

Liver Disease

Liver disease, including cirrhosis, used to be the second leading cause of death in patients with CF (after lung disease), accounting for about 2% of the deaths among people with CF. Experts predicted that as treatment for the lungs improved, and patients lived longer, more CF patients would develop liver disease; that is, as there were more adults, there would be more liver disease in CF patients. This has turned out *not* to be the case. It seems that most patients who will develop liver disease do so by their teens.

Reproductive System

The reproductive system is an area of concern virtually exclusively to teenagers and adults.

Men

Some 98% of men with CF are sterile, because of a blockage or incomplete formation of the *vas deferens*, the tube that takes sperm from the testicles to the penis. All other aspects of CF adult men's sex life is normal, but they cannot deliver sperm to their partners. Two percent of men with CF do not have this blockage, so you cannot assume that intercourse will not result in pregnancy. This may be good news for someone who wants to father children, or bad news for someone who thinks that CF alone is adequate male birth control. A semen analysis can be done to see if sperm are present. Men with CF have wondered if there was a way to get around the blockage of the *vas deferens*, since the sperm are made normally in the testicles, and just can't get out. Recently, a new high-tech microsurgical technique has been developed for *in vitro* fertilization, and has enabled a few men with CF-sterility to father children. This technique is called MESA, for microsurgical epididymal sperm aspiration. Here's how it works: using a special surgical operating microscope and tiny needle (because the structures are so small) a urologist aspirates (uses suction to pull out) some sperm from the man's epididymis (a crescent-shaped structure attached to the testicle). These sperm are then injected into one of the woman's eggs, which had previously been removed from her ovary and placed in a test tube. The injection technique is different from the usual in vitro fertilization procedures (not that *any* way of fertilizing a human egg outside the body can really be called "usual"). When in vitro fertilization is performed most often the egg and sperm are just put together, with the hope that they'll hit it off, and the sperm will enter the egg to fertilize it. But the sperm collected via MESA are generally not mature enough to fertilize an egg on their own, since they are removed before they have had a chance to take their normal maturing trip all the way through the epididymis. Since these somewhat immature sperm would not have much success at fertilizing an egg on their own, they are helped by being injected directly into the egg. The pregnancy rate with this technique may be as high as 50% per attempt. If the procedure works, and the egg is fertilized, the tiny several-cell embryo can be analyzed to see if it carries abnormal CF genes before it is implanted into the mother's uterus to grow and develop (the chances of the baby's having CF are shown in Table 11.1). The procedure is expensive ($10,000 in 1995), is not widely available, and is not covered by most insurance policies. Whether a couple where the husband has CF want to attempt this will depend on a number of factors, including: (1) Who will pay for it? (2) What will the couple do if the embryo is found to have two abnormal CF genes (most couples contemplating this procedure will decide to have the mother-to-be screened for the most common CF gene mutations beforehand)? (3) Is the father healthy enough to be able to help raise the child?

Women

The reproductive tract is fairly normal in most women with CF, although a fair proportion of women with CF may have irregular menstrual periods. Women with CF are able to get pregnant, and several hundred have carried their pregnancies to term, and had babies, most of whom have been healthy. It is probably a bit more difficult for a woman with CF to get pregnant than it is for one without CF, for a couple of reasons. The first factor that makes women with CF less fertile than normal is that the mucus in their cervix (the opening to the uterus) is—like most mucus in people with CF—extra thick and sticky, making it tough slogging for a sperm trying to swim from the vagina through that cervical mucus to get to the uterus (womb) to unite with an egg. In addition, if a woman's nutrition is poor, or if she is in poor health otherwise (as, for example, from severe lung disease), her periods may not be regular, and the periods may be *anovulatory* (meaning that no eggs are released). In 1994, in the United States, 58 women with CF delivered live babies, 14 had a therapeutic abortion, and 11 had spontaneous abortions (miscarriage or still birth).

As we discuss a little later in this chapter, the decision to have or not to have children is extremely important for any woman, particularly so for a woman with CF. Pregnancy can have a detrimental effect on the mother's health if her lungs were not in good condition at the onset of the pregnancy. (For most women whose lungs *are* in good shape, pregnancy does not usually seem to make the lungs worse than they would have been otherwise.)

Birth Control

For many excellent reasons (some discussed later in this chapter), women with CF often decide they do not wish to become pregnant. They certainly should not become pregnant unless and until their ability to take care of themselves (particularly their lungs) and their baby is solidly established. This means that birth control is essential for many women with CF. Not counting abstention (not having sex at all), the most effective birth control method is surgical: tubal ligation. Practically the only disadvantage is that if you change your mind, it will be difficult or even impossible to undo a tubal ligation. The pill is another reliable method of birth control that many women with CF have chosen, and have used safely and effectively. The pill has the further advantage of regulating menstrual periods— a relief to those many women with CF who had had irregular periods. It is theoretically possible that the pill may not work quite as well in women taking antibiotics. This possibility can be avoided by talking with your CF doctor or gynecologist and arranging a special schedule of only 3 or 4 days (instead of the usual 7) each month taking a "placebo" pill.

"Barrier" methods (diaphragms and condoms) are somewhat less effective than the other methods, mostly because they must be thought of and used each and every time a couple has intercourse. Condoms have the important advantage of providing excellent protection from sexually transmitted diseases, including AIDS. You should discuss the pros and cons of the various methods with your physician.

Vaginal Yeast Infections

Somewhere around 75% of *all* women will have a vaginal yeast infection some time in their lives. Women with CF are no exception, and probably have more of them than other women because of CF women's frequent use of antibiotics (see below). Women with CF would be expected to have more than their share of vaginal yeast infections (often referred to in the medical literature as *thrush* or *vulvo-vaginal candidiasis—Candida* being the most common yeast causing this infection). This is because being on antibiotics increases anyone's chances of getting this infection, since antibiotics kill bacteria, and that allows the yeast to multiply. One study from Australia showed this problem to be much more common in women with CF than women without CF, and for episodes of thrush to correspond to times they were taking oral antibiotics. Furthermore, diabetes also may make a woman more likely to develop a yeast infection, and more women with than without CF have diabetes. These infections are not dangerous, but can be extremely uncomfortable, causing terrible itching, and sometimes burning. These infections can usually be treated successfully with antiyeast cream placed in the vagina. Occasionally, an oral medication might also be needed. Women with CF who get these infections whenever they go on antibiotics can be helped tremendously by starting treatment with vaginal antiyeast medications as soon as they start their antibiotics.

OVERALL HEALTH

Many adults with CF find that they are able to do less and less as time goes on, mostly because of the worsening health of their lungs. This can be very difficult, particularly for people who used to be very active. Recurrent courses of IV antibiotics may be needed, and if they are carried out in the hospital these courses can have a huge impact on an adult's ability to continue to carry out a normal work and home life. Permanent IVs like Portacaths® and Mediports® (discussed in Chapter 7) can enable many adults to get their IV antibiotics at home, thus helping them to continue a relatively normal life.

One of the hardest parts for many people is getting used to using oxygen, something that was necessary for about 8% of all CF patients in 1994, most of them adults. People—especially children—may stare at you if have this greenish tubing wrapped around your ears and plugged into your nose. Different patients have handled this discomfort in different ways, from ignoring it to answering questions with a gentle explanation of what the oxygen tubing is for ("it's oxygen to help me breathe better because I have a lung problem"). Oxygen is discussed more in the Appendix B: *Medications.*

You may have less energy, and find you need to take more time to do things, and schedule more time for rest. Some people may be helped by getting a handicapped parking placard and license plates. If you belong to AAA, they can help get you the necessary forms; otherwise, contact your local driver's license bureau.

MEDICAL CARE

The training of physicians in the care of adult patients with CF is just now catching up with the tremendous improvement in longevity. Until very recently, CF was a disease of childhood, and physicians who were trained to care for adults were not taught about CF. Today, there are still too few internal medicine physicians (general medical specialists for adults) who have had training and experience in the problems and care of people with CF. Fortunately, however, there are more and more adult pulmonologists who have taken it upon themselves to become knowledgeable in the care of adults with CF, and medical training programs are beginning to pay more attention to the treatment of this important population. At present, the adult with CF generally has to rely on conscientious adult general medicine or pulmonary specialists who have taken the extra effort to educate themselves about CF (if it's possible to find one in your area), or continue to rely on the pediatricians and pediatric pulmonary physicians who have been the CF specialists for the longest time. Most CF centers have a program for their adult patients, and have physicians who are interested and knowledgeable in the care of adults with CF; in some centers these will be the pediatricians, and in others it will be internal medicine or adult pulmonary specialists.

Care at an approved CF center, with its team of experts, is very important. Studies in Europe, Australia, and North America have shown clearly that patients who receive their care at CF centers live longer than those whose care is not in centers; it's that simple. This is not to say that the general internist or family doctor isn't capable of participating in the care of adults with CF. Quite the contrary: the primary care physician can be a wonderful ally in maintenance of the health of people with CF just as with people without CF. But the CF care should be coordinated between the primary care doctors and the CF center, and not done to the exclusion of the CF center. It is quite important to insist that you have access to center care, particularly in this era when costs may be more important than patient health to some health care plans.

HEALTH AND DISABILITY INSURANCE

Health insurance is a very important issue, since medical care for any chronic illness, including CF, is so expensive. Once a person reaches adulthood, he or she is usually excluded from his or her parents' family insurance coverage. Some states have "over 21" laws, which extend health insurance and/or state programs to adults with certain chronic illness, including CF. Some employers have excellent employee health insurance, but some plans exclude anyone with a "preexisting condition," meaning that they don't pay any expenses related to a problem that you had before you joined the company, which of course would include CF. Some policies limit how much they pay for a particular illness; many have a lifetime limit to how much they will pay. You should find out if a hospitalization for CF at one time will count as the same "illness" as a previous hospitalization that was also due to CF. Some policies or certifiers are liberal in their interpretation, and might consider one pulmonary exacerbation (see Chapter 3, *The Respiratory System*) a separate episode of "bronchitis," "lung infection," or "pneumonia," and therefore pay for each of them, while others will be very strict and consider every episode to be part of CF, and be less willing to pay for multiple admissions.

Health Insurance When Changing or Leaving Jobs

If you want to change jobs, for any reason, you may be scared off by the new company's having a "preexisting condition" exclusion in its health insurance that won't pay for medical expenses associated with a preexisting condition for the first 12 months the person is working for the company and is covered by the new company's insurance. Don't let that stop you. There is a federal law, referred to as COBRA (standing for comprehensive omnibus budget reconciliation act), that requires that employees be allowed keep their medical insurance for 18 months after they stop working for an employer (unless they were fired for gross misconduct). That means you can start your new job, with the new insurance coverage, but retain your old insurance for the first 12 months. That way, if you have CF-related medical expenses within those first 12 months, the old company's policy will pay for them; then, once you've put in your 12 months, the new policy no longer excludes the preexisting condition. (There are some preexisting condition clauses that have a different 12-month exclusion: they won't pick up coverage of a condition until you've gone 12 months *without any medical expenses related to that condition*; those are very difficult to get around.)

That's the good news about COBRA and preexisting conditions. The bad news is that to continue your old insurance policy for the 12-month waiting time until the new one kicks in, you have to make the insurance payments yourself. This can amount to several hundred dollars a month, depending on the policy, and may be more than many patients can afford.

It is very important to look very carefully at insurance plans and possible exclusions before making decisions about employment. As we mentioned above, it is crucial to insist on being able to have access to a CF center for your care. Be certain that you will not be prevented from this specialized care. As this book goes to press health care reform bills are being considered in the United States Congress. If any of this legislation passes, it may well change what insurance companies are allowed to do in terms of excluding preexisting conditions, etc. Stay tuned, and check with your CF center. The center personnel are likely to be up to date on these regulations.

Unemployment

If you must stop working because of your health, there are some programs that can help with income, and some help specifically for medical bills.

Health Insurance If You Are Unemployed

The COBRA mentioned above is in force whenever you leave a job, whether it's to take another job (as discussed above), or to stop working entirely. In fact, if you are forced by your health to stop working, COBRA requires that you cannot lose your health insurance for 36 months after you stop working. Unfortunately, again, you *can* lose your health insurance if you can't pay for the premiums. People who have lost their jobs for health reasons may qualify for Medicare, which will pay some medical bills (but not prescriptions), but only after two years of being unable to work (!). So, some patients are caught in a difficult bind: too sick to work, unable to afford medical insurance, and with 24 months to wait until they can get Medicare. Some states have "over 21" programs that will pay for CF-related medical bills for people over 21 years old in this difficult 24-month waiting period. These programs are a big help, although they don't have unlimited resources, and have some arbitrary rules about what is and isn't covered. In Pennsylvania, for example, CF medical bills are covered (doctor's bills, most medications, etc.), but if you have CF diabetes, the state won't pay for your insulin or other diabetes-related expenses, even though the CF caused the diabetes. Your CF center staff is likely to be very knowledgeable about all these rules, and is there to help.

Social Security Disability Insurance

Everyone who is employed pays into the federal Social Security fund, designed to help people who become unable to work. If you become unable to work, you may be eligible to receive income from Social Security. The amount you receive depends on how long you've worked, and the amount of money you've put into the fund. A downside of this program is that—while it gives some income—it does not give health insurance for the first two years someone is on the program. After two years, you may qualify for Medicare, which is a form of health insurance (see above).

Some patients who have lost their jobs because of their health may qualify for public assistance (welfare), even if they are getting monthly Social Security Disability checks. For some, however, their income may be too high to qualify for public assistance. Your CF center social worker should be able to help you through the maze of public and private organizations set up to help. Or you can call your local Social Security office or Public Assistance office.

EDUCATION

Many adults with CF choose to continue their education beyond high school, and some attend trade schools, while many graduate from college and even get advanced degrees.

One of the main ways in which CF affects an adult's education is in the decision of whether to leave home to attend college. Leaving home is an exciting and valuable experience for many young adults, with CF or without. It is a time to establish one's independence and even to help "invent" a new personality. It can mean leaving unwanted parts of the past behind, and fitting in with a new set of friends. Unfortunately, for too many people with CF that has meant trying to leave CF behind: not wanting to be different, so not wanting to tell anyone about CF can also mean not doing treatments, not taking medicines, not taking care with nutrition, and so on. In too many cases it has been possible to ignore CF until it's been too late. There are far too many young adults who have let their health slide, and have realized what their parents and physicians had been saying all along about taking care of themselves only after they have suffered irreversible lung damage. Far too many adults have come to us and said, "I wish I had listened, and taken care of myself, but I thought I knew everything, and I never believed I could get sick. Now I wish I had it to do over again . . ."

Leaving home most often means leaving behind the people who perform daily chest physical therapy treatments, which, in turn, means that a replacement must be found (either a replacement person to help with the treatments or a replacement form of airway clearance, using a technique you can do on your own). Much of the chest physical therapy can be done oneself, especially if you use the Flutter (see Chapter 3, *The Respiratory System*) or percussor vest, or mechanical percussors with straps or extension handles, but some young adults feel more secure with a treatment performed by someone else, and may feel that their parents do the best chest PT. They are probably right. After all, it is very likely that no one cares as much about your health as you and your parents do. However, there are ways to get adequate help with chest PT. Many college health services will offer assistance in this realm. Some schools that have physical therapy students or respiratory therapy students may be able to arrange for these students to help give treatments. College students often have close friends who learn how to administer treatments. Others have placed more emphasis on an aerobic exercise program or on "huff" techniques that are easier to perform on oneself than the traditional chest physical therapy.

The Flutter (see Chapter 3) has freed many people from dependence on others for effective airways clearance treatments. Some CF physicians will accept 15–20 minutes each day of vigorous exercise as a substitute for chest PT. Whatever one chooses, it is extremely important to find some way to keep up with treatments, and not give in to the temptation to skip them in the excitement of being away on one's own, perhaps for the first time. There are always reasons to skip a treatment (test tomorrow, party tonight, etc.), and while it's fine to skip an occasional treatment, this cannot become a habit. A problem with many treatments, including chest PT and other airway clearance techniques, is that you may not feel much better after them; what's important is their cumulative effect over many days, weeks, and months. So you may well skip a treatment and not notice any dire consequences. If this happens, it's easy to let yourself slip into a habit of skipping treatments. Unfortunately, many people *have noticed* their lungs being worse from skipping treatments only after irreparable harm has been done to them. And then it's too late. So, it's important to try to keep up with all your treatments. It's also important to keep up with good nutrition, which many young adults have let slide when their parents (usually especially their moms) are not there to nag them.

While we're on the topic of nonhealthful temptations, it's important to mention two others, namely, smoking and drinking. It should be obvious (but isn't always) that smoking (cigarettes particularly, but also probably marijuana) is bad for anyone's lungs, and especially so if one has underlying lung disease like CF. There is definite evidence that second-hand cigarette smoke (that is, someone else is doing the smoking, and you're breathing in the extra smoke that just happens to be in the air around) is harmful to CF patients; it stands to reason that active smoking is that much worse. Smoking will absolutely disqualify you for a lung transplant if you should ever decide that you want one. Alcohol in moderation is probably not bad, but you should discuss it with your physician, because there are some medications, including some antibiotics, that interact badly with alcohol.

Many states have vocational rehabilitation offices or bureaus (OVRs or BVRs) that provide educational and occupational counseling and financial assistance for students after high school. These programs used to be extremely helpful, with some of them automatically paying college tuition for anyone with CF, but many are now suffering from slashed budgets, and may not be able to provide as much assistance as in years gone by. They may still be able to give helpful guidance on career selection, though, and are worth checking out. Your CF center social worker should be able to tell you about these resources, or you can call your state Department of Labor and Industry Office of Vocational Rehabilitation.

EMPLOYMENT

Men and women with CF have had—and succeeded at—many different kinds of jobs, including physician, CF research scientist, lawyer, race car driver (at least one woman!), basketball coach, school teacher, computer repair technician, farmer, homemaker, etc., etc. Cystic fibrosis may well influence one's career choices. It is important to consider your current physical condition and what your physical condition will be in several years as you make occupational plans. In general, a relatively sedentary job is better over the long haul than one that is physically demanding. This does not mean that a sedentary *life* is preferable, but rather that one should exercise during nonwork time. It also doesn't mean that physical labor is *bad,* but rather it makes sense to plan for a time when you might not be as strong as you are when you are starting employment. Then, if you should become ill or weakened, it would not jeopardize your job and would only affect your exercise regimen. Jobs involving constant exposure to dust, chemical fumes, or smoke should be avoided. If you're thinking about teaching school, especially younger children, you should keep in mind the possible danger of near constant exposure to an ever-changing array of respiratory viruses.

If someone is not able to continue to do full-time work, some employers may be able to offer part-time work. Some patients have been able to do some of their work at home, particularly with the help of a computer modem and/or fax machine.

The Americans with Disabilities Act (ADA) of 1990 is a very important law for people with CF to know about. This is a federal law that protects people with disabilities from being discriminated against, including in the workplace. What "disability" means for this law is different from what it may mean in other settings. There have been many people who have applied for Social Security Disability (see below) and have been denied those benefits because they weren't sick or "disabled" enough. Yet these people may still be covered by the ADA. For this law, the definition of a person with a disability is someone who

- "has an impairment that substantially limits one or more major life activities; or
- has a record of such an impairment; or
- is regarded as having such an impairment."

People with CF, even those who are not dreadfully ill, may qualify. Here's how: CF may be considered to give a "substantial limitation" to the "major life activities" of breathing, eating, or walking. This may be true even if with treatment, you breathe, eat, and walk well. *The disability determination must be made without considering the effects of treatments*. Even for someone who has absolutely no limitation from CF, the ADA may provide protection for you from the situation where an employer or union official *thinks* you're limited. Of course, if anyone (from CF or other cause) becomes too sick too work, then the employer can fire that person. But before an employer can fire you because you are unable to do your job, the ADA requires that "reasonable accommodation" be made to allow you to continue to work. This "reasonable accommodation" includes such things as job restructuring, changing work hours, and giving additional sick time (paid or unpaid). This might mean allowing you to start work later in the morning, to allow for morning chest PT. Unless there is something crucial about your job that requires it to be done very early, and doing it later would mean a hardship for your employer, you may be have the right to have your work hours changed. Another possible "reasonable accommodation" would be getting 2 weeks more sick leave for a hospital admission.

Applying for a Job

Patients often wonder what they should do about mentioning their CF in a job interview. Most lawyers and disability rights experts think it's not a good idea to volunteer the information during an interview. If you do mention your CF, and aren't offered the job, it will be hard to know (or prove) whether it was the employer's feelings about CF that caused you to lose the job. On the other hand, if you don't mention CF, and are offered the job, but then the job offer is withdrawn after the employer finds out you have CF, it's easier to prove that the offer was withdrawn because of CF, and that's illegal. If you are asked point blank during an interview if you have a disability, it gets tricky. Employers are allowed to ask if you will be able to do what's required for a specific job, but are not allowed to ask if you have a disability. If you tell an interviewer that it's illegal to ask if you have a disability (which is true), you could lose the job because of an "attitude" problem, whereas if you lie and say you don't have any problem, then you put yourself in a compromised position if and when it ever comes out that you have CF. In actual fact, in most cases, the question won't come up.

MARRIAGE AND FAMILY

About half of CF patients over 25 years of age marry, and most of these marriages succeed, with a lower divorce rate than in the general population. Decisions about raising a family are definitely difficult if one partner has a life-shortening disease that limits fertility. Women with CF have a more difficult time conceiving than women without CF, and 98% of men with CF are sterile. Careful consideration must be given to the potential parents' long-term health, and difficult issues must be faced such as the possible death of one parent, which would leave the other a single parent and the child or children with only one parent. If it is the woman who has CF, the possible effects of pregnancy on her health must be considered. Pregnancy has often caused dramatic deterioration in the health of women with CF if their lungs were not in excellent shape at the outset. Similarly, in women with severe lung disease, the chances of having a miscarriage, stillbirth, premature birth, or birth of an abnormally small baby are increased. In addition, both parents must keep in mind that raising a child is hard, tiring work: occasionally up all night with crying or minor illnesses, giving the child attention for much of the day, and being exposed to the many different viruses that all children bring home from daycare or school. These can be difficult stresses and strains on the parent with CF, especially if he or she is the one doing most of the child care. Finally, with either parent having CF, the baby might have CF. The child will have gotten one abnormal CF gene from the parent with CF, and whether he or she ends up with CF depends on whether the other parent passes on an abnormal CF gene as well. The chances of this happening are presented in Table 11.1. Because of the dangers to the mother and baby, a number of women with CF lung disease have been advised not to get pregnant, or to terminate a pregnancy. This can be hard advice to hear, and has made some women sad and/or angry, particularly if they had their hearts set on having children. Both partners must be willing to discuss all the issues around the important decision of whether to have children or not. It certainly is OK to decide *not* to have children.

Infant Feeding: Breast vs. Bottle

Women with CF who do have babies may be interested in breast-feeding their infants. Breast milk from women with CF is perfectly normal and healthful for the infants. Breast-feeding may put a strain on the mother, however, and may put both a nutritional and energy drain on her. If a woman is having trouble maintaining her own nutrition, breast-feeding may add to her difficulty of keeping her weight up. Bottle-feeding infant formulas will also provide excellent nutrition for the baby, and will spare the CF mother that extra calorie drain. It will also make it possible for both parents to share the joy (and work) of feeding, including middle-of-the-night feedings.

Many couples in which the husband has CF have decided to adopt children, and some have decided to have children through artificial insemination. New, expensive, high-tech methods have made it possible for a few men with CF to father children, as discussed earlier in this chapter.

Sex

Most couples with one partner with CF are able to have fulfilling intimate relations, including an active healthy sex life. As you've already learned, men with CF have blocked or incompletely formed *vas deferens,* making it as though they had had a vasectomy. They can have sexual intercourse normally, only no sperm come out. Similarly, although women with CF have more difficulty getting pregnant than women without CF, they too usually have normal sex lives. For both men and women, coughing spells can be disruptive during intimate times, and this may on occasion be a problem. Some CF patients with more advanced disease have a harder time breathing when they are lying flat on their backs. If this is a problem that interferes with sex, different positions can be used. Just as oxygen can help people breathe more easily when they exert themselves in other ways, it can also be helpful for people who otherwise become short of breath during intercourse. Other small adjustments can make a big difference to the partner with CF if he or she has advanced lung disease that has interfered with a couple's sex life: consider timing your sexual activities for when you feel good. Many people with CF lung disease are not at their best in the early morning before a good aerosol and airway clearance session, so sex first thing in the morning may not be such a good idea for such a person. Similarly, some people feel short of breath and tired after a big meal, so think about giving yourselves a while to digest before planning exertion of any kind, including in bed. Finally, an aerosol and airway clearance may help make sex less taxing for the CF patient, and therefore more enjoyable for both partners.

PSYCHOLOGICAL ISSUES

The overall psychological health of CF patients is excellent. Professionals have been impressed at the low rate of depression and the excellent ability to cope among CF patients, who have a life-shortening disease that—for some—makes employment difficult, decreases fertility, and presents so many physical and financial obstacles. Most patients do extremely well psychologically and emotionally. They are models of a very realistic, healthy, positive outlook.

Nevertheless, some patients with CF will be sad, and some will be depressed. These feelings can interfere with people's ability to work, to sleep, to function in many different ways. These feelings should not be ignored, because in most cases, they can be helped with counseling or medication. If you experience depression, or other difficult emotions that make it hard for you to carry on, you should let your doctor or social worker know, because you are certainly not alone, and there is an excellent chance that you can get effective help.

DEATH

This book contains a whole chapter on the difficult subject of death. We mention the subject briefly here because it is an area of particular concern to adults. More adults than children with CF die each year, and the death rate for adults is much higher than that for children (in 1994, 71% of CF patients who died were 18 years or older). However, perhaps surprisingly, the chances of dying at any given age do *not* seem to keep increasing for every year you age: In 1994, the mortality rate for 10-year-olds with CF was 0.012 (meaning that of every one thousand 10-year-olds with CF, about 12 died), while it was 0.054 for 20-year-olds, but only 0.047 for 30-year-olds, and 0.045 for 41-year-olds. Further, if you look at pulmonary function test (PFT) results to try to predict who will die, you find big differences between children and adults, in favor of the adults: for any given PFT number, a child with that number will be more likely to die than an adult with the same number. An example is the FEV_1 : about 27% of children 6–17 years old who had an FEV_1 between 30% and 40% of normal died within 2 years, while only 18% of those aged 18–44 years died within 2 years. The same difference holds between children and adults for most PFT values. Experts speculate that a child who has a low PFT (bad bronchial blockage) may be sicker and have somehow more rapidly worsening lungs than an adult who has taken up to 30 more years to develop the same amount of blockage. So, adults with CF, even with fairly severe lung disease, have staying power. Nonetheless, some do die, and adults with CF have to face the issue.

Adults may have spouses, children, and jobs to consider, and personal and financial affairs to get in order. Adults will also be forced to confront issues like life support when they are hospitalized, since federal and state laws now require any adult who is admitted to the hospital to be informed of his or her right to make "advanced directives." These are decisions about what medical treatments they will or will not accept, including "artificial ventilation, artificial feeding, and artificial hydration."

Adults may have to decide whether they want to consider lung transplantation. Many patients have found this decision to be the most difficult they've ever faced, and thinking about it to be among the most stressful tasks they've ever undertaken. The stakes are so very high, with possible positive outcomes so positive, and possible negatives so very negative (these are discussed at some length in Chapter 8, *Transplantation*). Add to this the seeming irreversibility of the decision and the time pressure patients have felt to make the decision, and you have a recipe for a difficult and emotional time. It *must* be stressed that either decision—for or against transplant—can be the right one for different people.

COMMUNICATING WITH OTHER ADULTS WITH CYSTIC FIBROSIS

Many people with CF are interested in meeting others who might be going through similar trials and tribulations. Some communication with other CF adults happens through the CF center, just through the coincidence of being in the clinic waiting room at the same time, or being hospitalized at the same time. CF center physicians, nurses, and social workers can give you names of other patients/families who have expressed a similar interest. (Of course, not everyone wants to get together with other patients.) Many local CF Foundation branches used to have get-togethers for families, but because of increased concern about sharing bacteria that may be dangerous along with sharing good times, there are many fewer of these social functions these days. Since it appears that physical *contact,* or extremely close proximity, is usually required for transmission of bacteria, some CF centers are encouraging their adults to avoid physical contact with other CF patients, and, for example, to forego the usual handshake when they meet other CF patients. There are several newsletters that are aimed particularly at (and put out by) adults with CF. Newsletters come and go, and are often driven by one dedicated person so your CF center or the CF Foundation may be able to give you up-to-date information on these newsletters. The opinions expressed in the newsletters do not always coincide with what CF physicians might believe, so we urge you to discuss treatment issues with your physician. We include here several newsletters that have been around for at least a few years:

- **iacfa Newsletter** (the Newsletter of the International Association of Cystic Fibrosis Adults; Barbara L. Palys, 82 Ayer Road, Harvard, MA 01451-1409; e-mail: bpalys@genesis.nred.ma.us)
- **CF Roundtable** (A publication of the United States Adult Cystic Fibrosis Association: USACFA Inc., P.O. Box 1618, Gresham, OR, 97030-0519)
- **NETWORK** (Published quarterly by Cystic Fibrosis Network, Inc.: CF Network, Inc., P.O. Box 204, Dublin, PA 18917-0204)

SUMMARY

Most patients with CF now live well into their adult lives. Adulthood with CF brings challenges of living independently, perhaps facing declining health and the possibility of dying, but also the satisfactions that can come with approaching life with a positive attitude, and succeeding at many different tasks in one's personal, family, educational, recreational, and career paths.

15

Death and Cystic Fibrosis

THE BASICS

1. Many people with CF think about death, and most will die of their CF, and not of old age.
2. People with CF do not choke to death on their mucus.
3. Death is not painful for people with CF.
4. Death is seldom sudden or unexpected for people with CF.

It has been stressed throughout this book how well people live with cystic fibrosis (CF) and how much better and longer their lives are now than they were just a few decades ago. Advances in treatment and the exciting research progress promise even better things to come. In the meantime, people do still die from CF. In fact, until a cure is found, it is probable that most people with CF will die from their disease, and not of old age. In order to dispel some common misunderstandings and fears about dying, this chapter will discuss what happens when someone dies from CF.

Most people who die from CF die because their lungs have become so damaged that they can no longer perform the work of bringing in oxygen and eliminating carbon dioxide. At this point, the level of these gases in the bloodstream will be inappropriate. All body tissues need oxygen to stay alive, so when the oxygen level is too low, life is impossible. When the carbon dioxide level rises, it acts first like a sedative and then like a general anesthetic, putting the person to sleep. If the carbon dioxide levels become extremely high, the person may sleep so deeply that the breathing efforts become very weak. This can happen to such a degree that the carbon dioxide builds up even further and the oxygen drops down even further, causing the person to die.

When someone's lungs are seriously damaged, both oxygen and carbon dioxide levels may be inappropriate; however, often one of these dominates. In some people, the low oxygen level is the factor that is most apparent in their final hours or days. When this is the case, unless something is done to alter the situation, it is an extremely uncomfortable condition. "Air hunger" is a term that is used to describe how someone feels if the oxygen level is too low. This condition is very distressing, both for the patient and for family and friends who find themselves unable to relieve the suffering. Fortunately, even when the lungs are so damaged that nothing can be done to prevent the person's death, most often something *can* be done to relieve that terrible feeling.

The other problem that can occur is that the carbon dioxide level can become dangerously elevated. In this case, the high carbon dioxide level serves as a sedative, and the patient is relaxed, often asleep for much of the time. These people are not suffering. As the condition progresses, the person may fall very deeply asleep, as though under a general anesthetic. In this situation, the person may be difficult or impossible to awaken, may not respond to people in the room, and may die in his or her sleep. This is more difficult for people who are watching and waiting with the patients than for the patients themselves, since they are not uncomfortable.

WHAT CAN BE DONE?

If someone's oxygen level is low enough to be causing terrible air hunger and distress, one relatively simple thing is to give more oxygen to breathe. Although this is an obvious thing to do, it is not always done, because of physicians' concerns about its effects on how the brain controls breathing. You'll recall from Chapter 3, *The Respiratory System,* that when someone's lungs are badly damaged, and the carbon dioxide level has been high for some time, a low oxygen level may become the brain's main signal to keep breathing. Conscientious physicians will be concerned that if extra oxygen is given, it may raise the blood oxygen level enough that the brain will respond by inhibiting the signal to breathe hard. Breathing will then get progressively shallower, and the carbon dioxide level will build higher, putting the patient to sleep, perhaps so deeply that he or she will die.

There are several fallacies in these concerns. The first is that even when someone's carbon dioxide level has been high for some time, receiving extra oxygen *rarely* lowers the breathing level. Sometimes it even improves it (probably just by giving needed oxygen to the breathing muscles). The second essential point is that at this time, the primary concern should be for the patient's *comfort,* and sedating the person slightly by allowing the carbon dioxide to build up may, in fact, be helpful. The extra oxygen may change the situation from one in which low oxygen dominates, making the patient suffer, to one in which high carbon dioxide dominates, making the patient sedated and comfortable.

Another treatment for people who are suffering from low oxygen levels is the careful administration of a medication that can relieve the anxiety and discomfort. Morphine is the best drug for this purpose and is extremely effective. Its main danger is that too much of it can oversedate people to the point where they fall so deeply asleep that they don't wake up. Given carefully, the drug is not likely to cause this problem, and is very likely to relieve otherwise unbearable suffering. Its effects are often like those just discussed of administering oxygen: morphine and/or oxygen can sedate someone whose oxygen levels are intolerably low, making that person much more comfortable. Each medication alone or in combination with the other may also oversedate. Almost always, if a person is likely to be dying, the primary concern should be for the person's comfort.

MYTHS ABOUT DYING WITH CYSTIC FIBROSIS

There are a number of widespread misunderstandings about dying with CF that are important to mention and correct.

Choking

"My child (or I) may choke on thick mucus and die."

It is certainly true that thick mucus is a problem for people with CF, and that some children and adults with CF have very hard coughing spells, where it can look (and feel) as though they won't be able to catch their breath. However, *people with CF do not die by choking on their mucus.* In fact, a sudden unexpected death in CF is extremely rare. People with CF do not go to bed well and die during the night.

Predictions

"Doctors know when a person with CF is going to die."

It *is* possible to know that someone is getting sicker and that his or her pulmonary function has been declining for several months. Some statistics enable physicians to say that someone with these numbers for PFTs has a 50% chance of dying within the next two years. There are no PFT results (or other test results) that can give a higher-than-50% likelihood of dying within the next two years. In extreme conditions, experienced CF physicians may be able to say that someone is so sick that he or she is not likely to live many more hours or days. *It is never possible to be definite about the timing of death.* Physicians who have worked with CF patients for any length of time have seen patients who they thought could not possibly make it *through the night,* pull through and recover sufficiently to live for months or even years longer. For this reason, many CF physicians believe that when someone is extremely ill and is unlikely to recover, it is still worth giving as much treatment as possible to enable the lungs to recover (usually IV antibiotics, aerosols, and postural drainage)—*if these treatments do not interfere with the patient's comfort*. Certainly, very invasive and uncomfortable procedures and treatments, such as using a tube in the trachea and a mechanical ventilator, are not justifiable if the chances of recovery are extremely small. On the other hand, relatively simple treatments such as IV medications, which might give a person the slight chance of recovery and which would not interfere with comfort, should be given.

Pain

"Dying from CF is very painful."

If someone is dying with a very low oxygen level, that sensation of suffocation can be terrible. That sensation can most often be lessened considerably, though, by giving oxygen, and sometimes a sedative, perhaps morphine. There is usually no physical pain.

"It's better to die at home than in the hospital."

The idea is appealing of dying among loved ones, in a familiar setting, without strangers being present and suffering intrusive treatments. This can be arranged in most hospitals, though. When the patients, family, and physician have discussed all these matters and agreed on the approach, the procedures and medications necessary to keep the patient comfortable can be handled much more readily in the hospital. For extreme circumstances, the support of the hospital staff can be very comforting to patients and their families. In some communities, Hospice may be able to provide many of the necessary services, medications, and support in the home.

"It's important to keep fighting."

Very often, when someone with CF is dying, that person has lived for many years (usually decades) with the disease, has done much to stay well (exercise, postural drainage treatments, medications, etc.), and has been recognized as fighting against the odds. Family, friends, and the patients themselves think of them as "fighters," in the very positive sense of that word. Too often, however, in a family's grief over losing a very special person, they may convey to that person the idea that they *must* keep fighting, and not give in. It is usually not intended this way, but the message may come across that if the patient dies, he or she has let down the family. Sometimes, after a long fight, patients may need permission to let go, and rest. They need to know that they don't have the burden of supporting their surviving family.

TRANSPLANTATION AND DYING

While the advent of lung transplantation for patients with CF has brought hope to many, and has extended the life of some, it has greatly complicated the dying process for many others. If someone is dying, and is also awaiting transplant, there can be conflicting goals: for the dying patient, it has been traditionally believed that the humane approach was to stress *comfort,* even if that meant fewer days of life. For the hopeful transplant candidate, the goal sometimes changes to extending life day-by-day as long as possible until donor organs become available. In some centers, this life extension has included measures as drastic as tracheostomy and mechanical ventilation (often in a center hundreds of miles from home). Patients and families can be in a very difficult bind: do they forego the chance of extended life—with renewed health—that transplant represents, in favor of a peaceful, calm, and relatively comfortable death, or do they forego that peace, calm, and comfort for the possibility of years more of good life? The 2-to-3- year waiting list for donor lungs has made this decision all the more difficult.

PATIENTS' CONCERNS ABOUT DYING

Adolescents and adults with CF (and occasionally younger children with CF) may worry about death. It is important for them to have someone to be able to talk with about these concerns. Very often they may be worried because a friend or acquaintance has died, and it may be reassuring for them to hear of ways in which they are different from the person who died, and that they are not in danger of dying soon. On the other hand, it may be that their concerns are very realistic, and that they are in fact close to the end of their lives. In either case, it is extremely important for them to be able to confide in someone, and express their fears, and have their questions answered.

It is tempting for people who care a lot about patients to reassure them, and to try to cheer them up and turn their thoughts away from death and dying. It's fine to look on the bright side of things as much as possible, but you don't do a child (or adult) a service by refusing to talk about worries on his or her mind. It may be that just listening and being supportive can relieve someone tremendously. Many people have thoughts and worries about their own death, and it is helpful for those thoughts to be discussed openly. *It is not helpful, however, to force a discussion of death on someone who is not ready for it.* Parents, close friends, physicians, and other personnel at the CF center may be the people chosen to share in this kind of discussion.

The questions that children have about death may range from whether they will be in pain (on this point they can be reassured) to whether they will see their dead relatives. A family's religious beliefs will have a strong influence on what they will want to tell children about those questions.

REACTIONS TO THE DEATH OF SOMEONE
WITH CYSTIC FIBROSIS

When a loved one dies, family and friends have many different kinds of feelings. Sadness and grief for the lost loved one, and for the suffering that he or she might have gone through, are often accompanied by feeling sorry for oneself for having to go on without the person who has died. There is also commonly a feeling of relief, especially if the death comes after a prolonged difficult period. This relief may cause guilt, but it is a perfectly normal and healthy feeling. Parents who have lost a child with CF may have some renewed sense of guilt for having "caused" the CF, or for not having done more for their child. Again, these feelings are normal, but must be balanced by the realization that *no one causes a genetic disease,* and that, in most cases, families have done an outstanding job in caring for their children. It may be time to remember that until recently, all children with CF died before school age, and if their child lived a good life beyond that, it represents an improvement, due in great part to the parents' treatment.

Parents with other children with CF may be especially sad to think that what one child has just gone through will be repeated for the surviving sibling(s). This may be true. It is also true that treatment continues to improve, and surviving children may be able to be spared some of what their sibling has just gone through.

Surviving brothers and sisters have complex reactions, which may be confusing to them. They will be sad, of course. They may have a frightening feeling that they were somehow to blame for their brother's or sister's death because of "bad thoughts" they had had. It is important for them to know that all children at some times wish that their siblings were dead, or out of the way, so that they can have their parents' attention and love. They might be feeling especially guilty because they had wished these things and had felt that their parents favored the sick child. They need to know that these thoughts are normal, and that they are not bad for thinking them, and that they did not cause their sibling's death. It can be helpful to point out ways in which the surviving child was special to the sibling who has died.

If the surviving sibling has CF, he or she may be especially frightened about his or her own fate. In this case it is helpful to point out any differences that could indicate a better prognosis for the surviving child, and to assure him or her that you and the physicians will do everything they can to keep him or her well for as long as possible. It is important to give the child the chance to express worries, however, and give reassurances that you'll be with him or her.

POSTMORTEM EXAMINATIONS (AUTOPSIES)

A physician may request permission for performing an autopsy. This is very difficult to think about. The postmortem examination is very important when it was not clear why the patient died. In these cases, important information may be discovered, which may make it somewhat easier for surviving family members and friends. It is also possible that something might be discovered that could benefit other children or adults with CF.

ORGAN DONATION

When someone has died, it can provide a small bit of comfort to know that he or she may still be able to help someone who is alive but suffering. Organ donations for transplantation may offer this solace. Cystic fibrosis patients have been able to donate their eyes to enable others to see, and their hearts to enable others with terminal heart disease to live.

RESEARCH

As everyone who is reading this book now knows, the basic defect for CF is just now becoming understood, and there is no cure for CF, but many scientists around the world are working toward these ends. In some cases, the research can only be carried out with tissues from someone with CF. This means that it may be possible for organs from someone with CF to be donated to a research laboratory, in order to help answer the questions about CF to help future generations of people with CF. The fact that many, many patients and their families have asked that their organs or tissue be donated for CF research has been part of the reason we've learned so much about CF, and have come so much closer to improved treatments, to the point where we can think about a *cure*.

16

Research and Future Treatments

THE BASICS

1. CF research has increased our understanding of CF, and given new treatments.
2. Basic researchers (researchers working in the laboratory) are now looking into the different CF gene mutations, how the CF cells interfere with salt and water transfer, how CF cells might be made to act like they didn't have CF, and how to cure CF cells with gene therapy.
3. Clinical researchers (researchers working with patients) are looking into new ways of fighting infection, decreasing airway inflammation, thinning CF mucus, and transferring healthy genes into CF patients' cells.
4. Both researchers and patients have responsibilities to continue CF research.
5. New treatments will soon be available for fighting infection, reducing inflammation, and thinning mucus, continuing to improve the outcome for patients.
6. One day, gene therapy may be possible, and may cure CF.

Despite the tremendous improvement in the quality and length of life of patients with cystic fibrosis (CF), and the almost incredible advances in our understanding of the basic defects in CF cells, there is still a long way to go in understanding the disease enough to improve the treatment for it. The only way treatment will improve is through research, just as the current achievements in treatment were derived from previous research. Research into the various aspects of CF has become one of the most exciting areas in all of science, with some of the most creative scientists being attracted from other fields and now directing their attention to solving the many problems of CF. This chapter reviews the main areas of current research interest and progress, and the direction for future research, and then discusses future treatments.

Research is divided into two categories–clinical and basic. Clinical research deals directly with people, examining the effects of diseases or treatments on individual patients or groups of patients. Basic research, sometimes called "bench research," concerns itself with tissues, cells, and even molecules, and not the whole person. Basic research provides the foundation for clinical research. Both are essential for a complete understanding and satisfactory treatment of any disease, including CF. In the current era of CF research, the lines between basic and clinical research have been blurred: basic scientists work on ways to alter cells, and to deliver genes to cells, in the laboratory, and these techniques are quickly applied to people, to see if genes can be delivered to the cells of living people and if their cells can be altered in safe, healthful ways.

BASIC RESEARCH IN CYSTIC FIBROSIS

Genetics

Since CF is a genetically determined disease, finding the CF gene in 1989 was an extremely important step toward unraveling the mysteries of the disease, and therefore getting closer to solving them. A new science, molecular genetics, has enabled scientists to take apart human chromosomes in the laboratory, and discover what individual tiny portions of the genetic material do. As you've already learned earlier in this book, scientists were able to use these techniques, and work their way along chromosome number 7, focus in on the section that contains the gene for CF, isolate the tiny portion of the genetic material that actually determines whether someone has CF or not, and work with it to determine the chemical events it directs. You've also seen that scientists have discovered that there are over 500 different ways that the CF gene can be abnormal and produce CF! Even with this huge number of different mutations, several percent of CF patients have genes that have not yet been identified.

Work will continue to identify *all* of the CF mutations. Right now, the 500-plus mutations identified account for about 90% of cases of CF. Until we can get closer to 95% or higher, genetic screening tests for CF won't be good enough for general use.

Work will also continue to try to unravel how the different defects (*mutations*) in the CF gene determine the different defects in the cell, and will focus on ways of manipulating the cell to make the genetically abnormal cell act as though it were normal.

Salt Transport and CFTR Function

Exciting research is being conducted in laboratories around the world to figure out exactly why chloride cannot be secreted normally through epithelial cells, why sodium seems to be *overabsorbed* through airway cells, why these defects lead to the problems that occur in the affected glands and organs, and, finally, what might be done to reverse these cellular transport abnormalities. It seems that the diuretic medication amiloride blocks some of the overabsorption of sodium, and the chemicals UTP (uridine triphosphate) and CPX may increase chloride secretion by cells. These possibilities are being studied actively in several laboratories.

You may recall from Chapter 1, *The Basic Defect,* that the CFTR protein is produced within the cell, then must fold into a particular shape so that it can be transported to the cell membrane, where it does its job of allowing chloride to exit the cell (see Figure 1.4). You may recall further that some of the CF mutations create a situation where the CFTR protein doesn't get to the cell membrane, but if it is artificially placed there by researchers, it is able to work, to a certain degree. Various chemicals and conditions have been identified that help get the protein from where it's made to where it belongs. These substances are referred to as "chaperones" or "chaperonins," and they are an active area of research. It is intriguing to think there may be chemicals which patients might be able to take as medications that could get the CFTR protein to the cell membrane in millions of airway cells when otherwise those proteins would be "stuck" in the interior of the cell where they do no good.

Infection

Studies are going on at a basic level to try to understand what makes it easier for bacteria, including *Pseudomonas aeruginosa,* to stick to CF airway cells and therefore set up infection. Once the factors that promote this airway cell *adherence* are identified, it may be possible to undo them. Even before the full understanding is reached, at least one laboratory is studying *dextran,* a substance that seems to cut down on the adherence of *Pseudomonas* to airway cells.

Substances called *maganins* are an exciting group of chemicals being studied for their possible use in fighting CF infections. The discovery of this group of chemicals that appear to have very potent antibacterial properties is an example of serendipity (defined by my copy of Webster's as "an apparent aptitude for making fortunate discoveries accidentally") in science. Here, the serendipitous finding came from a scientist who was doing research that involved abdominal surgery on frogs. After the surgery, the frogs' bellies were rather crudely sewn back up, without any attention to sterile technique, before the frogs were put back into the dirty water in their tanks. One day it dawned on the researcher that an amazing thing was happening, or rather *not* happening: these frogs with fresh surgical wounds were being put into water that was teeming with bacteria, yet the wounds were not getting infected! Why? It seemed that the frogs must be producing very effective antibacterial substances that kept them uninfected. It turns out that this is the case, and this class of chemicals with antibacterial action has now been identified (and named: maganins). Scientists hope that these chemicals might have usefulness in fighting human (including CF) infections, too.

The history of medicine and science is filled with similar serendipitous findings.

Tissue Needed for Continuing Research

Investigators in several CF research centers are working with CF tissues in laboratories to answer these critical questions. Progress has been phenomenally fast, and yet it could be even faster if it were not for several problems: it is difficult to obtain enough tissue to work with. Even now that there are genetically engineered animals with abnormal CF genes, they are not the same as humans with CF. That means, for much of the research, tissue must still come from people with CF. Nasal polyps that are removed because they've blocked up the nose can be used, and lungs and livers that are removed from CF patients who are getting transplants provide a rich source of tissue for research. Still more is needed. Organs can be used from patients who die, but very few patients or families are aware of this latter possibility, and often CF physicians hesitate to bring up this potentially painful topic to a grieving family around the time of the death of a patient.

CLINICAL RESEARCH IN CYSTIC FIBROSIS

General

Scores of clinical research projects related to CF are continually being conducted. They may deal with any one of the problems seen with CF or its treatment. Some of the projects involve very few patients, while others involve national cooperative efforts among dozens of researchers and hundreds of patients. This chapter will review only a few of the more important areas of research, for an all-inclusive list is beyond the scope of this book. We can consider several main avenues of research, and as you'll see, some of the investigations span the gap between clinical and basic research.

Respiratory Research

Airway Infection

New antibiotics are constantly being developed. As they are developed, their effect in patients must be tested. At any one time there are several clinical trials in which CF patients are given a course of treatment with a new antibiotic or a new combination of antibiotics to determine the effect on outcomes such as pulmonary function, the types and quantities of bacteria found in the sputum, exercise tolerance, and length of hospitalization.

Airway Fluid Composition

The background for this section can be found in Chapter 1, *The Basic Defect.* Scientists working on understanding how CFTR works and how it malfunctions in CF cells (leading to *de*creased secretion of chloride and *in*creased absorption of sodium through airway cells) have been able to identify some chemicals that affect these abnormalities, in individual cells in the laboratory. These include amiloride, which partly blocks the overactive sodium channel (Figure 16.1A) and UTP, which appears to increase chloride secretion, not through the CFTR chloride channel, but through one of the alternative channels that is known as the calcium-dependent channel (Figure 16.1B). Amiloride aerosols have been studied in a fairly large number of patients, and the results were disappointing: some early studies hinted at a benefit, while other studies have not been able to confirm these

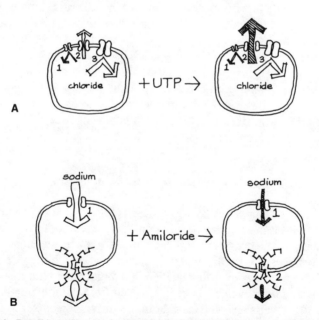

Figure 16.1. Possible treatments to alter airway fluid and salt contents. (**A**) The effect of UTP on chloride secretion is shown: UTP opens the calcium-dependent chloride channel, allowing chloride to leave the cell, even though CFTR remains closed or absent. (**B**) The effect of amiloride of sodium absorption is shown: amiloride decreases the amount of sodium brought out of the airway fluid through the cell, by decreasing the activity of the sodium pump. By increasing the amount of chloride and sodium that remains within the airways, the amount of fluid should also be increased, making for more watery, less thick secretions.

optimistic findings. Many researchers think that what might be needed is the *combination* of a sodium-absorption blocker (like amiloride) *and* a chloride-secretion enhancer (like UTP, or other chemicals that haven't reached the stage of clinical trials yet).

Airway Inflammation

Since inflammation within the bronchioles and bronchi is as important as the infection itself, research is now aimed at examining ways to decrease airway inflammation. (Important clinical studies have recently looked at the effect on pulmonary function of two different commonly used anti-inflammatory medications (prednisone and ibuprofen—see Appendix B: *Medications* and Chapter 3, *The Respiratory System,* for details).

Some of the inflammation in CF airways comes from the *proteases*—including elastase—released from the white blood cells that have been sent to fight infection. These proteases are chemicals that attack proteins, both the intended target—bacterial proteins—and also innocent bystanders—airway cell proteins. The airways of CF patients contain greater-than-normal amounts of proteases (especially elastase, which attacks elastin, an important structural lung protein) and proportionally less of the protease-neutralizing chemicals—*antiproteases* that the body usually produces to keep the proteases in check. The imbalance between elastase and the antiproteases in CF airways has been called the "elastase burden." There are now several different antiproteases that are being studied in CF patients. Studies with *alpha-1-antitrypsin (Prolastin®)* are under way, and several other antiproteases will soon be studied. The aim is to see if these drugs—taken by aerosol or IV—can decrease inflammation by decreasing the elastase in CF airways.

Airway Obstruction: Mucus-Thinning Agents

As you've heard many times, airway mucus is thick and sticky in people with CF, and therefore leads to airway obstruction. A large research effort culminated in the marketing of the drug DNase, which thins CF mucus in the test tube, and seems to help at least some CF patients in their day-to-day life. There are now at least two other drugs that are being studied that might do similar things. DNase works by degrading DNA that has been released from dying white blood cells. These white blood cells also add another important troublemaker to the airway secretions, namely, *actin*. Actin is the main substance in the skeleton of the white blood cells. Actin comes in long filaments, which—like the DNA—are to blame for a lot of the thickness and stickiness of CF airway secretions. Two substances—*gelsolin* and *thymosin β-4*—have been discovered that cut and untangle actin, and make CF mucus thinner (in the test tube). Eventually, studies will look at each of these drugs individually, and then in combination with each other, to see if they can safely thin mucus in CF patients.

Gene Therapy

As you read in Chapter 11, *Genetics,* gene therapy is placing a healthy gene into cells affected by an abnormal gene, and having that healthy gene take over the function of those cells. In CF, this would be getting a healthy CFTR gene into cells in order to correct the abnormalities in salt (sodium and chloride) and water traffic across the cell membranes. This would be most important in the lungs. Big strides have been made toward developing successful (safe and effective) gene therapy since the discovery of the CF gene in 1989: gene therapy *has worked* in the test tube, in individual CF cells, and it seems to have worked in CF mice. But it is a long way from here to having it work in human beings. Nonetheless, work continues, and most CF researchers think the day may come when gene therapy will provide a cure for CF.

Research is being conducted into a number of different questions regarding gene therapy, including:

- What is the best *vector* (or vehicle) to carry the healthy gene into CF cells? [The main vehicles being studied in 1996 are *adenovirus, AAV* (adeno-associated virus), and *liposomes* (specialized fat particles).]
- What is the best way to dampen the body's immune response to the virus (or other vehicle) so the body doesn't set up inflammation in response to gene therapy? Should this be done by modifying the body's immune system, or by designing a "stealth" virus that would not be recognized as "foreign" by the immune system, or perhaps by alternating two or more different families of viruses?
- Is there a way that gene therapy can be done once for a patient, or must it be done repeatedly?

There are currently many clinical trials going on around North America and Europe using various vectors to deliver healthy CF genes to the diseased cells of CF patients. Although these studies have the eventual *goal* of leading to gene therapy, it would be inaccurate to say that the trials going on now, and for the next few years, are actually *gene therapy* trials, because these trials are not really *therapy* (treatment): no one who goes into these current trials expects to be made more healthy by the trial. Rather, these are experiments to see if it is possible to get the healthy gene into cells in living CF patients, and to make the cells act as though they no longer have CF, while not causing harmful reactions. And the targeted cells are only a few. In many of the studies, the nose is the site targeted, while in a few others, it's a very small part of one lobe of one lung. The nose is used in so many of these studies because the cells lining the nose are the same as those lining the trachea and bronchi, and the inside of the nose is a lot easier to get to than the inside of the bronchi. Also, if there is inflammation or any other reaction, it should do less harm in the nose than in the lung. At any rate, even a wildly successful application of the gene transfer (the gene gets into the cells, the cells begin to conduct chloride and sodium normally, there is no inflammation, the viruses do not multiply and infect other cells), won't influence the patient-volunteer's health. So, we refer to these experiments as *gene transfer trials,* and try to avoid calling them "gene therapy," so that we don't give the mistaken impression of being a lot closer to a cure than we really are. Of course, *if* these trials are successful, there will then at some point in the future be trials of gene transfer to the whole of both lungs (perhaps by aerosol), with the hope of benefiting the volunteer's health. In fact, the prospect of eventual gene therapy has enabled us to talk of the possibility of a *cure* for CF for the first time since the disease was described half a century ago.

EXERCISE TOLERANCE

Exercise tolerance has its own category because it seems to be affected by many other factors, and seems to affect many other factors. Research into exercise has shown that exercise testing can be helpful in assessing a patient's progress before and after treatments of various kinds (hospitalization, exercise training programs, etc.). Exercise testing can also identify patients whose oxygen level may drop while they are active. Research in exercise tolerance has also led to the understanding that most patients with CF can exercise safely and receive the same benefits that their classmates and friends receive from a regular exercise program. Important research has also been done with regard to salt loss during exercise in the heat, leading to the recognition that people with CF can replace that salt perfectly well on their own without salt tablets or other forced salt replacement. More recent research showed that a patient's fitness level as measured in an exercise test correlated more closely than any other measure with the patient's likelihood of surviving for the next eight years. Future research will be directed at determining the type of exercise that is most helpful for patients with CF and whether exercise can improve lung function or delay its deterioration.

PSYCHOLOGY AND EDUCATION

Research studies in several centers are examining the psychological adjustment of patients with CF and their families. Several studies have shown that CF patients and their families are remarkably well-adjusted, and others are directed at understanding these strengths so that people with other chronic illnesses might benefit. Additional research is focusing on the best way to educate children with CF about their illness.

RESEARCH ETHICS

Investigators' Responsibilities

Many medical researchers feel a responsibility to do what they can to answer questions that will ultimately lead to better health and less suffering for people. They also have the responsibility of conducting their research so that its drawbacks are clearly outweighed by the potential benefits. (For basic research, the drawbacks are expenditure of limited research dollars and pain and suffering of laboratory animals, while for clinical research, the drawbacks are expense, patients' inconvenience, discomfort, and possibility of toxic side effects.) All federally funded research is evaluated for the balance of risks and benefits by Institutional Review Boards (sometimes called Human Rights Committees) of the hospital or university where the research is taking place.

Patients who are asked to participate in research must be given complete and understandable explanations of the research, including its possible risks and benefits. In most cases, patients or legal guardians must sign a "consent form," saying that they do understand, and that they are participating voluntarily.

Patients' Responsibilities

Patients and families have responsibility, first of all, to themselves. People have an absolute right to refuse to participate in research, for whatever reason they might have. It is worth mentioning, though, that for a disease like CF, where there is no animal that has the exact disease, and where there are relatively few patients with the disease (some 30,000 to 50,000 in the entire United States), it is essential that some people with the disease volunteer to help with research. If no one volunteers, the progress that is being made will come to a halt. Families who do participate in studies often feel that they reap large benefits from being a part of the research team that will eventually control CF. Yet, it is unfair for the burden of all the research studies to fall on a small group of people who participate time after time, while others never help. Patients associated with a large CF center are likely to have many research projects from which to choose, so they may easily participate in some, while skipping others. In 1994, 96% of CF centers participated in clinical research, and 33% of patients seen at these centers participated in at least one of these studies.

FUTURE TREATMENTS

There are a number of treatments that are currently under study, and it is possible to predict that these will be in use eventually. It is quite possible that other treatments that have not even been thought of may come to light over the next years.

Lung Therapy

Anti-infective Treatment

New anti-*Pseudomonas* antibiotics are continually being developed. Some of these antibiotics have already been employed successfully on a "compassionate-use" basis (this is when a not-yet-released drug can be used for a sick patient for whom no other drugs would work). It is conceivable that some of the other anti-infective avenues currently being investigated will lead to useful treatments. So, we might even see drugs derived from the *maganins* that frogs use so successfully. It is also possible that we'll see a therapeutic use for a preparation of dextran, or other agents that prevent the adherence of *Pseudomonas* to airway cells.

With the participation of many scientists and CF patients, clinical and basic research has helped answer many questions about CF and its treatment. The continued enthusiasm of researchers and patients will ensure the eventual success of understanding CF completely, developing optimum treatments and—one day—finding a cure.

Anti-inflammatory Treatment

The role for prednisone, ibuprofen, and perhaps other anti-inflammatory medications will continue to be worked out, and these drugs will likely find their niche in the treatment armamentarium for CF patients. It is likely that one of the now-experimental anti-inflammatory drugs, such as alpha-1-antitrypsin (Prolastin®), will also be employed to cut down on airways inflammation.

Mucus-Thinning Medications

Gelsolin and thymosin β-4 are likely to come into use, perhaps alone, perhaps together, perhaps together with DNase, in order to thin the airway secretions of CF patients.

Altering Airway Fluid and Salt Contents

We will probably see aerosol treatments with UTP and amiloride—or other medications that are designed to make the salt and fluid composition of CF airway secretions closer to normal (see Figure 16.1).

Gastrointestinal System: Liver

For the small number of patients with liver problems, it is likely that there will be wider use of ursodeoxycholic acid, and that it will be started earlier in patients who show any abnormalities of liver function. The technique of TIPS, discussed in Chapter 4, is also likely to be used in a few more patients.

SUMMARY

The participation of an ever-increasing number of superb scientists and CF patients has meant that both basic and clinical research has answered many questions about CF and its treatment. The research to date is paying off with improved treatment that will continue to improve the length and quality of CF patients' lives. The continued enthusiasm of researchers and patients will ensure that we will eventually understand CF completely, have optimum treatments and—one day— a cure.

17

The Cystic Fibrosis Foundation

THE BASICS

1. The CF Foundation (CFF) is the national organization that raises money to support CF research.
2. CFF research has been very helpful in increasing our understanding of CF, and should lead to better treatment.

The mission of the Cystic Fibrosis Foundation (CFF) is to fund the research to find a cure for cystic fibrosis (CF), as well as to improve the quality of life for people with CF by uncovering new means to treat and control this disease. Established in 1955 by a small group of parents and caregivers of CF-affected children, the CFF has grown into a voluntary health organization that, today, sponsors 112 specialty care centers and 10 distinguished research centers across the United States.

The medical/scientific program is the primary focus of the CFF. To ensure that its mission is met, the Foundation has fostered partnerships with caregivers, donors, volunteers and corporations, and is poised to take full advantage of the resources available.

FUND RAISING

The CFF receives no federal or state funds for its programs. Therefore, it fulfills the task of supporting medical research and care with its own fund-raising program. Fund raising is coordinated at the Foundation's national office and is implemented through a network of more than 56 chapters and branch offices across the country. These local fund-raising chapters, working with thousands of volunteers and staff, stage special events throughout the year—from black-tie dinners, to bowl-a-thons and the annual GREAT STRIDES walk.

The Foundation's national office has a list of fund-raising chapters, available upon request.

MEDICAL/SCIENTIFIC PROGRAM

Because research progress is the primary goal of the Foundation, a variety of funding mechanisms are used to support CF research, including multidisciplinary research centers, individual grants for basic and clinical research studies, graduate and postgraduate research training programs, and large-scale clinical trials to evaluate new CF treatments.

CFF Research Centers

In 1981, the CFF launched a program to establish a network of research centers focused on CF. The concept for these centers grew from the recognition that solving a complex disease like CF requires many scientists from different fields of research, working together to find the needed answers to cure this disease. This program is the first such initiative supported by a voluntary health organization and is endorsed by the federal government's National Institutes of Health (NIH).

By 1996, the number of research centers supported by the CFF reached 10. Scientists at these centers are studying many different aspects of the disease. Their research has resulted in such accomplishments as: identifying the CF gene and its protein product; determining abnormalities in the cells affected by the disease, and uncovering the mechanisms of lung infection and lung damage. Moreover, these centers have also been responsible for developing methods that will help scientists throughout the country pursue their own studies that will lead to new therapies to treat CF.

In 1993, in cooperation with the NIH, the Foundation established nine CF gene therapy centers. It is estimated that the combined federal and CFF commitment to these centers during their first five years will be in excess of $50 million. These "centers of excellence" are involved in developing new and effective delivery systems to administer normal copies of the CF genes to the airways of CF patients. They were the first federally established gene therapy centers dedicated to one disease. This major investment by the federal government reflects the confidence that individuals have for the prospects that gene therapy will cure CF.

Individual Research Grants

In addition to supporting a network of research centers, the CFF also recognizes the importance of stimulating and supporting research by individual scientists and institutions. To that end, the Foundation has been the sole catalyst for pushing the field of CF to the forefront of the scientific community by offering a number of avenues of research support.

1. *Research grants* provide support for pilot and feasibility projects ranging from basic laboratory investigations to clinical management of the disease. These grants are intended to enable investigators to obtain preliminary data so that they can competitively apply for support from other agencies.
2. *New investigator research grants* attract young scientists to the field of CF by supplying support while they are establishing their careers.
3. *Special research awards* are offered in response to special "Requests for Applications" by the CFF. The objective of these awards is to direct research efforts toward specific areas of CF-related research. The size of these awards can exceed $100,000 a year for up to three years for a single grant.
4. *Clinical research grants* provide support for studies to improve clinical management of CF, as well as to test various therapeutic approaches. As scientists unravel the basic defect that causes the disease, more and more opportunities exist for moving new drugs and products from the test tube to the bedside.
5. *The Harry Shwachman Cystic Fibrosis Clinical Investigator Award* provides the opportunity for young physicians to develop into independent clinical researchers. The award enables top candidates to have three years of active experience in CF-related studies.
6. *CFF/NIH Awards* fund highly meritorious CF-related research projects that have been approved by the NIH but cannot be supported by available funds. The CFF furnishes support for up to two years while investigators reapply to the NIH. As the NIH budget continues to shrink, the availability of this mechanism becomes increasingly important to the CF scientific community. It helps to ensure that research opportunities are not lost because of limited federal funds.

Fellowships

Training new investigators and caregivers to apply their talents to CF is a crucial priority of the Foundation. To that end, the CFF offers a variety of awards for individuals interested in CF-related careers.

1. *Research fellowships* offer postdoctoral training in basic or clinical research. Preference is shown to recent graduates or those just beginning their investigative careers.
2. *Clinical fellowships* provide up to two years of specialized academic training for new physicians with specialties in pulmonary or gastrointestinal medicine. These fellowships offer training on how to care for CF patients.
3. *Third-year and fourth-year clinical fellowships* provide additional years of research training for physicians who have committed themselves to specializing in CF care. This extra training will equip clinicians with the necessary background and tools to conduct the important research needed to bring and end to CF.

4. *The Dr. Leroy Matthews Award* supports outstanding newly trained pediatricians and internists to pursue clinical proficiency in CF-related subspecialties for up to six years.
5. *Student traineeships* are available to undergraduate and graduate students in the biomedical sciences as an introduction to the field of CF research.

Peer Review

To ensure that it invests in the best and most promising research, the CFF has established a model system for carefully reviewing each proposed project. Research applications are carefully reviewed by a committee of scientific experts where it is judged on the quality of the science and its potential importance to understanding CF.

The Foundation also devotes considerable effort to monitoring scientific advances in many different diseases and encouraging scientists to become involved in CF-related research. This is accomplished through special scientific meetings, interaction with professional societies, and preparation of materials for the scientific community at large. The Foundation's annual North American Cystic Fibrosis Conference attracts thousands of scientists and caregivers from around the world to discuss the latest advances in CF research and care. This forum encourages collaboration and provides a high level of information exchange.

The Foundation's efforts have contributed to a dramatic increase in the overall scientific interest in the field of CF among leading researchers. This has been evident in the increased number of research studies submitted to, and supported by, the Foundation and the NIH, as well as the actual advances made toward understanding the disease.

CLINICAL RESEARCH

The Foundation's Clinical Research Program, established in 1983, supports treatment-oriented research. The CFF has initiated many large-scale clinical trials involving thousands of people with CF. These studies have provided important information that has helped to refine CF care.

The program's intent is twofold. The first purpose is to support individual research studies, submitted through the Foundation's grants program, with research to be conducted through the network of CFF care centers. Through this mechanism, the Foundation has helped to carry out studies on the effects of exercise and nutrition on lung function.

The second part of the program involves large-scale clinical trials which are developed and managed by the Foundation and its medical advisors. These studies require the participation of many CFF care centers and hundreds of individuals with CF to evaluate new CF therapies. These trials generally represent the final stage of studying promising new treatments before their translation into standard medical care.

In addition, the CFF works closely with the pharmaceutical industry to promote the development of new therapies. Clinical data provided by the CFF Patient Registry (a confidential database) on every patient seen in the care center network is an invaluable resource for drug testing in CF patients. The data provide information leading to patient selection and trial design. Further, it keeps track of important factors after the drugs are approved by the Food and Drug Administration.

CYSTIC FIBROSIS FOUNDATION CARE CENTERS

The CFF Care Center Program is a nationwide network of more than 112 medical institutions (see Appendix F) where individuals with CF and their families can seek diagnosis, comprehensive specialized care, and long-term follow-up from professionals knowledgeable in the latest treatment advances in CF. Most centers are associated with major medical schools and teaching hospitals and offer a range of outpatient and inpatient services. As part of this care network, centers must meet specific CFF requirements in terms of staff, facility, and service. Centers are regularly reviewed by the CFF Center Committee. Staff at these care centers have specialized training related to CF. In addition, the Foundation keeps these professionals up to date on research and advances in care through special meetings and publications.

The CFF care center network is a key source for care and support of individuals with CF and their families. In addition, these centers are an important resource for research on CF and provide the environment for conducting clinical research on new treatments. Further, the CFF care centers are an important part of the education and training of health professionals who are interested in CF.

The center network of the Foundation has been heralded as being one of the finest models for taking care of patients with a chronic disease. The existence of these centers has greatly contributed to the improvement in the life expectancy and the quality of life for CF patients.

PARTNERSHIP WITH THE NATIONAL INSTITUTES OF HEALTH

Beyond the Foundation, research related to CF is also funded by the NIH, the leading supporter of biomedical research in the world. The CFF has carefully designed its programs to complement those CF-related programs of the NIH. In addition, the Foundation interacts regularly with the staff of the NIH to identify additional research opportunities related to CF and to encourage scientific interest in these areas. The Foundation's efforts have led to a series of NIH research meetings on CF and to a dramatic increase in the NIH support of CF studies. In 1996,

NIH support of CF-related research was more than $40 million. The Foundation will continue to work closely with the NIH to identify research opportunities and to support promising new studies.

OTHER FOUNDATION EFFORTS TO IMPROVE QUALITY OF LIFE

The Foundation's Public Policy and Consumer Affairs Programs address legislation and social concerns affecting individuals with CF. The CFF actively participates in developing and monitoring legislation at the federal and state levels to promote and protect the needs of people with CF and their families. One emphasis has been to advocate for increased federal investment in biomedical research. Activities include testifying on Capitol Hill in support of enhancing the budget of the NIH and orchestrating national letter-writing campaigns to Congress and the Administration. In turn, the NIH supports CF research that complements Foundation initiatives.

Several other health-care issues are also at the forefront of the Foundation's public policy agenda. The CFF continually strives to eliminate "preexisting condition" clauses from all health insurance programs. Another key Foundation platform is the effort to guarantee a "point-of-service" option in all health care packages so that individuals with CF may consistently receive care at accredited CFF care centers. Elimination of lifetime caps is also of paramount importance to the CF community. Eliminating maximum lifetime capitations from health insurance policies will help to ensure that families will not be destroyed financially as they deal with the complexities of this disease. Another issue that is also attaining heightened status is genetic discrimination; the CFF supports legislation to eliminate genetic discrimination in the workplace for adults with CF.

The CFF Consumer Affairs Program strives to address the practical and psychosocial issues surrounding individuals with CF and their families. Through direct contact with CFF staff and through educational pamphlets, individuals with CF and their families can obtain information on health care, insurance and managed care, college planning, state-supported "over-21" programs, and employment.

DIRECTIONS FOR THE FUTURE

Although it is impossible to predict when medical research will provide the answers needed to control CF, the CFF is approaching the future with an increasing sense of optimism, challenge, and vigor. It will continue its emphasis on research to understand CF and to develop therapies that will further improve the life of individuals with CF. This strategy will also continue to stimulate new and innovative research and to involve outstanding scientists in this effort.

To support its aggressive medical/scientific plans, the CFF is implementing new approaches to raising funds at the local and national levels. To be even more effective, the Foundation also seeks to involve more members of the community in its chapters and care centers.

The future directions of the CFF will continue to be shaped by its ultimate goal—to find a cure for cystic fibrosis. The outlook for individuals affected by this disease grows brighter every day. The ingredients necessary to reach this goal—the base of scientific knowledge, the research technologies, and the medical/scientific manpower—are now available. Research continues to progress as the Foundation seeks the answers needed to conquer this disease.

APPENDIX A

Glossary of Terms

aerosol A mist for inhalation, usually containing medicine. Aerosol mists may be made by an air compressor that blows air through a *nebulizer*, which contains liquid medicine, or may come from a handheld spray can.

airways The tubes that carry air in and out of the lungs. These tubes begin with the nose and mouth and include the trachea (windpipe), bronchi, and bronchioles.

alveoli The air sacs of the lung where gas exchange takes place.

anastomosis A surgically created junction between two structures. An example of an anastomosis is the junction formed between the donor and recipient airways during a lung transplant.

anorexia Loss of appetite.

anticoagulant A drug that prevents blood clots.

atelectasis Incomplete expansion of a portion of the lung, usually caused by mucous plugging.

BAL An abbreviation for bronchoalveolar lavage.

b.i.d. An abbreviation meaning "twice a day."

baseline One's normal state of health. The baseline or usual level of functioning includes a number of considerations, such as the amount of cough, exercise tolerance, and breathing effort. One's baseline health is often referred to for comparison. For example, after a pulmonary exacerbation, the goal of treatment is to return someone to his or her baseline state of health.

bicarbonate An acid-neutralizing juice that is normally produced by the pancreas.

biopsy A small tissue sample of an organ. For example, after liver transplantation, the physician may wish to examine a piece of the transplanted liver; the piece obtained is known as a biopsy sample. "Biopsy" can also be used as a verb: taking the small piece of the organ is called a biopsy.

blood gas The level of oxygen and carbon dioxide in the bloodstream, especially in the arteries. The term "blood gas" is also used to refer to the test and to the actual measurement of oxygen and carbon dioxide.

bronchi The tubes through which air travels between the trachea and the bronchioles.

bronchioles The smallest airways, connecting the bronchi to the alveoli. These airways differ from the bronchi in that they are smaller and have no cartilage to support them.

bronchoalveolar lavage Washing a fluid (usually sterile salt water) into a small airway through a bronchoscope and then sucking the fluid back into a container. The fluid mixes with cells and other materials in the airway and allows them to be examined in the laboratory.

bronchoscope An instrument that allows someone to look into the trachea and airways. There are two major types of bronchoscopes. The "rigid" bronchoscope is a steel tube that is placed through the mouth and into the trachea and airways. The "flexible" bronchoscope is a softer rubber and plastic bronchoscope that can be placed into the trachea and airways through either the mouth, nose, or endotracheal tube.

bronchoscopy   Looking into the airways using a bronchoscope.

bronchus   Singular of bronchi.

cardiopulmonary bypass   A heart-lung machine, used during cardiac surgery temporarily to take the place of the heart and lungs.

cardiovascular system   The heart and blood vessels.

central line   A kind of intravenous catheter that extends into a very large vein, or even into the heart.

cilia   The tiny hairs in the nose, trachea, and bronchi, which, through their coordinated movement, help keep the airways clean.

clubbing   An abnormal shape to the tips of the fingers and toes, which is associated with many different conditions, including cystic fibrosis.

cyst   A fluid-filled sac.

dehiscense   The breakage of an anastomosis.

diaphragm   The main breathing muscle. The diaphragm is located at the bottom of the lungs, and separates the chest from the abdomen.

digestion   The process of breaking foods down into particles that are small enough to be absorbed through the intestinal wall into the bloodstream.

donor   A person donating tissue for transplantation; the person from whom a transplanted organ comes.

ectasia   Abnormal distention or enlargement. Bronchi*ectasis* is abnormal widening of the bronchi.

-emia   A suffix meaning "in the blood." Thus, hypox*emia* means lower than normal oxygen level in the blood.

enzymes   Chemicals that help perform biologic processes in the body; "enzymes" usually refer to digestive enzymes, which are the chemicals formed in the pancreas which break down food into absorbable particles.

esophagus   The tube that connects the mouth to the stomach.

fellow   A physician in training for a subspecialty. A fellow has completed medical school, internship, and a specialty residency.

fibrosis   Scarring.

flaring   Nasal flaring.

gas exchange   The process of bringing oxygen into the bloodstream and removing carbon dioxide.

gastrostomy   A surgical opening through the abdominal wall into the stomach. A tube is placed through this opening, which allows feedings to be given through the tube.

GE reflux   Gastroesophageal reflux. A process in which fluid moves backward from the stomach into the esophagus.

graft   Tissue from one person placed into a second person. An example is a lung graft, in which a lung from one person (donor) is placed into a second person (recipient).

heart failure   A condition in which the heart is not able to pump its full load of blood, resulting in the backup of fluid. Heart failure is *not* heart stoppage.

hemoptysis   Coughing up blood.

hep lock   (*see* Glossary of Drugs in Appendix B). An intravenous needle whose end can be plugged while it is not being used for medication administration.

hyper   A prefix meaning "more than normal." Thus, a *hyper*active child is more active than normal.

hyperalimentation   This term literally means "overfeeding," but actually refers to the method of giving extra nutrition through an IV.

hypo   A prefix meaning "less than normal." Thus, *hypo*xia means less oxygen than normal.

IM   Intramuscular. A way of administering medicine by injection into the muscle.

immunosuppression   Decreasing the immune response, usually using medications known as immunosuppressives.

intern   A physician who has graduated from medical school, and is training in a medical specialty such as pediatrics, internal medicine, family medicine, or surgery.

internal medicine   The branch of medicine dealing with the general health of adults.

internist   A medical specialist in internal medicine (not to be confused with an *intern*).

-itis   A suffix meaning "inflammation." Thus, bronch*itis* means inflammation of the bronchi.

IV   Intravenous. This can mean the way a drug is given (IV) or the actual tubing used to give the drug ("the IV").

jejunostomy   A surgical opening made through the abdominal wall into the jejunum. This opening is used to hold a tube for feedings, as is a gastrostomy.

jejunum   The second part of the small intestine.

larynx   The part of the upper airway that contains the vocal cords—the "voice box."

lobe   The largest division of the lung. The right lung has three lobes and the left has two.

lumen   The inside of a tube. The lumen of the bronchial tubes is where the air flows.

lymphocyte   A type of white blood cell. Lymphocytes are important in immune function and are involved in rejection of grafts.

mucociliary escalator   A mechanism for keeping the lungs clear. Particles get trapped in the mucus, and the cilia move the mucus out of the lungs.

mucous   Having properties like mucus. ("Mucus" is a noun; "mucous" is an adjective.)

mucus   The slimy fluid secreted in many glands of the body, and whose function appears to be to protect and lubricate.

nasal flaring   Widening of the nostrils with each breath (often abbreviated, "flaring"). This is a sign that someone is working harder than normal to breathe.

nebulizer   A device used with an air compressor that directs the compressed air past liquid medication, lifting the medication into a mist ("aerosol") for inhalation.

NG tube   Nasogastric tube. A tube that passes through the nose into the stomach. This tube is used for feeding someone who can't eat, for continuous feeding during sleep, or for the administration of other substances such as medicines.

panresistant   Resistant to all tested antibiotics.

peak   The highest level that a drug reaches in the bloodstream.

PFT   Pulmonary function test.

pneumothorax   Collapsed lung caused by a hole in the lung. Air escapes from the lung through this hole, collects within the chest, and presses in on the lung.

pulmonary exacerbation   An episode of worsening of the lung disease, usually caused by worsened bronchial infection.

pulmonology   The branch of medicine dealing with breathing problems.

recipient   A person receiving tissue for transplantation.

reflux   The backward movement of fluid; this term is often used to refer to *gastroesophageal reflux*.

rejection   The body's attempt to destroy transplanted tissue. Rejection is carried out by lymphocytes, which are immune cells capable of causing damage to foreign cells.

resident   A physician who has completed medical school and is undertaking further training in a medical specialty.

resistant   This term means "not killed by" when used to describe bacteria's relation to an antibiotic. For example, the statement, "*Pseudomonas* bacteria are resistant to penicillin," means that, in the laboratory, penicillin does not readily kill *Pseudomonas*.

respiratory failure   The condition in which blood oxygen levels are too low and blood carbon dioxide levels are too high.

retracting   The pulling in of skin between the ribs with each breath, indicating hard breathing.

saline   Salt water (see Appendix B).

sedation   A state of reduced excitement, anxiety, and (often) a state of mildly reduced consciousness. A variety of drugs are used to produce sedation, and are commonly used to decrease anxiety during medical procedures.

segment   The second largest division of the lung. Each lobe is divided into several segments.

sensitive   This term means "killed by" when used to describe bacteria's relation to an antibiotic. For example, the statement, "*Strep* bacteria are sensitive to penicillin," means that, in the laboratory, penicillin kills *Strep*.

specialty (or medical specialty)   One of the main branches of medical practice in which physicians can become trained and qualified. The specialties are pediatrics, internal (adult) medicine, obstetrics/gynecology, surgery, psychiatry, and family medicine. Physicians may focus their skills and training in more specialized areas, called *subspecialties,* such as pediatric pulmonology, cardiology, and neurosurgery. (A pediatric pulmonary specialist must first become a pediatrician; a neurosurgeon must first become a surgeon.)

sputum   Mucus from the lungs which is coughed up and spit out.

stenosis   Narrowing. In transplantation, stenosis can occur at an anastomosis, for example, where a donor bronchus is attached to the recipient bronchus.

stoma   A hole, usually one created purposely by a surgical procedure. This word is often used as a suffix: tracheo*stomy* is a hole made in the trachea; gastro*stomy* is a hole through the abdominal wall into the stomach.

toxicity   Harmful effect(s). This term is often used to refer to the undesirable effects of a medication.

TPN   Total parenteral nutrition. This term refers to nutrition given through an IV (same meaning as *hyperalimentation*).

trachea   The tube that carries air from the mouth and throat into the chest, where it connects with the bronchi from each lung.

tracheostomy   A hole placed in the trachea.

trough   The lowest level that a drug reaches in the bloodstream (this level is found immediately preceding a dose of the drug).

ventricle   One of the two main portions of the heart. The right ventricle pumps blood through the lungs, and the left ventricle then pumps the blood to the rest of the body.

APPENDIX B

Medications

Your physician knows the most about your treatment needs and will prescribe the best medications for you. *No medications should be taken without the advice of your physician.* Contact your physician if you have questions about the medications described.

INTRODUCTION

This appendix is organized according to the systems of the body; for example, the antibiotics used to combat lung infection are discussed under *Respiratory System Medications: Lungs*, and digestive enzymes are discussed under *Gastrointestinal and Digestive System*. There is a separate category for medications used specifically for people who have gotten an organ transplant. For each medicine discussed, there is information on how the drug is taken as well as possible side effects or dangers.

The most common method of taking the drugs described in this Appendix is by mouth. Some medicines can be given by injecting them into a vein (IV, for *intravenous*) or into a muscle (IM, for *intramuscular*). Others can be taken as *aerosols*, and breathed into the lungs, or sniffed into the nostril, while still others may be applied directly to the skin.

A word about side effects: Every medicine has *potentially* serious side effects. There is *no* drug that has only good effects, and absolutely no dangers. However, all the drugs discussed here have passed numerous tests, which, to most doctors and scientists, will mean that the drug's benefits outweigh their risks. Most people are able to take most of the medicines in this book without experiencing any serious problems. The "undesirable effects" noted for each drug are not meant to frighten you but to help you be as well informed as possible about your medications.

Drug names (generic names and the trade names given by the drug companies) are listed in the *Glossary of Drugs* at the end of *Appendix B*.

RESPIRATORY SYSTEM MEDICATIONS

Lungs

Antibiotics

Antibiotics are drugs used to fight infections caused by bacteria. They do not kill other kinds of germs, such as viruses and fungi. There are many different families of antibiotics, several methods of taking antibiotics, and certain unwelcome effects with which you should be familiar. These areas are all discussed below.

Perhaps two introductory words should be said about antibiotics and undesirable effects: the first is that antibiotics kill or control bacteria; that is their job, and they are usually very good at it. However, antibiotics can't tell good bacteria from bad. Everyone does have some good bacteria in the body, especially in the mouth and intestines. Among other things, these good bacteria keep people from becoming overrun with funguses and yeasts. Sometimes while someone takes antibiotics, the good bacteria are killed along with the bad. When this happens, a yeast infection can take hold, with a cheesy-looking material in the mouth or vagina. The condition is referred to as *thrush* when it occurs in the mouth. Generally, these yeast infections are easily dealt with, but your doctor needs to know about them in order to prescribe the right medicine (usually nystatin). The same problem of killing the good bacteria can also cause trouble in the intestines, and some patients develop diarrhea from antibiotics.

The last point to mention is that with the availability of so many new medicines, it is possible that new side effects can appear that have not been seen or recorded. If you develop *any* disturbing symptoms or problems shortly after you've started taking a new antibiotic, it may be from the new drug and you should let your doctor know about it.

Penicillins

This family was first used in the early 1940s and was one of the earliest groups of drugs to be used to fight infection in people. The number of drugs included in this family has grown tremendously over the past 30 years. New members of the penicillin family keep appearing, so it is impossible to list them all. Although the members of the penicillin family have distinct, individual personalities, there are a number of shared characteristics. The most important of these is that if you are allergic to any one penicillin, there is a strong chance that you will be allergic to all of them.

1. *PENICILLIN* The first in its family (as you might have guessed from the name), this drug kills many germs, especially *Streptococcus (Strep)* and *Pneumococcus* (the "pneumonia germ"). These bacteria are not the major problem bacteria for CF patients. The most common causes of CF patients' bronchial infections are *Haemophilus, Staphylococcus (Staph)*, or *Pseudomonas*, and penicillin is usually not effective in treating these infections.
   How taken: Penicillin can be given by mouth, by IV, or IM.
   Undesirable effects: Allergic reactions to penicillin can be mild, but can also be very serious. Any of the drugs in this family can cause a reaction in someone who is allergic to penicillin. Penicillin injections are painful. Other than these two problems, penicillin is remarkably gentle to the human body while being brutally hard on the unwelcome bacteria.
2. *AMPICILLIN* Ampicillin kills *Haemophilus* (also called *H. flu*) in addition to the bacteria which penicillin kills. It does not usually kill *Staph* or *Pseudomonas*.
   How taken: Ampicillin is most commonly taken by mouth. It can also be given by IV or IM injection.
   Undesirable effects: Loose stools are fairly common in people taking oral ampicillin. A skin rash may appear in some people, too, even if they are not actually allergic to the penicillins.
3. *AMOXICILLIN* This is a slightly different version of ampicillin; it kills the same bacteria, but is given only by mouth, and is less likely to cause diarrhea.
4. *AUGMENTIN* This combines amoxicillin with another chemical, clavulanic acid, and makes it effective against *Staph* in addition to the usual bacteria which are killed by amoxicillin.
5. *METHICILLIN, OXACILLIN, NAFCILLIN* These three drugs have been modified so that they kill *Staph* very well. They do not usually kill *Haemophilus* or *Pseudomonas*.

How taken: These drugs are used mostly by IV, but can also be given IM. Oxacillin and nafcillin have some effect if taken orally (but not as much as cloxacillin or dicloxacillin, discussed next).

Undesirable effects: These drugs are irritating to the tissues where they are injected. They can cause discomfort as they go into a vein.

6. *CLOXACILLIN, DICLOXACILLIN* These are also good anti-*Staph* drugs, used only by mouth. Otherwise they are similar to the other anti-*Staph* penicillins.

7. *CARBENICILLIN, TICARCILLIN, PIPERACILLIN, MEZLOCILLIN, AZLOCILLIN* These are anti-*Pseudomonas* drugs. They generally do not kill *Staph*, but they do kill *Haemophilus*.

How taken: Almost always given IV. They can be given IM, but most people feel this is not a practical way to administer the drugs over the relatively long period of time (1–3 weeks or longer) for which they are usually used. Carbenicillin can also be given by mouth for treating bladder infections, but none of the drug gets to the lungs if it's taken by mouth. Therefore, orally, it is not effective in treating CF *Pseudomonas* bronchial infections. Occasionally, these drugs are given by inhalation.

Undesirable effects: In addition to the possibility of allergic reactions in people who are allergic to penicillin, and the irritation these drugs can cause when they are injected, there are some other problems which occasionally arise. These medicines can make liver tests appear abnormal; fortunately, however, the problem is only with the lab result and not with the liver itself. The liver continues to function normally, and if the medicine continues to be given, the tests will return to normal. These antibiotics can also interfere with the function of platelets (blood cells which are responsible for proper clotting of blood).

8. *TIMENTIN* This combines ticarcillin with clavulanic acid, the way Augmentin combines it with amoxicillin, to make the ticarcillin effective against *Staph* in addition to *Pseudomonas* and *Haemophilus*.

9. *ZOSYN* This is similar to Timentin, in that it takes an anti-*Pseudomonas* penicillin—piperacillin, in this case—and combines it with a chemical (tazobactam in this case) that enables the drug to kill *Staph* in addition to *Pseudomonas*.

Sulfa Drugs

These were the first antibiotics ever used to fight infections in people, and they still have many uses.

1. *SULFISOXAZOLE* This drug can help in some infections with *Haemophilus,* but it is of little use in fighting *Pseudomonas.*

How taken: By mouth.

Undesirable effects: Problems with this drug are not common. Some people have allergic skin reactions.

2. *TRIMETHOPRIM-SULFAMETHOXAZOLE (TMP-SMX)* This is a combination of two drugs. Trimethoprim is not a sulfa drug, but the combination is quite effective in treating several kinds of bacteria, usually including *Haemophilus*. It is not usually effective for infections caused by *Staph* or *Pseudomonas.*

Aminoglycosides

This family includes gentamicin, tobramycin, neomycin, kanamycin, amikacin, and netilmicin. Many kinds of *Pseudomonas* infections can be treated effectively with these drugs, especially with gentamicin, tobramycin, amikacin, and netilmicin. These drugs seem to be particularly helpful in killing *Pseudomonas* if they are given with an anti-*Pseudomonas* penicillin.

How taken: Almost always given by aerosol, or IV or IM injection since these antibiotics are not absorbed well into the bloodstream if they are taken by mouth. Shots into the muscle with these drugs are not as painful as with the penicillins.

Undesirable effects: The two main problems with these drugs are their effects on the kidney and the ears. These problems are usually (but not always) avoidable if the blood levels of the drug are checked and dosages adjusted to keep the blood levels in what is considered to be the safe range. (Levels do not need to be checked if gentamicin or tobramycin is used by inhalation, since almost none of the drug gets absorbed into the bloodstream from the bronchi.) The kidney problems are usually just abnormal lab results, and are not uncomfortable for the patient. The ear problem is worsened hearing. The harmful kidney effects almost always disappear if the drug is stopped (or the dosage reduced). If the drugs are continued after the hearing or kidney damage has begun, there can sometimes be serious and permanent damage.

Chloramphenicol

This is one of the most powerful and effective antibiotics available for use in CF patients. It kills *Haemophilus,* some *Staph,* and another family of bacteria called anaerobes (bacteria that live without oxygen). It generally does not kill *Pseudomonas.* Despite this fact, it often is helpful in CF patients whose main infection seems to be *Pseudomonas.* It is not known if this is because those patients have other bacteria which are not found on culture (like the anaerobes, which are difficult to culture in the lab). Because of its serious side effects, it should never be taken without your doctor's direct instruction.

How taken: By mouth or IV.

Undesirable effects: This drug has developed a bad reputation because of some real dangers and because of a lot of misuse. Some pharmacists who are not aware of its benefits in CF patients may even try to convince you not to take it! There are two main problems with chloramphenicol, both having to do with the body's production of blood: in rare instances (less than one case in 40,000 courses of treatment), the production of blood cells may be shut off completely and irreversibly. If this happens, it is nearly always fatal. Another much more common blood-production problem is that, in many people, taking large doses for more than 2 weeks can result in the slowing down of the production of blood cells and lead to anemia. This problem is very different from the complete shut off of blood production, for this slow production always returns to normal after the drug is stopped. Most doctors check blood counts in their patients on "chloro" to detect if blood cell production is slowing down. There are a few other less common, nuisance-type problems, including a tingling feeling in the fingers and some rashes. Rarely, it can cause blurry vision and very rarely, blindness. Most of the serious problems with chloramphenicol have arisen when it is used inappropriately. Furthermore, there is strong evidence that this drug can be extremely effective in treating patients with CF lung infection when other antibiotics have not helped. Most CF doctors feel that the strong chances of its helping to stop or limit lung damage outweigh the small chance of a serious problem with it. However, it has become difficult to obtain because it is rarely used in non-CF patients.

Cephalosporins

This family of antibiotics is growing even faster than the penicillins. Most members of this family are helpful in combatting infections with *Strep, Staph,* and *Haemophilus.* Some of the newest members of this family have some activity against *Pseudomonas.* To preserve space, only a few of the more commonly used cephalosporins are listed here (but a more complete listing is in the glossary).

How taken: Cephalexin and cefaclor are both taken by mouth only. Cephalothin, cephaloridine, ceftazidime, and ceftaxime are given only by injection (IM or IV).

Undesirable effects: About one-third of people who are allergic to penicillins will also be allergic to cephalosporins. Other problems are fortunately not common, but include diarrhea or other stomach/intestinal upset.

Erythromycin

These drugs are most commonly substituted for penicillin in people who are allergic to penicillin. They kill *Strep,* many *Staph* and *Haemophilus,* and several other bacteria which aren't big problems in CF. They do not kill *Pseudomonas,* but may decrease the inflammation caused by *Pseudomonas.*

How taken: Erythromycins are most often taken by mouth, but IV forms are also available.

Undesirable effects: Abdominal cramping is sometimes an effect of these drugs, and some years ago there was a scare about liver damage with some erythromycin preparations. It now seems that liver damage is not very likely with this medicine.

Tetracyclines

The tetracyclines were among the first drugs available which had any effect against *Pseudomonas.* They are no longer as helpful as they once were because many bacteria have become resistant to their effects. There are still some *Pseudomonas, Staph, Haemophilus,* and *Strep* bacteria that are sensitive to tetracyclines.

How taken: The tetracyclines are usually taken by mouth, but can be given by IV or IM injection.

Undesirable effects: The main undesirable effect of tetracycline, one that's known to those CF patients in their 30s, is that if it's given to people between the ages of approximately 4 months and 8 years, it can permanently stain their teeth a grayish/brownish/yellow color. Twenty years ago, physicians knew about the tooth problem, but often didn't have any other antibiotics to give, so they had to use a tetracycline. Fortunately, today there usually is another antibiotic available, and tetracycline should almost never be used in young children. Other side effects include allergic reactions, intestinal upset, and a rash that is made worse by being exposed to the sun.

Quinolones

This family of antibiotics has some activity against *Pseudomonas* in the lung, even when the drugs (especially ciprofloxacin) are taken by mouth.

How taken: Several of these medications can be taken by mouth.

Undesirable effects: Remarkably few side effects have been recognized with these antibiotics. To date, intestinal upset has been seen occasionally. Another problem seems to be that bacteria become resistant to the quinolones very soon after the patient starts to take them (within a week or two). Young animals given these drugs have developed some problems with the cartilage in their joints, so most physicians are reluctant to prescribe the drugs for young children. These drugs may also cause a skin rash with sun exposure.

Imipenem

This drug has activity against *Pseudomonas, Staph, and Haemophilus,* and seems relatively safe and efective.

How taken: This drug is given by IV.

Undesirable effects: Imipenem can make the vein tender, and may cause nausea, particularly while it is running in.

Aztreonam

This drug is one with some anti-*Pseudomonas* activity; it seems to be safe and effective.

How taken: Aztreonam is taken by IV injection.

Undesirable effects: The side effects of this drug have been few and not very serious. They have included diarrhea, nausea, allergic reactions, and tenderness at the site of injection.

Bronchodilators ("Asthma Medicines")

Some people with CF also have asthma, or a condition like asthma, where the bronchi can become partly blocked for a time when the bronchial lining becomes inflamed and swollen and the muscles surrounding the bronchi squeeze down. Bronchodilators are medicines that open (dilate) the bronchi by relaxing the muscles around them. The medicines are effective in treating bronchospasm once it starts and help to prevent it from occurring. Some of these drugs can be taken by inhalation, some by injection (either IM, IV, or under the skin), some by mouth, and some by several different methods. Bronchodilators seem to help some people with CF, while not being effective in others.

Beta-Agonists

This is the name applied to a class of very helpful bronchodilators, including albuterol and others.

How taken: These drugs are best taken by inhalation (either from a handheld cannister-type nebulizer—usually called a *metered-dose inhaler,* or just *MDI,* or from the air-compressor type of aerosol machine). They can also be taken by injection or by mouth (pills or liquids), although the beneficial effects tend to be less and the side effects more than if they are used by inhalation.

Undesirable effects: The three main undesirable effects of this class of drugs are (1) shakiness, which often goes away with continued use of the drugs; (2) overactiveness (getting "hyper"), a fairly uncommon side effect; and (3) stimulation of the heart, causing it to speed up, which can be somewhat annoying. It may also cause an irregular heartbeat, which can be dangerous. Dangerous effects are uncommon if the drugs are taken by mouth or by inhalation. In the 1960s, a number of deaths were reported in patients with asthma who used their handheld nebulizers of beta-agonists too much. It's not clear what caused these deaths, but there are two likely reasons: it may have been the chemical used to make the aerosol, and not the bronchodilator itself; or, it may have been that patients got such good relief from the inhalations that they didn't see their doctor for a very serious asthma attack, but instead kept puffing on their aerosols, even when the effect lasted a shorter and shorter time. When they finally did try to go for help, they were too sick. Today, the vehicle for delivering the aerosol is safer. However, there is still a danger if a patient with asthma or CF tries home-prescribed antibiotics, bronchodilators, etc. While they may seem to work at first, they can lead to serious consequences. Talk to your doctors about medicine changes, in order to avoid dangerous combinations or dosages, and to avoid overlooking a serious problem for which you should be seen.

Theophyllines

This family of bronchodilators is a large and excellent one. However, there may be some confusion dealing with dosages and preparations, since almost every drug company has its own version of theophylline, with a similar name but different dosage. In addition, people process theophyllines at different speeds. In one person, 100 mg may reach a good level in the bloodstream and stay there for a long time, while in another, it may give only a low level and be gone quickly. For this reason, doctors often like to check a blood level of theophylline, to see if someone needs more or less than the average to reach a level in the bloodstream that is effective and safe.

Some theophyllines are short-acting, and are eliminated from the body quickly. Others are released slowly, and stay in the body longer. The short-acting theophyllines usually need to be given 4 times a day (about every 6 hours), while the slow-release or sustained-release kind can be given 3 times a day (every 8 hours), or even (especially for older children, adolescents, and adults) twice a day, and still keep a good blood level for many hours.

How given: Theophylline can be given in the vein ("aminophylline"), or by mouth as a liquid, tablet, or capsule. There are preparations that can be given rectally, like an enema. Usually the rectal kind is not as safe, since it's harder to predict just how much will be absorbed into the bloodstream.

Undesirable effects: There are two main side effects: some people get stomach upset with this family of medicines, and may lose their appetite, or even vomit. Nausea or vomiting can be important signs that the person is getting too much theophylline. People with CF may be more likely than other people to have this stomach upset with theophyllines. Some children also become agitated or overactive when they get too much of this drug. These side effects are quite common. However, if the drug is started (or restarted) at a very low dose, then raised very slowly, most people will be able to tolerate relatively high levels of the drug. A very large overdose can cause seizures (convulsions), a danger which, fortunately, is rare. These drugs are used much less frequently than they were ten years ago.

Anti-inflammatory Medications

Steroids

Steroids, also called "corticosteroids," are cortisonelike drugs whose name strikes fear in the hearts of many people because of the serious side effects caused by improper use. Actually, steroids can be extremely useful and very safe if used properly. In fact, everyone's body makes these drugs themselves and they are extremely important in maintaining health. They are very potent agents for decreasing inflammation and swelling within the bronchi (and elsewhere). In asthma, they also seem to increase the sensitivity of the body to the effects of the beta drugs. The inhaled, nonabsorbed steroids have become *the* "front-line" treatment around the world for people with asthma. It's not yet clear if they will also be helpful for people with CF.

How taken: Steroids can be taken by mouth (pills or liquid), by IV injection, or by inhalation. The inhaled steroids, beclomethasone, triamcinolone, and others, affect the bronchi by *preventing* inflammation and bronchoconstriction, much more than by reversing inflammation and bronchoconstriction once they've started. Almost none of the inhaled steroid is absorbed into the bloodstream, so it has very little toxic effect on the rest of the body. There are many different schedules for taking steroids. They can be given several times a day, once a day, or once every other day. They can be given for a brief period—a 3- to 5-day "burst"—or for months. The schedule depends on the drug being used, what it is being used for, and the characteristics and needs of the person taking it.

Undesirable effects: There are many possible effects including greatly increased appetite and swelling ("chipmunk cheeks"), acne, slowed growth in height, increased possibility of developing diabetes, eye cataracts, bone brittleness, and difficulty in fighting infection. In general, the lower the dose and the shorter the length of time steroids are given the less likely one is to develop side effects. When these drugs are used by mouth or injection for longer than a week, the body begins to detect them and seem to say, "Well, we don't need to make any more of our own." If the drug is then stopped abruptly, the body is left without the protection of its own steroids. For this reason, if steroids are required for more than 6 or 7 days, you can't suddenly just stop the drug; instead, you need to reduce (taper) the amount you take over several days or even weeks (depending on how long you've been on them, and how used your body has become to receiving them from an outside source) so that your body gradually gets used to the idea of having to make steroids on its own again. If the drugs are used for less than a week, they can be stopped abruptly with an extremely small likelihood of side effects. Another way to get around most of the side effects is to take the drugs every other day. This gives the body a day to recover between doses. In some cases, when steroids are really needed, a patient may not be able to tolerate being off them for that in-between day.

Cromolyn and Nedocromil

These drugs don't actually relax the muscles around the bronchi, but may be very effective in preventing certain bronchoconstricting chemicals from being released in the body. They seem to help about 60% of patients with asthma or asthmalike conditions. There is no way of telling which patients will be helped by them, except by trying.

How taken: These drugs are almost always taken by inhalation, either from a liquid aerosolized in a regular air compressor/nebulizer, or—most commonly—from a handheld metered-dose inhaler.

Undesirable effects: A few patients may have some bronchial irritation from these medicines if they are inhaled in the powdered form. Otherwise, they are unlikely to cause any trouble.

Mucolytics

Lysis means destruction or decomposition of a substance, so *muco*lytics are drugs that destroy or break down mucus. Since much of the lung trouble in CF has to do with extra-thick mucus, a completely safe and completely effective mucolytic for the lung would be wonderful.

There isn't such a drug now. However, there's one that comes closer than anything previously available. When one drug, DNase (Pulmozyme®) is put in a glass test tube with CF lung mucus, it breaks down the mucus, making it much more watery, and easier to move. It seems to help some patients, and even has improved lung function in several hundred patients over a period lasting six months. Other patients have not had measureable improvements in pulmonary function, but have *felt* better. Very few patients are harmed by it. Not everyone with CF is helped by it, and it is impossible to predict who will benefit. It is extremely expensive ($12,000 per year).

How taken: This drug is always given by inhalation.

Undesirable effects: A very few patients with very severe lung disease, and a large amount of thick mucus, may have trouble handling that mucus if it is suddenly all liquefied at once. This is uncommon.

Mucomyst® (Acetylcysteine)

This is another mucolytic, one that's been in use for decades. Like DNase, it is highly effective in breaking down CF mucus, *in the test tube.* Unlike DNase, it does seem to have adverse effects on a number of patients. In many people, this drug causes bronchial irritation with production of more mucus. In others, it causes bronchospasm. Some physicians prescribe an aerosolized bronchodilator along with Mucomyst® to try to prevent bronchospasm. Mucomyst® smells like rotten eggs and is expensive.

Oxygen

Most people with CF don't need any more oxygen than the amount that is in the regular air around us. Air is 21% oxygen, and at sea level this generally provides plenty of oxygen for most people's bodies. If the lungs are severely affected by disease, or when someone is at high altitude—including in a commercial airliner, whose cabins are pressurized to be like an altitude of 5,000–8,000 feet—or when someone with moderate lung disease is exercising, it may be difficult for enough oxygen to enter the bloodstream. In these cases, people can breathe extra oxygen—air with 25%, 30%, 40% or more oxygen. When someone's blood oxygen level is very low, it is remarkable how much better a little extra oxygen can make him or her feel.

How given: Oxygen can be kept in metal cylinders of different sizes. Small "B-cylinders" are about $3\frac{1}{2}$ inches across and 16 inches high, and weigh about 6 pounds when full. If someone is using 5 liters/minute (see below), these cylinders last 44 minutes. Other cylinders are as follows:

Cylinder time (at 5 liters/min)	Size (inches)	Weight (full)
B: 44 min	$3\frac{1}{2} \times 16$	6 lb
D: 70 min	$4\frac{1}{4} \times 20$	10 lb
E: 2 hr	$4\frac{1}{4} \times 30$	14 lb
M: 11 hr	$7\frac{1}{8} \times 46$	82 lb
G: 17 hr	9×51	127 lb
K: 23 hr	9×55	150 lb

Oxygen can also be stored in liquid form. Liquid oxygen tanks hold much more oxygen in the same space than oxygen gas. Different sized tanks of liquid oxygen are also available:

Cylinder time (at 5 liters/min)	Size (inches)	Weight (full)
Stroller: 3½ hr	13½ oval	9.5 lb
L-30: 86 hr	12 × 35	120 lb

One other way of giving extra oxygen in the home is with an oxygen extractor or concentrator, which takes in regular room air and gets rid of the parts of air that are not oxygen (mostly nitrogen), resulting in almost pure oxygen. This method is expensive, and the machines are fairly bulky and somewhat noisy, but for someone who needs oxygen much of the time, it may be cheaper and more convenient than using many small tanks.

Just how much extra oxygen you breathe depends on how the oxygen gets from the tank to your lungs. The main methods are mask and nasal cannula. The mask takes the pure oxygen from the tank and mixes it with varying amounts of room air to deliver 25%, 30%, 35%, 50%, or even 100% oxygen. Nasal cannulas, which consist of a flexible plastic tube with two short plastic prongs at the end that stick a short way into the nostrils, can deliver different amounts depending on how high you set the flow of oxygen from the tanks: for every liter per minute of oxygen flow, you add about 3–4% oxygen above room air. That means that if the flow is set at 4 liters/minute, you get $4 \times 3 = 12\%$ or so above room air (room air has 21% oxygen), or $12 + 21 = 33\%$ oxygen. There are some newer methods which some adults are finding more convenient and less noticeable to other people than the old methods. These include nasal cannulas which come through eyeglasses (and therefore have just a little bit of tubing sticking out the end of the eyeglass nosepiece), and oxygen through a tiny tracheostomy (a small hole placed surgically in the neck; this way, the tubing can go under the clothes, and the tracheostomy itself can be hidden under a turtleneck or scarf). Other methods include oxygen tents, which surround the whole upper body; oxygen hoods, which surround the whole head; and single nasal tubes (with one thin tube going into the nostril). Most of these last methods are useful mainly for babies, and therefore are not used very much in CF, since babies with CF usually don't need extra oxygen.

Amount needed: Your doctor may want to do a "blood gas" or check a "pulseox" to see how much oxygen you have in your blood before he or she decides whether you need extra oxygen. The blood gas test involves taking blood from an artery (usually the radial artery, at the wrist), and is therefore somewhat more painful than most blood tests, which are usually taken from a vein (closer to the skin surface than arteries). However, if some lidocaine or other local anesthetic—like EMLA cream—is used, this is not a painful test, and it can be very important. The pulseox is a less painful (and slightly less informative) test you've probably had done when you've done PFTs. This shines light through the finger and the computer calculates your blood oxygen level. To understand how much extra oxygen is needed, you have to understand how the brain directs breathing. This is discussed in Chapter 3, *The Respiratory System.*

Undesirable effects: The main danger of oxygen is giving so much that it turns off the signal to breathe. Oxygen is also very dry, even when it's been humidified (as it should always be before it's breathed), and can make the mouth and nose uncomfortably dry. Too much oxygen can be toxic to lung tissue (this is not a problem with less than 40% oxygen). The problem you might have heard of concerning eye damage from oxygen is true only in premature babies.

Addiction: Some people worry that once they start on oxygen they'll become addicted in the way that someone gets addicted to morphine or heroin. This does not happen. People whose lungs are bad enough that they need extra oxygen feel much better when they take that oxygen, and they won't want to stop taking it while their lungs are still in that condition. But if the lung disease improves, and extra oxygen is not needed any more, people don't continue to desire the extra oxygen because the body is now supplying it. If the lungs cannot improve, the person will continue to want to use the oxygen, but this is not an addiction.

Other worries about oxygen. Some people worry that needing oxygen is a bad sign—"the beginning of the end," or some such. It certainly *does indicate* that someone's lungs are in worse shape, but many people need oxygen for a few days or weeks, and then are able to get back to doing well without extra oxygen.

Cough Medicines

There are two main kinds of medicines that usually are referred to as "cough medicines." One of these is the expectorants. Expectorants are intended to make it easier to bring up mucus from the lungs. This is a good idea, but unfortunately these drugs don't work. The other kind of cough medicine is the cough suppressant, that is, a drug which controls the cough center in the brain, and says, "don't cough, no matter what is in the lungs that needs to come up." This is usually a terrible idea, especially for someone with CF. Some drug preparations are available which combine these two types of cough medicine, which have opposite goals! In the majority of cases, including most patients with CF, cough is an important defense mechanism that keeps the lungs clear of substances that shouldn't be there. Cough is a sign that something is wrong, but efforts should be directed at what is wrong. If someone is coughing because of bronchospasm, a bronchodilator will relieve the bronchospasm, and thus stop the cough; in a sense, it is a good kind of cough medicine. Similarly, if someone with CF is coughing because infection in the bronchi has gotten out of control, antibiotics are probably needed; they may control the infection and thus stop the cough. Other kinds of cough medicines are rarely useful.

UPPER AIRWAY

Polyp Medicines

Many people with CF have nasal polyps, which are growths of extra tissue (not cancer) in the nose. Usually these cause no problems except mild stuffiness, but they can get large enough to be seen at the end of the nose or block one side of the nose so you can't breathe through it. A few medicines have been used to shrink polyps, and some people feel that they work. These medicines include antihistamines, decongestants (like Neo-Synephrine), and steroid sprays (like Beconase, Vancenase, and Nasalide). A person with nasal allergy symptoms may also be helped by some of these same nasal sprays.

Sinus Medicines

On x-ray examination, most CF patients appear to have abnormal sinuses. Usually this bothers the radiologist more than the patient. Occasionally, there can be actual sinus infection (sinusitis), which may be a nuisance to the patient. In these cases, doctors may prescribe a decongestant and/or antibiotics.

Allergies

Allergies can cause problems with either the upper respiratory system (stuffy sneezy nose) or lungs (congestion, wheezing) or both. CF patients are somewhat more likely than people without CF to have allergies. It is often very difficult to tell if an upper or lower airway problem is caused by infection or by allergy. Complicating the matter is that either one can probably make the other worse, so that constriction of the bronchi from a pollen allergy will make it harder to clear mucus from the bronchi, and make it easier for infection to get out of control.

Antihistamines

Histamine is a chemical that is released from white blood cells in response to different things including irritation and allergy. Its release can cause many of the problems we associate with allergies: runny nose, itchy nose, constricted bronchi, hives. Antihistamines do not stop the release of histamine from the blood cells, but they do help to block its action in the nose, skin, etc.

How taken: These are most commonly taken by mouth but can be given by injection.

Undesirable effects: The most common and often the most troublesome side effect from these drugs is drowsiness. They can also cause a dry mouth.

Decongestants

These drugs are supposed to make the nose less stuffy. Although they are used by millions of people, there is not very much scientific evidence that they work. Some decongestant nasal sprays can temporarily open blocked nostrils. If they are used for more than a few days, they can cause "rebound" inflammation and blockage of the nose that is just as bad as the inflammation the cold caused.

Allergy Shots

This is a very controversial topic. Most pulmonary specialists feel that allergy shots may be helpful for nasal allergies but not for bronchial allergies (asthma), while many allergists feel that they sometimes can be helpful for asthma too. There is nothing about CF which makes someone more or less likely to respond well to allergy shots than anyone else.

THE HEART

The heart is not directly affected by CF, and most people with CF have very good hearts. Therefore, there usually is no need for heart medications. However, if someone's lungs become badly diseased (from CF or any other cause), the heart may not be able to pump all the necessary fluid through the diseased lungs. When this happens, two types of medicines are sometimes used: diuretics and digitalis.

Diuretics

These drugs help the kidneys get rid of extra fluid that may have built up in the body because of the heart's inability to pump all of the fluid. Most doctors agree that when someone has heart failure because of severe lung disease, it is very important to cut down on the amount of fluid that the heart is asked to pump. This is accomplished through restricting the amount of salt and fluid consumed and through careful use of diuretic medicines.

Furosemide

How taken: Furosemide (Lasix) can be taken by mouth (tablet, liquid) or by injection (either IM or IV).

Undesirable effects: Furosemide causes the body to lose potassium in addition to other salts and this can upset the body's salt balance if used in high doses every day for too long. This effect can be lessened by an every-other-day schedule in people who tolerate this schedule. The drug can also do too much of a good thing—in eliminating too much excess fluid, it may actually dehydrate the patient. Furosemide has been associated with some cases of hearing problems, which are usually reversible. Occasionally, someone who is allergic to sulfa drugs may be allergic to furosemide.

Spironolactone (Aldactone)

This drug is less powerful than furosemide, but keeps the body from losing potassium.

How taken: Oral tablets.

Undesirable effects: Any diuretic may cause excess loss of water (dehydration) and salt balance problems. Spironolactone may also give some gastrointestinal (GI) upset. A rash is sometimes seen. It may cause breast enlargement and/or impotence in men. These effects are nearly always temporary and disappear when the drug is stopped.

Thiazides

How taken: These diuretics are usually taken by mouth (tablet; although a liquid preparation is also available). Rarely they may be given by IV, but not by IM injection.

Undesirable effects: These are quite safe and usually there are no problems. Textbooks do list many possible reactions, including GI upset, dizziness, fatigue, headache, anemia, weakness, muscle spasms, gout.

Digitalis

This drug has been known for centuries and is very effective in making the heart contractions stronger. It is not clear whether it is helpful in people whose heart problems are mainly caused by lung problems.

How taken: Digitalis preparations can be taken by mouth (tablets or liquids) or by IV injection.

Undesirable effects: Too much digitalis can be very dangerous and can cause heart beat irregularities, confusion, visual problems, vomiting, diarrhea, headache, weakness.

GASTROINTESTINAL AND DIGESTIVE SYSTEM MEDICATIONS

The main problem in the gastrointestinal and digestive system is the thick mucus that blocks the ducts of the pancreas and prevents the digestive chemicals *(enzymes)* from reaching the intestines where they mix with the food that has been eaten. If these digestive enzymes are not available, the food cannot be digested, that is, broken down into particles small enough to be soaked up into the bloodstream through the wall of the intestine. As a result, a lot of the food (especially the fat) will not be available to the body and will pass out into the stools. Most (but not all) CF patients have this problem. Another gastrointestinal problem is that the intestines' own mucus is very thick which can sometimes lead to blockage of the intestines.

Digestive Enzymes

These enzymes come from the pancreas of animals. They have changed what used to be a serious, even fatal, problem into a nuisance problem. With enzyme type and dosage properly adjusted, most CF patients are able to absorb the majority of what they eat (even the fat). Thus, they are able to get the nutritional value from the food which would be lost without the enzymes. Enzymes are discussed fully in Chapter 6, *Nutrition.*

Anti-acid Drugs

Excess stomach acid can cause several different types of problems in anyone, and at least one additional problem if someone has CF. Too much acid can destroy the old kind of digestive enzyme medicines, although this is much less a problem with enteric-coated enzymes. Too much acid can also help cause ulcers. Occasionally, the stomach acid can reflux (go backward) up into the esophagus causing heartburn (the burning discomfort felt when the esophagus becomes irritated from acid). Drugs that prevent the stomach from making too much acid, or drugs which neutralize the acid once it is made, may be helpful for any of these problems.

Cimetidine

Cimetidine (Tagemet) is one of the most prescribed drugs in the world, largely because it is very effective in decreasing the production of stomach acid.
How taken: Cimetidine is almost always taken by mouth, in a tablet, or liquid, usually before meals and before bed.
Undesirable effects: This is a very safe drug. Mild diarrhea, headache, or swelling of breasts have been seen in people taking cimetidine, but none of these problems is common.

Ranitidine

Ranitidine (Zantac) is a close relative of cimetidine, and is newer. It can be taken at a lower dose, less frequently, with comparable effects to cimetidine.

Omeprazole

This is a powerful drug that shuts off the stomach's production of acid.

Undesirable effects: This is a safe drug. Mild diarrhea and headache occur in some people taking the medicine.

Various Antacids

These medicines, taken by mouth as chewable tablets or the more effective liquid form, do not influence how much acid is produced by the stomach, but they can neutralize the acid once it's formed.

Antireflux Drugs

Several drugs may be helpful for patients with gastroesophageal reflux.

Cisapride

Cisapride may help reduce gastroesophageal reflux by two of its effects: it strengthens the grip of the muscle at the bottom of the esophagus, and it increases the speed with which the esophagus and stomach empty, leaving less there to back up into the esophagus.

Undesirable effects: This is a very safe drug. Mild diarrhea is about the only side effect, and even it is not very common.

Reglan

This drug has been in use longer than cisapride, and does about the same things.

Undesirable effects: This drug can also give diarrhea. Its most worrisome side effect is that it can cause abnormal movement of the face and tongue. If the medicine is not stopped when this symptom appears, it can become permanent.

Anticonstipation Medicines

Constipation is seldom a problem in patients with CF, but it does occur occasionally. Failure to pass any stool can be an important sign of a dangerous intestinal obstruction called meconium ileus in a newborn infant and DIOS (distal intestinal obstruction syndrome) in someone older.

Dietary Fiber

Someone who has difficulty passing bowel movements may benefit from increasing the amount of fiber in the diet. Foods high in fiber include fruits and some vegetables; bran is an especially good source of fiber. Breakfast cereals with bran should have at least 4 grams

(g) of dietary fiber per serving to be effective (this information is included on the side-panel of the cereal box; if the information isn't there, it's likely that there is very little fiber in the cereal).

Enzymes

Before more drastic measures are undertaken, it usually helps to make sure the digestive enzyme dose is appropriate, since very bulky poorly digested stools may make blockage more likely.

Mineral Oil

On some occasions a physician may prescribe oral mineral oil to help pass stools.

Bowel Stimulants

If someone is not completely blocked up, some medications which stimulate intestinal contractions may help the bowels to empty. Senekot is one such laxative.

Enemas

With more blockage, enemas may be needed to help wash out the lower intestines. Generally, several types of enemas can be used in different situations. Always check with your doctor to be sure it's safe to use an enema, and to find out which kind.

Gastrografin Enemas

Severe intestinal obstruction is a serious matter that used to be treatable only with surgery. Fortunately today, many cases can be treated in the hospital with special enemas. Gastrografin is a substance which can be used for an enema, and has several useful properties. It shows up on x-ray, so the radiologist can see the outline of the bowel to make sure there is not another problem causing intestinal blockage, and to make sure the enema is going far up into the intestines so that it will work. It's very slippery, allowing it to slip by the blockage. It also acts like a sponge, pulling in lots of fluid from the rest of the body to help make the stools stuck in the bowel become more watery and easier to move out.

How performed: These enemas always must be done where there is x-ray equipment and a radiologist. This usually means they are done in the hospital. Most children who need them are sick enough to need to be in the hospital anyway.

Undesirable effects: These enemas are somewhat uncomfortable, as is true of any enema, but they can provide prompt relief from the abdominal pain from intestinal blockage. The main danger of this procedure is that so much fluid is pulled into the bowel from the rest of the body that the patient can become dehydrated. For this reason, most doctors will not perform this procedure on an infant unless the baby has an IV line in place, with fluids running in.

Miscellaneous

1. GoLYTELY. A salty liquid which can be drunk in large quantities to "flush out" the intestines.
2. COLACE. A stool softener.
3. LACTULOSE (CEFULAC, CHRONULAC). Medicines taken by mouth that pull fluid into the intestines to help make the bowel contents more watery, and easier to move.

Antibloating Medications

Some patients with CF have trouble with abdominal bloating. This may be caused by the thick mucus in the intestines, which can surround little air bubbles, which does not let the little bubbles get together to make a single bubble that is big enough for a burp. Some drugs containing simethicone (Mylicon, Silain) may help dissolve some of that mucus and allow a gentle upwards or downwards explosion of that air, relieving the pressure and discomfort. These drugs are taken by mouth (tablets or drops) and are very safe.

Liver Medications

Occasionally, patients with CF liver disease may need to take even more vitamins than usual. There is also a new drug (*Actigall,* or ursodeoxycholic acid) that might help liquefy the secretions that otherwise block the smallest ducts within the liver and gallbladder.

Vitamins

These are not really drugs, and should be a regular part of the diet. Four vitamins (A, D, E, K) are "fat-soluble," meaning that they dissolve in fat and are only absorbed in the body when fats are absorbed. Thus, patients who have trouble absorbing fats may have low levels of these vitamins. For this reason, most nutrition experts agree that CF patients should probably receive supplements of these vitamins, at least some of the time. Vitamin D can probably be supplied from regular multivitamin preparations, but vitamin K, vitamin A, and vitamin E need to be taken separately. Your physician may periodically check your blood levels of the various vitamins. Some people feel quite well, and yet are deficient in several vitamins. For the vitamin E, most preparations you can buy will not work for someone who has trouble absorbing fats, and a form which is partly dissolvable in water needs to be used.

Growth and Appetite Stimulants and Supplements

Hormones

Most of the drugs used to stimulate appetite and growth are anabolic steroids and androgens (male hormones). They are widely used, but have not been conclusively shown to be safe or effective in patients with CF.

How taken: These hormones can be given by injection or taken by mouth.

Undesirable effects: These are too numerous to list completely, are worrisome, and can actually result in stopping growth sooner than it would have stopped naturally (as these hormones increase bone growth, they also close the growth plate of the bones—the part of the bones where growth takes place—more quickly than normal). Other undesirable effects include fluid retention, hirsutism (increased hairiness), baldness, various genital disturbances (too big, too little, too excitable, not excitable enough), acne, sleeplessness, liver disease, nausea, ulcerlike symptoms, and finally, disqualification from the Olympics.

Diet Supplements

Many different kinds of diet supplements are available, from vanilla milk shakes and ice cream sundaes to expensive "elemental" (predigested) formulas. These are discussed in Chapter 6, *Nutrition.* These supplements usually have high calorie contents. They seem to be helpful in some people, while in others, the number of calories taken in with the supplements is balanced by the number of calories not eaten in the regular meals. Some programs have been successful in helping patients gain weight and height by running nighttime feedings of these dietary supplements through a stomach tube while the patients sleep. Such a program, of course, should never be undertaken without your doctor's knowledge and cooperation.

How taken: Some of these can be sprinkled on top of regular meals; some can be eaten between meals. Others are designed to be given through a tube (mostly because they taste so bad, but also because they can be given very slowly while the patient sleeps).

Undesirable effects: The supplements may interfere with normal mealtime appetite. The tube feedings require a tube which can be somewhat uncomfortable and/or inconvenient. Several tubes can be used, including a nasogastric tube, which goes through the nose ("naso-") into the stomach ("gastric"), and is usually put in each evening and removed in the morning. Another kind of tube is a permanent tube placed by a surgical operation which makes a hole or stoma in the wall of the abdomen directly into the stomach (a gastrostomy tube) or into the second part of the small intestine, the jejunum (a feeding jejunostomy tube). Possible problems from these nighttime feedings include overfilling the stomach.

TRANSPLANT-RELATED DRUGS

Anti-Rejection Drugs

Steroids

(See above for more on steroids.) Steroids decrease inflammation, and they are important tools in preventing and fighting acute rejection (see Chapter 8, *Transplantation*).

Antilymphocyte Drugs

Lymphocytes are the white blood cells most responsible for rejection, so specific antilymphocyte drugs have been sought: if you decrease the rejection caused by the lymphocytes without interfering with other white blood cells trying to fight infection, that would be ideal.

Cyclosporine. This is the first very successful antilymphocyte drug used to help treat and prevent rejection.

How taken: This drug can be taken IV or by mouth.

Undesirable effects: This drug can cause high blood pressure, kidney damage, seizures, shakiness, hairiness, and excessive growth of the gums. Too much may lead to infection.

Tacrolimus (FK-506). This drug is similar to cyclosporine, but may be a bit more effective.

How taken: This drug can be taken IV or by mouth.

Undesirable effects: This drug can cause high blood pressure, kidney damage, seizures, shakiness, hairiness, and headache. Too much may lead to infection.

"Antimetabolites"

These drugs interfere with the body's ability to make white blood cells, so there are fewer cells around to reject an organ. (Of course, that also means there are fewer white blood cells to fight infection.)

Azothioprine (Imuran).

How taken: This drug can be taken IV or by mouth.

Undesirable effects: The main side effect is too much of its desired effect, that is, the white blood cell count getting too low and therefore the body not being able to fight off infection. The platelet count may also go too low, and—since platelets are needed for proper clotting of blood—there can be abnormal bleeding.

ATG (antithymocyte globulin). This is an antibody made by horses and directed against human lymphocytes.

How taken: This drug is taken by IV.

Undesirable effects: The drug can cause fever and "flu"-like symptoms, including headache.

OKT3. This is a "bioengineered" antilymphocyte drug.

How taken: This drug is taken IV.

Undesirable effects: The drug can cause fever and "flu"-like symptoms, including headache.

GLOSSARY OF DRUGS

This glossary is a partial list of drugs which can be found under both their generic and trade names. Drugs that are discussed in this appendix contain references to the appropriate section. For example, PenVee K is a form of the antibiotic penicillin, which is discussed under *Lungs: Antibiotics: Penicillins.*

Accelerase   (triacylglycerol lipase) A digestive enzyme with bile salts (*see* page 306).

Accurbron   A theophylline (*see* page 299).

acetylcysteine   A mucolytic (*see* page 301).

Actifed   (triprolidine hydrochloride + pseudoephedrine hydrochloride) A decongestant/antihistamine combination (*see* page 304).

Actigall   (ursodeoxycholic acid). A bile salt now used to treat CF liver disease (*see* page 309).

acyclovir   An antiviral drug.

ADEK   A multi-vitamin that includes vitamins A, D, E, and K.

Adrenalin   (epinephrine) A bronchodilator (*see* page 298).

Aerobid   An inhaled steroid (*see* page 299).

Aerolate Jr. and Sr.   Theophylline bronchodilators (*see* page 299).

Afrin   (oxymetazoline hydrochloride) A decongestant (*see* page 304).

albuterol   A beta-agonist bronchodilator (*see* page 298).

Aldactone   (spironolactone) A diuretic (*see* page 305).

Allerest   A decongestant/antihistamine (*see* page 304).

Alupent   A beta-agonist bronchodilator (*see* page 298).

amantadine   A medication that can help control infection with the influenza virus.

Amcill   (ampicillin) An antibiotic (*see* page 294).

amikacin sulfate   An aminoglycoside antibiotic (*see* page 295).

Amikin   Amikacin sulfate, an aminoglycoside (*see* page 295).

Aminodur   A theophylline bronchodilator (*see* page 299).

aminophylline   A theophylline bronchodilator (*see* page 299).

amoxicillin   An antibiotic (*see* page 294).

Amoxil   Amoxicillin (*see* page 294).

Amphojel   (aluminum hydroxide gel) An antacid (*see* page 306).

amphotericin   A drug used to fight infection caused by funguses.

ampicillin   An antibiotic; an effective antibacterial agent (*see* page 294).

Ancef   (cefazolin sodium) A cephalosporin antibiotic (*see* page 296).

Aquamephyton   A vitamin K preparation (*see* page 309).

Aquasol A   A vitamin A preparation (*see* page 309).

Aquasol E   A vitamin E preparation (*see* page 309).

Asbron   A theophylline bronchodilator (*see* page 299).

Atgam   An anti-thymocyte globulin for fighting organ rejection (*see* page 310).

Atrovent   A kind of bronchodilator.

Atuss   A cough medicine that includes a cough-suppressant, an antihistamine, and a decongestant (*see* page 304).

Augmentin   (amoxicillin/clavulanate potassium) An antibiotic (*see* page 294).

Avazyme   (chymotrypsin) A digestive enzyme, useful only for digesting protein, and not fat
(*see* page 306).

Azactam   (*see* Aztreonam *below*).

azlocillin   An anti-*Pseudomonas* antibiotic (*see* page 295).

Azmacort   (triamcinolone acetonide) An inhaled corticosteroid (*see* page 299).

azothioprine   An antimetabolite, for fighting organ rejection (*see* page 311).

Aztreonam   An anti-*Pseudomonas* antibiotic (*see* page 298).

bacampicillin HCl   An ampicillin (*see* page 294).

Bactrim   (trimethoprim-sulfamethoxazole) A combination antibiotic (*see* page 295).

Bactrim DS   Double-strength Bactrim (*see* Bactrim).

Basaljel   (aluminum carbonate gel) An antacid (*see* page 306).

beclomethasone dipropionate   An inhaled corticosteroid (*see* page 299).

Beclovent   (beclomethasone dipropionate) A corticosteroid (*see* page 299).

Beconase   (beclomethasone dipropionate) A nasal steroid spray often used for polyps or nasal
allergies (*see* page 303).

Beepen-VK   (penicillin) An antibiotic (*see* page 294).

Benadryl   (diphenhydramine hydrochloride) An antihistamine (*see* page 304).

Betapen-VK (penicillin V potassium) An antibiotic (*see* page 294).

Biaxin (clarithromycin) an erythromycin antibiotic (*see* page 297).

Bicillin (penicillin G benzathine) An injectable (IM) penicillin (*see* page 294).

Bilezyme A digestive enzyme combination containing protein-digesting enzymes but no fat-digesting enzymes. Also contains bile salts (*see* page 306).

Bilogen A digestive enzyme that contains protein-digesting enzymes but no fat-digesting enzymes. Also contains bile salts (*see* page 306).

bisacodyl A laxative (*see* page 308).

bran A very rich source of dietary fiber. Taken in pure form, it tastes like rabbit food, but is very effective (*see* page 307).

Brethine (terbutaline sulfate) A beta-agonist bronchodilator (*see* page 298).

Bricanyl (terbutaline sulfate) A beta-agonist bronchodilator (*see* page 298).

Bristagen (gentamicin) An aminoglycoside antibiotic (*see* page 295).

Bristamycin An erythromycin (stearate) antibiotic (*see* page 297).

Bronchobid Duracaps A combination bronchodilator drug that includes theophylline and ephedrine, related to the beta-agonists (*see* page 298).

Broncholate Capsules A combination bronchodilator including theophylline and ephedrine (*See* Bronchobid *above*).

Brondecon (oxtriphylline + guaifenesin) A bronchodilator and "expectorant" combination. The bronchodilator is oxtriphylline, a close relative of theophylline (*see* page 299). The expectorant is called guaifenesin (*see* page 303).

Brondelate Same as Brondecon.

Bronitin Mist An adrenaline inhaler.

Bronkaid A bronchodilator that contains theophylline (*see* page 299), guaifenesin, and expectorant (*see* page 303).

Bronkaid Mist An adrenaline inhaler.

Bronkodyl A theophylline (*see* page 299).

Bronkolixir A combination bronchodilator that contains theophylline, ephedrine sulfate (related to beta-agonists) (*see* page 298), guaifenesin, an expectorant (*see* pages 303), and phenobarbital. Phenobarbital is a potent sedative whose proper use is in people with psychiatric illness to control agitation, anxiety, and insomnia, and as a seizure medication in patients who have epilepsy. It is useless as a bronchodilator. (In this particular preparation, all of the medications are in such low doses that they do neither good nor harm anyway.)

Bronkometer (isoetharine mesylate) A form of a $beta_2$-bronchodilator for inhalation (*see* page 298).

Bronkosol (isoetharine HCl) A beta-agonist bronchodilator, for use in an aerosol (*see* page 298).

Bronkotabs A combination theophylline bronchodilator, ephedrine (*see* page 298), guaifenesin (*see* page 319), and phenobarbital (*see* Broncholixir).

carbenicillin An anti-*Pseudomonas* antibiotic (*see* page 295).

Ceclor (cefaclor) A cephalosporin antibiotic (*see* page 297).

cefaclor A cephalosporin antibiotic (*see* page 297).

cefadroxil A cephalosporin antibiotic (*see* page 297).

Cefadyl (cephapirin sodium) A cephalosporin antibiotic (*see* page 297).

cefamandole A cephalosporin antibiotic (*see* page 297).

cefazolin An analogue of a cephalosporin antibiotic (*see* page 297).

Cefobid A cephalosporin antibiotic with some effect against *Pseudomonas* (*see* page 297).

cefoperozone A cephalosporin antibiotic with some effect against *Pseudomonas* (*see* page 297).

cefotaxime A cephalosporin antibiotic (*see* page 297).

cefoxitin An analogue derivative of a cephalosporin antibiotic (*see* page 297).

cefprozil A cephalosporin antibiotic (*see* page 297).

ceftazidime An anti-*Pseudomonas* cephalosporin (*see* page 297).

Ceftin cefuroxime

Cefulac (lactulose) An anticonstipation medication (*see* page 309).

cefuroxime A cephalosporin antibiotic (*see* page 297).

Cefzil cefprozil

Celbenin (sodium methicillin) An anti-*Staph* antibiotic (*see* page 295).

Cenalax An anticonstipation drug (*see* page 307).

cephalexin A cephalosporin antibiotic (*see* page 297).

cephaloglycin A cephalosporin antibiotic (*see* page 297).

cephaloridine A cephalosporin antibiotic (*see* page 297).

cephalosporins A family of antibiotics (*see* page 296).

cephalothin A cephalosporin antibiotic (*see* page 297).

cephapirin A cephalosporin antibiotic (*see* page 297).

cephradine A cephalosporin antibiotic (*see* page 297).

Cerose A combination of various cough medicines (*see* page 303).

Cerylin A combination theophylline bronchodilator (*see* page 299) and guaifenesin expectorant (*see* page 303).

chloramphenicol An antibiotic (*see* page 296).

Chloromycetin (chloramphenicol) An antibiotic.

Chlor-Trimeton (pseudoephedrine sulfate + chlorpheniramine maleate) An antihistamine (*see* page 304).

Choledyl (oxtriphylline) A bronchodilator closely related to theophylline (*see* page 304).

cimetidine An antacid preparation (*see* page 306).

Cipro A quinolone antibiotic (*see* page 297).

ciprofloxacin A quinolone antibiotic (*see* page 297).

cisapride An antireflux medication (*see* page 307)

Claforan A cephalosporin antibiotic (*see* page 297).

clarithromycin An erythromycin antibiotic (*see* page 297).

Cleocin (clindamycin) One of the aminoglycoside antibiotics (*see* page 295).

clindamycin An antibiotic.

clotrimazole An anti-yeast medication, used for vaginal yeast infections.

cloxacillin An anti-*Staph* penicillin (*see* page 295).

Cloxapen (cloxacillin) A penicillin.

cod liver oil A traditional source of vitamins A and D whose main advantage is its bad taste (*see* page 309).

codeine A cough suppressant (*see* page 303).

coffee A caffeine-containing popular drink. Caffeine is also found in Coca-Cola, Pepsi, and in some cases serves as a bronchodilator (*see* page 298).

Colace (docusate sodium) A stool softener (*see* page 309).

colistin A very potent antibiotic, a relative of the aminoglycosides. Given intravenously it can have severe side effects including headaches and kidney damage (*see* page 295).

Coly-Mycin S (colistin sulfate) An antibiotic.

Contac An antihistamine and decongestant (*see* page 304).

Co-Pyronil (pyrrobutamine compound) An antihistamine and decongestant combination (*see* page 304).

Coricidin An antihistamine and decongestant (*see* page 304).

Cotazym (pancrelipase) A pancreatic digestive enzyme (*see* page 306).

Cotazym-B A digestive enzyme with bile salts (*see* page 306).

Cotazym-S An enteric-coated pancreatic enzyme (*see* page 306).

co-trimoxazole A combination antibiotic (trimethoprim-sulfamethoxazole) (*see* page 295).

Co-Tylenol A combination of decongestant, antihistamine, and cough suppressant with acetaminophen (*see* pages 303, 304).

Creon (pancreatin) An enteric-coated pancreatic enzyme (*see* page 306).

Criticare A nutritional supplement and formula that is very low in fat and whose protein is predigested (*see* page 310).

cromolyn An inhaled medicine used to prevent bronchospasm (*see* page 300).

cyclacillin "Twin brother" of ampicillin; an effective antibacterial agent (*see* page 294).

Cyclapen cyclacillin

Decadron (dexamethasone) A steroid (*see* page 299).

Declomycin (demeclocycline) A tetracycline antibiotic (*see* page 297).

Delatestryl (testosterone enanthate) A male hormone sometimes used to stimulate growth and appetite (*see* page 309).

Deltasone (prednisone) A steroid sometimes used to decrease bronchial inflammation (*see* page 299).

Demazin (chlorpheniramine maleate + phenylephine hydrochloride) A combination antihistamine-decongestant (*see* pages 303, 304).

demeclocycline A tetracycline antibiotic (*see* page 297).

Demerol (meperidine [pethidine] hydrochloride) A narcotic painkiller and sedative.

Depo-Testosterone A male hormone (testosterone) in injectable form sometimes used as a growth and appetite stimulant (*see* page 309).

De-Tuss A combination cough medicine and antihistamine (*see* pages 303, 304).

dexamethasone A steroid that is sometimes taken by aerosol inhalation (*see* page 300).

dextromethorphan (DM) A cough suppressant (*see* page 303).

Dianabol (methandrostenolone) An anabolic and male sex hormone sometimes used for growth and appetite stimulant (*see* page 309).

dicloxacillin sodium An anti-*Staph* penicillin (*see* page 295).

digitalis A drug that strengthens heart contractions (*see* page 305).

digitoxin A digitalis drug (*see* page 305).

digoxin A digitalis drug (*see* page 305).

Dilaudid (hydromorphone hydrochloride) A narcotic that is occasionally used for pain and for cough suppression.

Dimetane (brompheniramine maleate) A combination cough medicine, antihistamine, and decongestant (*see* pages 303, 304).

Dimetapp Similar to Dimetane.

diphenhydramine hydrochloride An antihistamine (*see* page 304).

disodium cromoglycate Cromolyn; used in treatment of bronchial asthma (*see* page 300).

diuretics Medications that increase the kidneys' production of urine, and thus help rid the body of excess fluid (*see* page 305).

Donatussin (chlorpheniramine maleate + phenylephrine hydrochloride + guaifenesin) A combination cough medicine, antihistamine, and decongestant (*see* pages 303, 304).

Dorcol (guaifenesin + phenylpropanolamine hydrochloride + dextromethorphan hydrobromide) A cough medicine that includes a decongestant and a cough suppressant (*see* pages 303, 304).

doxycycline A tetracycline antibiotic (*see* page 297).

Dristan   A decongestant (*see* page 304).

Dynapen   (dicloxacillin) An anti-*Staph* antibiotic (*see* page 295).

dyphylline   A form of theophylline bronchodilator (*see* page 299).

E-Mycin   An erythromycin antibiotic (*see* page 297).

EES   (erythromycin ethylsuccinate) An erythromycin antibiotic (*see* page 297).

Elixicon   (theophylline) A theophylline bronchodilator (*see* page 299).

Elixophyllin   A form of theophylline bronchodilator (*see* page 299).

EMLA cream   A local anesthetic that can be put on the skin to numb a site for IV needle placement.

Ensure   A calorie supplement (*see* page 310).

Entolase   An enteric-coated digestive enzyme (*see* page 306).

Entolase-HP   An enteric-coated digestive enzyme (*see* page 306).

enzymes   Catalysts of chemical reactions; (*see* page 308).

ephedrine   Sometimes used as a bronchodilator (*see* page 298).

epinephrine   Adrenalin. Often used as an emergency bronchodilator, similar in some of its action to the "beta-agonists" (*see* page 298), but with more effect on the heart (speeds it up).

Erythrocin   An erythromycin antibiotic (*see* page 297).

erythromycin   A family of antibiotics (*see* page 297).

ethacrynic acid   A diuretic (*see* page 305).

fiber   An important component of the diet (*see* page 307).

Fleet enemas   Occasionally used for treating constipation (*see* page 308).

Fortaz   (ceftazidime) A cephalosporin antibiotic (*see* page 297).

furosemide   A diuretic (*see* page 305).

Gantrisin   (sulfisoxazole) A sulfa antibiotic (*see* page 295).

Garamycin   (gentamicin) An aminoglycoside antibiotic (*see* page 295).

Gastrografin   (meglumine diatrizoate) A substance that is occasionally used in the hospital for an enema (*see* page 308).

Gaviscon   (aluminum hydroxide + magnesium carbonate) An antacid (*see* page 306).

Gelusil   (aluminum hydroxide + magnesium hydroxide + simethicone) An antacid (*see* page 306).

gentamicin   An aminoglycoside antibiotic (*see* page 295).

Geocillin   An oral form of the antibiotic carbenicillin. The oral form of the medicine is not effective for lung disease (*see* page 295).

Geopen   An injectable form of carbenicillin (*see* page 295).

GoLYTELY   A salty liquid which can be drunk in large quantities to "flush out" the intestines (*see* page 309).

guaifenesin   an expectorant (*see* page 303, "Cough Medicines").

Halotestin   (fluoxymesterone) A male sex hormone sometimes used for growth and appetite stimulation (*see* page 309).

heparin   An anticoagulant; that is, a drug which prevents clotting of the blood. This is very useful when used in very small amounts in a needle in a vein. It can keep the blood from clotting up the needle so that the needle can be used for a long time for administration of IV antibiotics.

heparin lock   A needle which is inserted in the vein and periodically rinsed out with heparin solution. This enables the needle to be used for administration of intravenous antibiotics on an intermittent basis. Once rinsed out, the needle can be plugged up and just taped to the arm without any extra tubing connected to it, leaving the arm free.

Hep-Lock   The dilute heparin solution used in a heparin lock.

hetacillin An antibiotic related to ampicillin (*see* page 294).

Hexadrol (dexamethasone) A steroid sometimes used to decrease bronchial inflammation (*see* page 299).

Hycodan (hydrocodone bitartrate) A combination cough medicine that contains a cough suppressant (*see* page 303).

Hycotuss (hydrocodone bitartrate + guaifenesin) A multi-ingredient cough medicine which includes a cough suppressant (*see* page 303).

hydrocodone bitartrate A narcotic sometimes used as a cough suppressant (*see* page 303).

hydrocortisone A steroid occasionally used in different forms to decrease bronchial inflammation (*see* page 299).

Ilozyme (pancrelipase) A pancreatic enzyme (*see* page 306).

imipenem An anti-*Pseudomonas* antibiotic (*see* page 298).

Intal cromolyn sodium (*see* page 300).

ipecac A medicine used to induce vomiting (usually used after a child has accidentally ingested a poisonous substance).

isoetharine A bronchodilator drug taken by inhalation (*see* page 298).

isoproterenol An inhaled bronchodilator (*see* page 298).

Isuprel (isoproterenol) A bronchodilator taken by inhalation (*see* page 298).

kanamycin An aminoglycoside antibiotic (*see* page 295).

Kantrex (kanamycin) An antibiotic (*see* page 296).

Keflex (cephalexin) A cephalosporin antibiotic (*see* page 297).

Keflin (cephalothin sodium) A cephalosporin antibiotic (*see* page 297).

Kefzol (cefazolin sodium) A cephalosporin antibiotic (*see* page 297).

lactulose An anticonstipation medication (*see* page 309).

Lanophyllin A form of theophylline bronchodilator (*see* page 299).

Lanoxin (digoxin) A type of digitalis (*see* page 305).

Larotid (amoxicillin) An antibiotic (*see* page 294).

Lasix (furosemide) A diuretic (*see* page 305).

Ledercillin (penicillin G procaine) A form of penicillin (*see* page 294).

Lincocin (lincomycin HCl) An antibiotic.

lincomycin An antibiotic not commonly used in CF.

Lufyllin (dyphylline) A theophylline bronchodilator (*see* page 299).

Maalox An antacid (*see* page 306).

Marax (ephedrine sulfate + theophylline + hydroxyzine HCl) A combination drug including a theophylline bronchodilator (*see* page 299) and another bronchodilator.

Maxair (pirbuterol) A beta-agonist bronchodilator (*see* page 298).

Medihaler-EPI An inhaled form of epinephrine or adrenalin (*see* page 298).

Medihaler-ISO (isoproterenol sulfate) An inhaled bronchodilator with isoproterenol (*see* page 298).

Metaprel (metaproterenol sulfate) A beta-agonist bronchodilator (*see* page 298).

metaproterenol sulfate A beta-agonist bronchodilator (*see* page 298).

methacycline A tetracycline antibiotic (*see* page 297).

methicillin sulfate An anti-*Staph* antibiotic (*see* page 294).

methyltestosterone A male sex hormone, sometimes used as a growth and appetite stimulant (*see* page 309).

metoclopramide A drug that increases the movement of foods through the gastrointestinal tract and which may decrease gastroesophageal reflux (*see* page 307).

Mezlin (mezlocillin) An anti-*Pseudomonas* antibiotic (*see* page 295).

milk of magnesia   There are several different preparations: antacids (*see* page 306), and laxatives which are used as an anticonstipation preparation (*see* page 307).

Minocin   (minocycline HCl) An antibiotic (*see* page 297).

minocycline   A tetracycline antibiotic (*see* page 297).

misoprostol   An anti-acid medication (*see* page 306).

mucolytics   Chemicals that break up mucus (*see* page 300).

Mucomyst   (acetylcysteine) A mucolytic (*see* page 301).

Mycostatin   (nystatin) A drug that kills yeast infections, which can appear when a patient is taking antibiotics. Mycostatin is occasionally prescribed when a child is taking antibiotics.

Mylanta   (aluminum hydroxide + magnesium hydroxide + simethicone) An antacid (*see* page 306).

Mylicon   (simethicone) An antibloating drug (*see* page 309).

Nafcil   (nafcillin sodium) An antibiotic.

nafcillin   An anti-*Staph* antibiotic (*see* page 294).

Naldecon   A decongestant antihistamine combination (*see* page 304).

Nebcin   (tobramycin sulfate) An aminoglycoside antibiotic (*see* page 295).

nedocromil   An inhaled anti-inflammatory medication closely related to cromolyn (*see* page 300).

neomycin   An aminoglycoside antibiotic (*see* page 295).

Neo-Synephrine   (phenylephrine HCl) A decongestant (*see* page 303).

netilmicin   An aminoglycoside antibiotic (*see* page 295).

Novahistine   A combination of many ingredients, used for coughs and cold symptoms (*see* pages 303, 304).

nystatin   Used to fight yeast infections which can appear when a patient is taking antibiotics.

omeprazole   An anti-acid drug (*see* page 307).

Omnipen   (ampicillin) An antibiotic (*see* page 294).

Organidin   (iodinated glycerol) An expectorant (*see* page 303).

oxacillin   An anti-*Staph* antibiotic (*see* page 294).

oxtriphylline   A theophylline bronchodilator (*see* page 299).

oxytetracycline   A tetracycline antibiotic (*see* page 297).

Pancrease   (pancrelipase) An enteric-coated digestive enzyme (*see* page 306).

pancreatin   A digestive enzyme (*see* page 306).

pancrelipase   A digestive enzyme (*see* page 306).

Panmycin   (tetracycline) An antibiotic (*see* page 297).

Papase   A drug with some enzyme activity (*see* page 306).

Pediamycin   (erythromycin ethylsuccinate) An erythromycin antibiotic (*see* page 297).

Pediazole   (erythromycin ethylsuccinate + sulfisoxazole acetyl) A combination antibiotic that contains erythromycin and a sulfa drug (*see* pages 295, 297).

penicillin   An antibiotic (*see* page 294).

Pen-Vee-K   A penicillin antibiotic (*see* page 294).

phenylephrine hydrochloride   A medication sometimes used in aerosols. It constricts blood vessels and may therefore cut down on swelling in the bronchi, by decreasing the blood flow to the bronchi.

piperacillin sodium   An anti-*Pseudomonas* antibiotic (*see* page 295).

Pipracil   (piperacillin) An antibiotic.

pirbuterol   A beta-agonist bronchodilator (*see* page 298).

Pneumovax   The so-called "pneumonia vaccine." This is useful for children who have a particular deficiency in their body defenses which enables them to become infected with a germ called pneumococcus, such as children with sickle-cell disease. Many physicians feel that it is of no particular value to patients with cystic fibrosis.

Polycillin (ampicillin) An antibiotic (*see* page 294).

Polycose A high-calorie diet supplement (*see* page 309).

Poly-Histine A cough and cold preparation (*see* pages 303, 304).

Polymox (amoxicillin) An antibiotic (*see* page 294).

polymyxin-B An antibiotic.

polymyxin-E An antibiotic, also known as colistin, that is effective against *Pseudomonas*; however, it is often difficult to tolerate.

prednisolone A steroid used to decrease inflammation (*see* page 299).

prednisone A steroid used to decrease inflammation (*see* page 299).

Prilosec (omeprazole) An anti-acid drug (*see* page 306).

Primaxin (imipenem) An antibiotic with some activity against *Pseudomonas* (*see* page 298).

Principen (ampicillin) An antibiotic (*see* page 294).

Propulsid (cisapride) An anti-reflux drug (*see* page 307).

Prostaphlin (oxacillin sodium) An anti-*Staph* penicillin antibiotic (*see* page 294).

Proventil A beta-agonist bronchodilator (*see* page 298).

prunes One of the best sources of dietary fiber, especially effective in combatting constipation (*see* page 307).

Quibron A bronchodilator preparation that contains several different drugs, including theophylline and an expectorant (*see* page 299).

quinolones A family of antibiotics (*see* page 297).

ranitidine A medication that decreases the stomach's production of acid (*see* page 306).

Reglan metoclopramide (*see* page 307).

ribavirin An aerosol medicine which can help control some viral bronchial infections, especially bronchiolitis caused by RSV (respiratory syncytial virus).

Robitussin (guaifenesin) A cough preparation consisting of an expectorant (*see* page 303).

Rondec (carbinoxamine maleate + pseudoephedrine HCl) A cough and cold preparation (*see* pages 303, 304).

saline Salt water.

Senekot (senna) An intestinal stimulant (*see* page 308).

Silain (simethicone) An antibloating drug (*see* page 309).

Slo-Phyllin Gyrocaps A long-lasting theophylline bronchodilator (*see* page 299).

sodium chloride Salt.

Somophyllin A theophylline preparation (*see* page 299).

Spectrobid A type of penicillin closely related to ampicillin (*see* page 294).

spironolactone A diuretic (*see* page 305).

Staphcillin (sodium methicillin) An anti-staph antibiotic (*see* page 295).

steroids Very potent drugs which are similar to the chemicals made in the body in the adrenal glands. They are very powerful and can be used safely for a short period of time for some purposes such as decreasing bronchial inflammation (*see* page 299). They are often employed for other purposes too, including growth and appetite stimulation (*see* page 309).

sulfamethoxazole A sulfa antibiotic (*see* page 295).

Sulfatrim A combination antibiotic trimethoprim-sulfamethaxozole (*see* page 295).

Sus-Phrine (epinephrine) A bronchodilator medication with some beta-agonist activity. It is used only by injection, and primarily for treating serious allergic reactions or an asthma attack (*see* page 298).

Sustacal A nutritional supplement formula (*see* page 310).

Sustaire　A theophylline bronchodilator (*see* page 299).

Tagamet　(cimetidine) An anti-acid drug (*see* page 306).

Tazidime　ceftazidime (*see* page 297).

Tedral　A combination drug which includes some theophylline bronchodilator (*see* page 299).

Tegopen　(cloxacillin sodium) An anti-*Staph* penicillin (*see* page 295).

terbutaline sulfate　A beta-agonist bronchodilator (*see* page 298).

Terramycin　(oxytetracycline) A tetracycline antibiotic (*see* page 297).

Testionate　A male steroid hormone used for growth and appetite stimulation (*see* page 309).

testosterone　The primary male hormone (*see* page 309).

Tetra-BID　A tetracycline antibiotic (*see* page 297).

tetracycline　An antibiotic family (*see* page 297).

Theobid　A theophylline bronchodilator (*see* page 299).

Theo-Dur　A theophylline bronchodilator (*see* page 299).

Theolate　A theophylline bronchodilator (*see* page 299).

Theophyl　A theophylline bronchodilator (*see* page 299).

theophylline　A family of bronchodilators (*see* page 299).

Theospan　A theophylline bronchodilator (*see* page 299).

ticarcillin　An anti-*Pseudomonas* penicillin (*see* page 295).

tilade nedocromil　(*see* page 300).

Timentin　An anti-*Pseudomonas* and anti-*Staph* antibiotic (*see* page 295).

tobramycin　An aminoglycoside antibiotic (*see* page 295).

Tornalate　(methanesulfonate) A beta-agonist bronchodilator (*see* page 298).

triamcinolone　An inhaled steroid (*see* page 299).

Triaminic　(phenylpropanolamine HCl + pheniramine maleate + pyrilamine maleate) A cold preparation (*see* page 304).

trimethoprim　An antibiotic usually found in combination with a sulfa drug (*see* page 295).

Tussionex　A cough mixture including an antihistamine, a narcotic cough suppressant (*see* page 303).

Tuss-Ornade　A cough medicine which also contains a decongestant and a cough suppressant (*see* pages 303, 304).

Ultrase　A pancreatic enzyme supplement (*see* page 306).

Vancenase　(beclomethasone dipropionate) A nasal steroid spray (*see* page 303).

Vantin　A cephalosporin antibiotic (*see* page 296).

Veetid B-Cillin　(penicillin) An antibiotic (*see* page 294).

Velosef　A cephalosporin antibiotic (*see* page 296).

Ventolin　(albuterol sulfate) A beta-agonist bronchodilator (*see* page 298).

Vibramycin　A tetracycline antibiotic (*see* page 297).

Viokase　(pancreatin) A digestive enzyme (*see* page 306).

Vipep　A nutritional supplement formula (*see* page 310).

Virazole　ribavirin

Vital　A nutritional supplement formula (*see* page 310).

Vivonex　A nutritional supplement formula (*see* page 310).

Winstrol　(stanozolol) A sex steroid hormone (*see* page 309).

Wycillin　(penicillin) An antibiotic (*see* page 294).

Zantac　(ranitidine) Helps to decrease the stomach's production of acid (*see* page 306).

Zymase　A digestive enzyme (*see* page 306).

APPENDIX C

Airway Clearance Techniques

POSTURAL DRAINAGE TECHNIQUES*

Infants

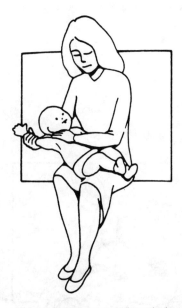

Figure 1. Draining anterior apical segments.

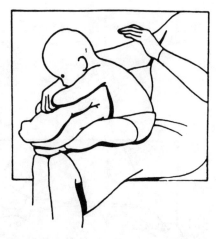

Figure 2. Draining posterior apical segments.

*The material presented here has been reproduced with the kind permission of Dr. Beryl Rosenstein from his excellent booklet, *The Johns Hopkins Hospital Cystic Fibrosis Patient Handbook* (Beryl Rosenstein and Terry S. Langbaum, editors).

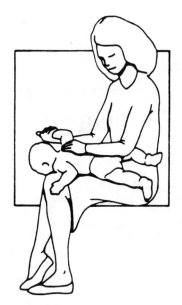

Figure 3. Draining right posterior segment.

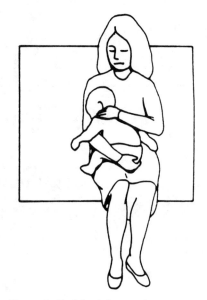

Figure 4. Draining left posterior segment.

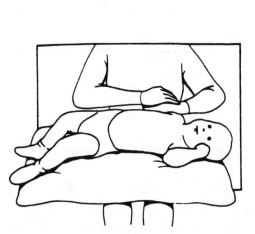

Figure 5. Draining anterior segments.

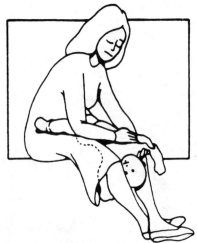

Figure 6. Draining right middle lobe.

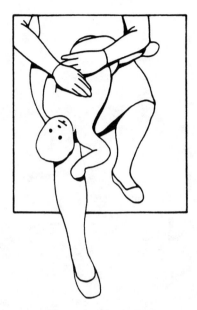

Figure 7. Draining left lingula.

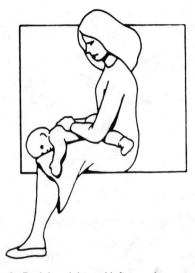

Figure 8. Draining right and left superior segments.

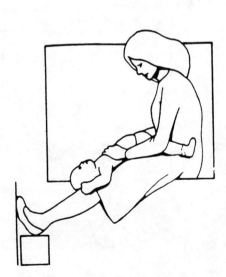

Figure 9. Draining anterior basal segments.

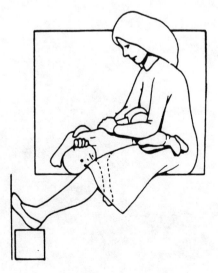

Figure 10. Draining left lateral basal segment.

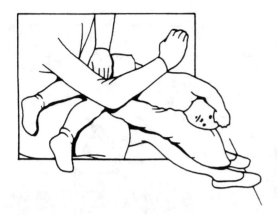

Figure 11. Draining right lateral basal segment.

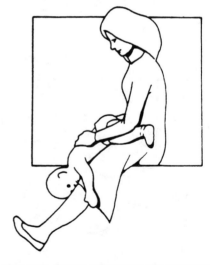

Figure 12. Draining posterior basal segments.

Toddlers

The following points will be helpful in performing postural drainage.

- Clap one minute—vibrate five exhalations—vibrate while huffing two to three times, cough, repeat once.
- Each session should last a maximum of 30 to 40 minutes.
- Always do treatment sessions *before* meals.
- Two to three sessions per day are usually recommended.

Other Considerations

Children may become frightened initially when given postural drainage. As this treatment is very important, you should be encouraged not to apologize or sympathize for having to give this form of treatment. Children should understand, to the best of their ability, why the treatment is being done and accept it as part of the daily routine. Children should be encouraged to talk and sing, as this helps them to breathe. Children should not be offered rewards for future treatments. The drainage should be done with as little fuss as possible.

Your child does not need to dislike the time spent in physical therapy. You can make this time a pleasant, quiet opportunity to spend in conversation, or you can provide entertainment by playing records or tapes, or by doing drainage in front of the television.

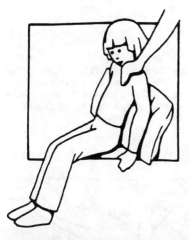

Figure 13. Upper lobes, apical segments. *Sitting:* Lean back against pillow (30° angle) and clap below collar bone in front with cupped hands.

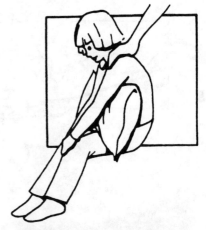

Figure 14. Upper lobes, posterior segments. *Sitting:* Lean forward onto pillow (30° angle) and clap behind collar bone on the back. The fingers usually go a little over shoulders.

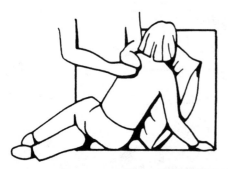

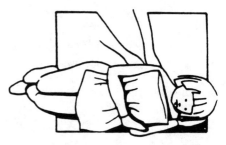

Figure 15. Left upper lobe. *Bed elevated 45°:* Head up, lying on right side. Place pillow in front, from shoulders to hips, and roll slightly forward onto it. Clap over left shoulder blade.

Figure 16. Right upper lobe. *Lying on left side:* Place pillow in front, from shoulders to hips, or roll slightly forward onto it. Clap over right shoulder blade.

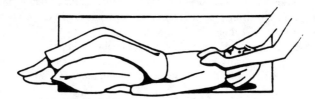

Figure 17. Upper lobes, anterior segments. *Lying flat on back:* Place pillow under knees and clap just below where you clapped on apical segment.

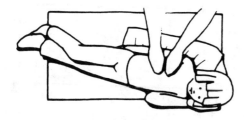

Figure 18. Right middle lobe. *Lying on left side:* Place pillow behind from shoulders to hips (30° tilt) and roll slightly back onto it (one-quarter turn). Clap over right nipple.

Figure 19. Left lingula. *Lying on right side:* Place pillow behind, from shoulders to hips, and roll slightly back onto it. Clap left nipple (30° tilt).

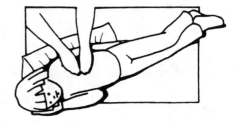

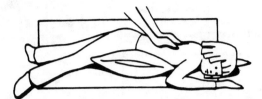

Figure 20. Lower lobes, superior segments. *Bed flat:* Lying on stomach with pillow under stomach, clap at area of shoulder blades (apex of lower lobes).

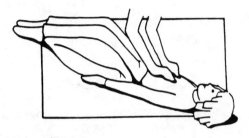

Figure 21. Lower lobes, anterior segments. *Lying on back:* Place pillow under knees and clap on lower ribs (45° tilt).

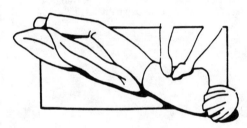

Figure 22. Lower lobes, left lateral. *Lying on right side:* Knees bent, clap at lower ribs, keeping spine straight (45° tilt).

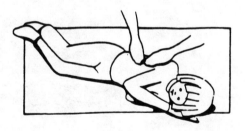

Figure 23. Lower lobes, right lateral. *Lying on left side:* Knees bent, clap at lower ribs, keeping spine straight (45° tilt).

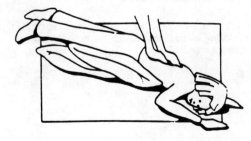

Figure 24. Lower lobes, posterior segments. *Lying on stomach:* Place pillow under hips and stomach to make spine straight (45° tilt). Clap at lower ribs (stay off spine).

Self Segmental Bronchial Drainage

Self Segmental Bronchial Drainage

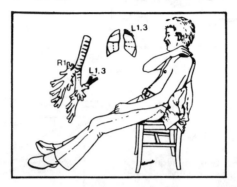

Figure 25. Sit on a chair and lean backward on a pillow at a 30° angle. Clap with a cupped hand over the area between the clavicle (collarbone) and the top of the scapula (shoulder blade). The area for clapping shown in the diagram is for the *apical*-posterior segment of the left upper lobe, *L1,3*. The *apical* segment of the right upper lobe, R1, is drained in the same position, with clapping on the right side. **Upper lobes:** apical segments: *1;* apical-posterior segment; left: *L1,3;* apical segment; right, *R3.*

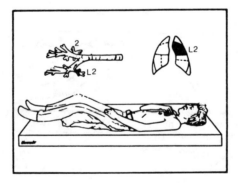

Figure 26. Lie flat on your back (supine) on a bed or drainage table. Clap between the clavicle (collarbone) and nipple. The area for clapping shown in the diagram is for the *anterior* segment of the left upper lobe, *L2.* **Upper lobes:** anterior segments: *2.*

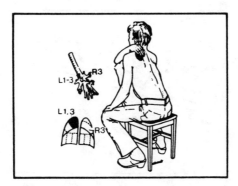

Figure 27. Sit on a chair leaning forward over a folded pillow at a 30° angle. Clap over the upper back. The area for clapping shown in the diagram is for the apical-*posterior* segment of the left upper lobe, *L1-3.* The posterior segment of the right upper lobe, *R3,* is drained in the same position with clapping on the right side of the upper back. **Upper lobes:** posterior segments: *3,* posterior segment; right: *R3;* apical-posterior segment, left: *L1-3.*

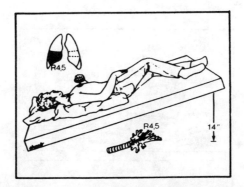

Figure 28. The foot of the table or bed is elevated 14 inches (about 15°). Lie head down on the left side and rotate 1/4 turn backward. A pillow may be placed behind and back (from shoulder to hip). The knees should be flexed. Clap over the area of the right nipple. Women should use a cupped hand with the heel of the hand under the armpit and the fingers extending forward beneath the breast. The area for clapping of the right *middle lobe, R4,5,* is shown in the diagram. **Right middle lobe:** *R4,5;* lateral segment: *R4;* medial segment: *R5.*

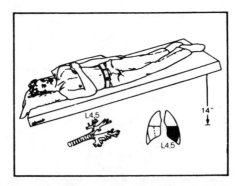

Figure 29. The *lingular* segment of the left upper lobe, *L4,5*, is drained by lying in a head-down position on the right side and rotating 1/4 turn backward. Clap over the area of the left nipple. Women should use a cupped hand with the heel of the hand under the armpit and the fingers extending forward beneath the breast. A pillow may be placed behind the back for support. **Lingular segment, left upper lobe:** *L4,5;* superior segment: *L4;* inferior segment; *L5.*

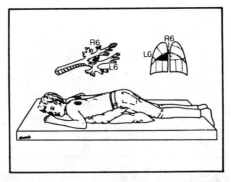

Figure 30. Lie on your abdomen on a bed or table which is in a flat position with two pillows under your hips. Clap over the middle part of the back at the tip of the scapula (shoulder blade) on either side of the spine. The area for clapping of the *superior* segment of the left lower lobe, *L6*, is shown in the diagram. The *superior* segment of the right lower lobe, *R6,* is done in the same position, with clapping on the right side. **Lower lobes:** superior segments, *6.*

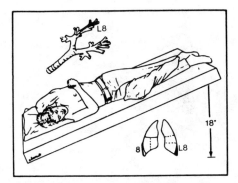

Figure 31. The foot of the table or bed is elevated 18 inches (about 30°). Lie on your side at a 90° angle in the head-down position with a pillow under your knees. Clap with a cupped hand over the lower ribs just beneath the axilla (armpit). The area for clapping shown is for drainage of the left *anterior basal* segment, *L8.* To drain the right *anterior basal* segment, *R8,* lie on your left side in the same position and clap over the right side of the chest. **Lower lobes:** anterior basal segments, *8.*

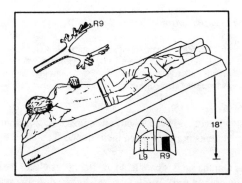

Figure 32. The foot of the table is elevated 18 inches (approximately 30°). Lie on your abdomen, head down, and rotate 1/4 turn upward from a prone position. Flex your upper leg over a pillow for support. Clap over the lower ribs. The area for clapping shown in the diagram is for the draining of the *right lateral basal* segment, *R9.* To drain the *left lateral basal* segment, *L9,* lie on your right side in the same position and clap over the lower ribs on the left side of the chest. **Lower lobes:** lateral basal segments, *9.*

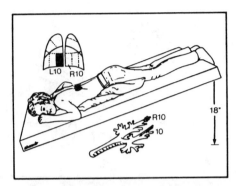

Figure 33. The foot of the bed or table is elevated 18 inches (about 30°). Lie on your abdomen, head down, with a pillow under your hips. Try to clap over the lower ribs close to the spine. The area for clapping shown in the diagram is for drainage of the *posterior basal* segment of the left lower lobe, *L10*. For drainage of the *posterior basal* segment of the right lower lobe, lie in the same position and try to clap over the lower ribs on the right side of the chest. This is a difficult area for some individuals to reach and you may want to obtain assistance in clapping in this position. **Lower lobes:** posterior basal segments, *10.*

FLUTTER TECHNIQUE

The Flutter technique has been very successful for children, adolescents, and adults, and is done independently. A simple piece of equipment is needed, namely, the Flutter device. It can be purchased from Scandipharm, Inc. (22 Inverness Center Parkway, Birmingham, AL 35242) or through many different pharmacies, including the national CF Foundation's pharmacy services.

The device (as you may recall from Chapter 3) is

a hand-held device, small enough to carry around in your pocket, that looks a little like a kazoo. It has a stainless steel ball in it that vibrates up and down (flutters, you might say) as you blow into the tube. The vibrations are transmitted backward down through the patient's mouth into the trachea and bronchi, where they shake the mucus free from the bronchial walls.

Instructions for its use are as follows:

Sit with your back straight and head slightly tilted back so that your throat and windpipe are wide open. Some patients prefer to place their elbows on a table to help keep them from slouching.

Hold the Flutter so that the stem is parallel to the floor (this places the cone at a slight angle, enabling the ball to flutter and roll). You'll then try slightly different positions and see which gives you the most vibrating in your chest.

The inhalation step (breath in) is very important. Take in as big a breath as possible. Then HOLD that breath for at least 2 to 3 seconds.

Then, at the end of the breath-hold, place the Flutter in your mouth and begin to exhale at a constant speed. You should NOT breathe out as fast as you can, but try different speeds of blowing out, and see which speed makes the most fluttering feeling in your chest, and helps you clear mucus best. While you're blowing out, keep your cheeks flat (don't let the vibrations be wasted on your cheeks; instead you want them to go to your lungs). While you're learning, you might hold your cheeks lightly with your other hand to keep them from vibrating.

Exhale as much air as possible. Really squeeze it out to help clean those small airways. This is a maximum effort (remember, not maximum hard blast, but maximum long breath out).

Leave the Flutter in your mouth and take in another big breath (through your nose) and repeat the whole Flutter breath several times.

Now, remove the Flutter, take in a big breath, hold it for 2 to 3 seconds, and "huff" out a breath, holding your mouth and throat open, and cough.

OTHER TECHNIQUES

The following techniques are used more in Europe than in North America. What follows is just a brief description of each, along with the name, address, phone, and fax for an expert from the International Physiotherapy Group for Cystic Fibrosis (IPG/CF). This group has dedicated itself to educating people interested in airway clearance for patients with CF.

PEP Mask

For the PEP mask (*positive* expiratory *pressure*) technique, the patient breathes through a special mask that has an exhale-valve that requires some air pressure to open. It is thought that this expiratory pressure is transmitted back down the airways and helps to prop them open during the exhalation, allowing mucus to be pushed out along with the air (remember that usually during exhalation, the airways tend to narrow a little bit, so this keeps them open wider than they would normally be). Contact:

Meret Falk and Mette Kelstrup
Physiotherapists
Department of Physiotherapy
Rigshospitalet
DK-2100 Copenhagen
Denmark
Phone: 45-35-453545
Fax: 45-35-456717

Active Cycle of Breathing

This technique has three phases, *breathing control* (quiet breathing), *thoracic expansion* (deep breaths in), and *forced expiration* or *huffs* (quick, strong—but never violent—breaths out, with the mouth and throat open). Contact:

Jennifer Pryor and Barbara Webber
Physiotherapy Department
Royal Brompton Hospital
Sydney Street
London SW3 6NP
United Kingdom
Phone: 44-171-351-8056
Fax: 44-171-351-8950

Autogenic Drainage

Autogenic drainage involves a series of breaths controlled so that some are done with very little air in the lungs, some with a medium amount, and some with the lungs filled almost to capacity. This technique requires instruction by someone very skilled in its use before it can be effective in mobilizing mucus. Contact:

J. Chevallier, P.T.
Zeepreventorium
5, Koninkluke Baan,
B8420 De Haan
Belgium
Phone: 32-59-233911
Fax: 32-59-234057

EXERCISE

Many people believe that vigorous exercise may be helpful to loosen mucus and to keep bronchi clear. Certainly, hard exercise, or laughing or crying, often result in a coughing spell that brings up mucus, even in people who do not raise mucus during the traditional PD treatments. Since there is not yet any scientific evidence that exercise can successfully replace the time-honored PD treatments, it is best to encourage patients to be very active *and* to do their treatments. (Exercise is discussed at greater length in Chapter 10, *Exercise*.)

APPENDIX D

Some High-Calorie Recipes

PASTA POT
by Stefani Czekaj

2 pounds ground meat
2 medium onions, chopped
1 clove garlic, minced
1 (14 ounce) jar spaghetti sauce
1 (16 ounce) can stewed tomatoes
3 ounces canned or fresh mushrooms
8 ounces shell or spring macaroni
3 cups sour cream
8 ounces Provolone cheese, shredded
8 ounces Mozzarella cheese, shredded

Cook beef in skillet; drain excess fat. Add onions, garlic, spaghetti sauce, stewed tomatoes and mushrooms. Simmer 20 minutes. Meanwhile, cook macaroni according to package directions; drain and rinse in cold water.

Pour shells in deep casserole, cover with tomato meat sauce. Spread sour cream over sauce and add Provolone cheese. Top with Mozzarella cheese. Cover casserole and bake at 350° for 35–40 minutes. Uncover and bake until cheese melts and browns.

Yield: 10 servings
1 serving: 613 calories

* For higher calories use cheeses made with whole milk.

FETTUCINI ALFREDO
by Kevin Helmick

1 (8 ounce) package fettucini, uncooked
½ cup melted butter
¾ cup grated Parmesan cheese
4 tablespoons half and half
salt and pepper

Cook pasta according to package directions; drain well. In warm serving dish combine butter, cheese, half and half, salt and pepper. Add pasta to mixture. Gently toss to coat all fettucini. Top with Parmesan cheese.

Yield: 4 servings
1 cup: 450 calories

SPINACH PASTA
by Peggy Tommarello

½ cup vegetable oil
1 tablespoon butter
1 teaspoon salt
1 teaspoon basil
2 cloves garlic, halved
1 package frozen spinach, cooked
½ pound small shells, cooked and drained
1 (6 ounce) can grated Parmesan cheese

Saute first 5 ingredients; add cooked spinach. Mix well. Saute for 7–10 minutes. Add cooked pasta and then the Parmesan cheese. Stir until pasta is coated; heat thoroughly. Serve hot.

Yield: 6 servings
1 serving: 363 calories

VEGETABLE PIZZA

2 packages crescent rolls
2 (8 ounce) packages cream cheese, softened
1 cup mayonnaise
2 teaspoons onion powder
2 teaspoons dry dill, crumbled
2 cups chopped broccoli
2 cups chopped cauliflower
1 green pepper, chopped
2 tomatoes, diced and drained
2 medium carrots, shredded

Unroll and pat crescent rolls onto a cookie sheet to make crust. Bake at 350° until light golden brown. Cool. Combine the cream cheese, mayonnaise, onion powder, and dill. Spread over cooled crust. Top with the broccoli, cauliflower, green pepper, and tomatoes. Place shredded carrots on top. Cut in small triangles to serve.

Yield: 12 servings
1/12 recipe: 272 calories

SHRIMP SPREAD

8 ounces cream cheese, softened
1 small onion, diced
¼ cup mayonnaise
1 (6 ounce) can mini shrimp
½ tablespoon lemon juice
¼ teaspoon garlic powder
½ tablespoon Worcestershire sauce
¾ cup cocktail sauce

Mix all ingredients except cocktail sauce. Refrigerate for at least one hour. When ready to serve, mound cheese mixture in middle of plate. Pour cocktail sauce over the mound of cheese. Serve with a favorite cracker. (Crabmeat can be substituted for the shrimp.)

Yield: 24 servings
¹⁄₂₄ recipe: 60 calories

ARTICHOKE PIZZAZZ
by Karen Ketyer

1 (14 ounce) can artichoke hearts, drained and chopped
1 cup grated Parmesan cheese
1 cup shredded Mozzarella cheese
1 cup mayonnaise
2 tablespoons chopped green onion
1 dash garlic powder

Combine all ingredients and put in a 1½ quart casserole dish or quiche pan. Bake at 350°, for 25–30 minutes. Serve hot with a sturdy cracker.

Yield: 1 quart
¹⁄₂₀ recipe: 88 calories

PEANUT BUTTER ROUND-UPS
by Amanda Ogden

1 cup shortening
1 cup granulated sugar
1 cup brown sugar, firmly packed
2 eggs
1 cup peanut butter
2 cups all-purpose flour
½ teaspoon salt
2 teaspoons baking soda
1 cup quick rolled oats

Mix the ingredients one at a time in order of recipe; mix well. Place a teaspoonful of mixture on cookie sheet. Press with fork. Bake at 350° for 10–12 minutes.

Yield: 6 dozen balls
1 ball: 85 calories

DOUBLE CHOCOLATE WALNUT BROWNIES
by Annette Lucas

1 cup (2 sticks) butter or margarine
4 squares (4 ounces) unsweetened chocolate
2 cups granulated sugar
3 eggs
1 teaspoon vanilla extract
1 cup sifted all-purpose flour
1½ cups coarsely chopped walnuts
1 (6 ounce) package semi-sweet chocolate pieces

In medium saucepan, melt butter and chocolate squares over moderate heat. Remove from heat. Gradually beat in sugar with a wooden spoon until combined. Add 1 egg at a time, beating well after each egg. Stir in vanilla. Gradually add flour; mixing well. Stir in 1 cup walnuts. Spread mixture into a greased 9 × 13 × 2 inch pan. Combine remaining walnuts with chocolate pieces; sprinkle over top of brownies, pressing down lightly. Bake at 350° for 35 minutes or until top springs back when lightly pressed with fingertip.

Yield: 24 squares
1 (2 inch) square: 200 calories

LEMON BARS
by Louise Bauer

1 cup (2 sticks) butter
2 cups all-purpose flour
3 tablespoons granulated sugar
2 (8 ounce) packages cream cheese
2 cups powdered sugar
2 small packages lemon pudding and pie filling (not instant)
1 medium container Cool Whip
chopped nuts

Combine butter, flour, and sugar like a pie dough. Pat into bottom of jelly roll pan or cookie sheet. Bake at 325° for 15 minutes. Cool.

Blend cream cheese and powdered sugar with electric mixer. Spread on cooled crust.

Cook pudding according to package directions. Spread on top of cream cheese layer. Let gel. Cover with Cool Whip and sprinkle with chopped nuts, if desired. Cut into bars to serve.

Yield: 24 bars
1 bar: 260 calories

MILKY WAY CAKE
by David Orenstein

1 pound of Milky Way bars
1 cup buttermilk (or plain yogurt)
3 sticks margarine
½ teaspoon baking soda
4 eggs
2 teaspoons vanilla
2½ cups flour
½ cup chopped nuts
2 cups granulated sugar
2 cups powdered sugar

Melt about 11 ounces of the candy bars and 1 stick margarine in double boiler until smooth; set aside. Cream granulated sugar and 1 stick margarine; add eggs 1 at a time, beat until smooth; add flour, buttermilk (or yogurt), and baking soda. Add milky way mix, 2 teaspoons vanilla, and nuts. Bake in greased and floured bundt pan or angel food pan for 1 hr 20 min at 325°.

Frosting: Melt remaining candy bars (about 5 ounces) and the other stick of margerine in double boiler until smooth, add little vanilla and powdered sugar until desidered thickness, add a little milk if necessary. This cake should be stored in the fridge, but it probably won't need to be stored long!

Yield: 12 servings
1 serving: 705 calories

SCOTCHEROOS
by Renee Exler

1 cup light corn syrup
1 cup granulated sugar
1 cup peanut butter
6 cups Rice Krispy cereal
1 cup semi-sweet chocolate chips
1 cup butterscotch morsels

Cook corn syrup and sugar over medium heat in saucepan until sugar is dissolved; stir frequently. When mixture starts to boil remove from heat, and stir in peanut butter; mix well. Add

Rice Krispy cereal; stir until well coated. Press mixture into buttered 9 × 13 × 2 inch pan. Set aside.

Melt chocolate and butterscotch morsels over low heat; stirring constantly. Spread over cereal mixture. Allow to cool, then cut into 1 × 2 inch squares.

1 × 2 inch square: 96 calories

CHEESECAKE SQUARES
by Amanda Ogden

1 (14 ounce) can sweetened condensed milk
½ cup lemon juice or 2–3 lemons squeezed
1 tablespoon grated lemon rind
⅔ cup shortening
1 cup brown sugar, firmly packed
1¾ cup all-purpose flour
1 teaspoon salt
1½ cups quick cooking oats

Blend milk, juice, and rind with electric mixer until thick; set aside.

Mix together shortening and sugar. Combine flour and other dry ingredients. Blend into shortening mixture. Blend in rolled oats. Place half of the oats mixture into a 9 × 13 × 2 inch pan and press and flatten down. Spread the lemon mixture over the oats mixture. Cover with remaining oat mixture, patting lightly. Bake at 375° for 25–30 minutes. Cool and cut into bars.

Yield: 24 squares
1 square: 203 calories

HEATH BARS
by Jane Strange

50–60 soda crackers
¼ cup butter, melted
1 cup (2 sticks) butter
1 cup dark brown sugar, firmly packed
1 (12 ounce) package milk chocolate chips
1 cup chopped nuts

Line large cookie sheet with tin foil; spread with melted butter. Place the crackers on buttered cookie sheet.

In medium sauce pan cook sugar and 1 cup butter until dissolved; stirring constantly. Allow sugar and butter to boil. Pour mixture over crackers. Bake at 375° for 7 minutes. Remove from oven and sprinkle with chocolate chips. As the chips melt, spread to smooth out. Sprinkle with nuts. Place in refrigerator to cool. Cut into bars to serve.

Yield: 24 bars
1 bar: 236 calories

KID PLEASIN' CHOCOLATE MOUSSE

1 (6 ounce) package chocolate instant pudding mix
3 cups cold whole milk
1 cup frozen whipped topping, thawed
12 cream-filled chocolate sandwich cookies, crumbled
8 cream-filled chocolate sandwich cookies, whole

Combine pudding mix and milk in a small mixing bowl; beat at low speed of an electric mixer until blended. Beat at low speed an additional 2 minutes. Fold in ½ cup whipped topping and cookie crumbs. Spoon mousse into 8 (6 ounce) dessert dishes. Cover and chill.

Garnish each serving with a drop of remaining whipped topping and a whole cookie just before serving.

Yield: 8 (6 ounce) servings
⅛ recipe: 276 calories

MIRACLE PUDDING
by Brenda McCullen

2 small packages chocolate instant pudding
1 (14 ounce) can sweetened condensed milk
1 large container Cool Whip

Prepare pudding according to package directions. Combine remaining ingredients with pudding and mix well. Refrigerate until chilled. Any flavor pudding may be used.

Yield: 8 servings
⅛ recipe: 513 calories

PUPPY CHOW
by Brenda McCullen

1 stick (½ cup) butter
1 (12 ounce) package chocolate chips
½ cup peanut butter
8 cups Rice Chex or Crispix cereal
2 cups powdered sugar

Melt the first three ingredients in a medium saucepan. Place the cereal in a large plastic container and add the melted mixture. Shake sealed container until all the cereal is coated. Add the powdered sugar.

Yield: 12 servings
¹/₁₂ recipe: 500 calories

FRUIT PIZZA
by Clare Jean Haury

1 package yellow cake mix
¼ cup water
¼ cup margarine, softened
2 eggs
¼ cup packed brown sugar
½ cup pecans, chopped
2 packages Dream Whip®
fresh fruit

Grease and flour two 12" pizza pans. Combine half the cake mix and all other ingredients except the pecans, fruit, and Dream Whip®. Mix well. Add remaining cake mix and mix well. Fold in nuts. Divide evenly between the 2 pans and spread to the edges. Bake at 350° for 15–20 minutes. Cool. Prepare Dream Whip according to directions on package. Top each cake with one package of Dream Whip and add sliced fresh fruit to decorate.

Yield: 12 servings
¹/₁₂ recipe: 350 calories

APPENDIX E

The History of Cystic Fibrosis

Some highlights in the history of cystic fibrosis are as follows:

1705 A book of folk philosophy states that a salty taste means that a child is bewitched.

1857 *The Almanac of Children's Songs and Games* from Switzerland quotes from Middle Ages: "Woe is the child who tastes salty from a kiss on the brow, for he is hexed, and soon must die."

1938 Andersen first describes CF, calling it cystic fibrosis of the pancreas.

1946 di Sant'Agnese and Andersen report using antibiotics to treat CF lung infection.

1953 di Sant'Agnese and colleagues describe the sweat abnormality in CF.

1955 First review of use of pancreatic enzymes.

1959 Gibson and Cook describe a safe and accurate way to do sweat testing.

1964 Doershuk, Matthews, and colleagues describe a modern comprehensive treatment program.

1978 First use of enteric-coated pancreatic enzymes.

1981–1983 Description by Knowles and colleagues and Quinton and coworkers of electrolyte transport abnormalities.

1989 Tsui, Riordan, and Collins discover CF gene.

1990 Correction of chloride transport defect in CF cells in culture by adenovirus-mediated gene transfer.

1992 First trials of gene transfer in living people with CF.

Modified from Taussig LM. *Cystic Fibrosis*. Thieme-Stratton Inc., New York, 1984.

APPENDIX F

Cystic Fibrosis Care Centers and Chapters in the United States

Alabama

Birmingham

UAB Cystic Fibrosis Center
The Children's Hospital
University of Alabama at Birmingham
1600 7th Street, South
Birmingham, AL 35233

Appts: (205) 939-9583

Center Director:

Raymond Lyrene, M.D.
(205) 934-3574 or
(205) 939-9583
Fax: (205) 975-5983

Mobile

USA Children's Medical Center
P.O. Drawer 40130
1504 Spring Hill Avenue
Mobile, AL 36640-0130

Appts: (334) 343-6848

Center Director:

Lawrence J. Sindel, M.D.*
(205) 343-6848
Fax: (205) 343-5708

*Preferred Mailing Address:

Pulmonary Association of Mobile, P.A.
3732A Dauphin Street
Mobile, AL 36608

Arizona

Phoenix

Cystic Fibrosis Center
Phoenix Children's Hospital
909 E. Brill Street
Phoenix, AZ 85006

Appts: (602) 239-6925

Center Director:

Peggy J. Radford, M.D.
(602) 239-5778
Fax: (602)239-2996

Tucson

Tucson Cystic Fibrosis Center
St. Luke's Chest Clinic
Arizona Health Sciences Center
1501 N. Campbell Avenue, Room 2340
Tucson, AZ 85724

Appts: (520) 694-7450

Center Director:

Wayne J. Morgan, M.D.
(520) 626-7780
Fax: (520) 626-6970

Arkansas

Little Rock

Arkansas Cystic Fibrosis Center
Arkansas Children's Hospital
800 Marshall Street
Little Rock, AR 72202-3591

Appts: (501) 320-1018

Center Director:

Robert H. Warren, M.D.
(501) 320-1006 or
(501) 320-1007
Fax: (501) 320-3930

Adult Program Director:

Paula Anderson, M.D.
(501) 686-5525

California

Long Beach

Cystic Fibrosis Center
Memorial Miller Children's Hospital
2801 Atlantic Avenue
P.O. Box 1428
Long Beach, CA 90801-1428

Appts: (310) 933-3290

Center Director:

Eliezer Nussbaum, M.D.
Fax: (310) 933-2541

Satellite Center:

Ventura County Medical Center
3400 Loma Vista Road
Ventura, CA 93003

Appts: (805) 652-6124

Director:

Chris Landon, M.D.

Los Angeles

Cystic Fibrosis Comprehensive Center
Children's Hospital of Los Angeles
4650 Sunset Boulevard
Mail Stop #83
Los Angeles, CA 90027-6016

Appts: (213) 669-2287 (direct line)
         (213) 660-2450 (hospital)

Center Director:

C. Michael Bowman, M.D., Ph.D.
(213) 669-2101
Fax: (213) 664-9758

Adult program:

University of Southern California
Ambulatory Health Care Center
1500 San Pablo Boulevard
Los Angeles, CA 90033

Appts: (213) 342-5100

Director:

Bertrand Shapiro, M.D.
Fax: (213) 342-8605

Satellite Center:

Kaiser-Permanente Southern California
13652 Cantara Street
Panorama City, CA 91402

Appts: (818) 375-2909 (ask for Linda
Barraza—open to members of
the Kaiser-Permanente Health
Plan only)

Director:

Allan S. Lieberthal, M.D.
(818) 375-2412
Fax: (818) 375-4073

Outreach:

Cedars Sinai Medical Center
8700 Beverly Boulevard
Los Angeles, CA 90048

Appts: (310) 855-4433

Codirectors:

C. Michael Bowman, M.D., Ph.D.
(children)
Andrew Wachtel, M.D. (adults)
Fax: (310) 967-0145

Oakland

1. Kaiser Permanente Medical Center
Attn: Gail Farmer, R.D.
Department of Pediatrics
280 West MacArthur Boulevard
Oakland, CA 94611

Appts: (510) 596-6906 (ask for Gail
Farmer)

Center Director:

Gregory F. Shay, M.D.
(510) 596-6596
Fax: (510) 596-6147

(Kaiser has four locations—call Gail
Farmer for information)

2. Pediatric Pulmonary Center
Children's Hospital - Oakland
747 - 52nd Street
Oakland, CA 94609

Appts: (510) 428-3305

Center Director:

Nancy C. Lewis, M.D.
Fax: (510) 428-3123

Orange

Cystic Fibrosis and Pediatric Pulmonary
Care, Teaching, and Resource Center
Children's Hospital of Orange County
455 South Main Street
Orange, CA 92668

Preferred Mailing Address:

P.O. Box 5700
Orange, CA 92667

Appts: (714) 532-8317

Center Director:

David Hicks, M.D.
(714) 997-3000, ext. 8616
Fax: (714) 289-4072

Palo Alto

Stanford Cystic Fibrosis Center
Lucile Packard Children's Hospital at
  Stanford
725 Welch Road
Palo Alto, CA 94304

Appts: (415) 497-8841 (scheduling)
         (415) 497-8845 (coordinator)

Center Director:

Richard Moss, M.D.*
(415) 723-5191
Fax: (415) 723-5201
E-mail: ma.rbm@forsythe.stanford.edu

*Preferred Mailing Address:

Department of Pediatrics G309
Stanford University Medical Center
300 Pasteur Drive
Stanford, CA 94305-5119

Satellite Center:

California Pacific Medical Center
Department of Pediatrics
2340 Clay Street, Room #325
San Francisco, CA 94115

Director:

Karen A. Hardy, M.D.
(415) 923-3434
Fax: (415) 923-3506

Sacramento

Cystic Fibrosis and Pediatric Respiratory
  Diseases Center
University of California at Davis School of
  Medicine
Department of Pediatrics
2516 Stockton Boulevard
Sacramento, CA 95817

Appts: (916) 734-3112

Center Director:

Ruth McDonald, M.D.
(916) 734-3189
Fax: (916) 456-2236

Adult Program Director:

Carroll Cross, M.D.

San Bernardino

Brian Wesley Ray Cystic Fibrosis Center
San Bernardino County Medical Center
Department of Pediatrics
780 East Gilbert Street
San Bernardino, CA 92415-0935

Appts: (909) 387-8155 or
         (909) 387-7705

Center Director:

Gerald R. Greene, M.D., M.P.H.
Fax: (909) 387-0565

San Diego

San Diego Cystic Fibrosis and Pediatric
  Pulmonary Disease Center
UCSD Medical Center
200 West Arbor Drive
Mail Code 8448
San Diego, CA 92103-1990

Appts: (619) 294-6125

Center Director:

Michael Light, M.D.
Fax: (619) 296-3758

San Francisco

Cystic Fibrosis Center
University of California at San Francisco
Room M650
505 Parnassus Avenue
San Francisco, CA 94143-0106

Appts: (415) 476-2072

Center Director:

Gerd J.A. Cropp, M.D., Ph.D.
(415) 476-2072
Fax: (415) 476-4009

Adult Program Director:

Michael S. Stulbarg, M.D.
(415) 476-5993
Fax: (415) 476-9531

Satellite Center:

Valley Children's Hospital
Pediatric Pulmonary and Respiratory
   Care
3151 N. Millbrook, Suite 121
Fresno, CA 93703

Appts: (209) 228-6363

Director

R. Sudhakar, M.D.
Fax: (209) 224-6933

Colorado

Denver

Denver Children's Hospital
1056 East 19th Avenue
Box B395
Denver, CO 80218-1088

Appts: (303) 837-2522

Center Director:

Frank J. Accurso, M.D.
Fax: (303) 837-2924
E-mail: accurso.frank@tchden.edu

Adult Program Director:

David Rodman, M.D.
University of Colorado
(303) 270-7047
Fax: (303) 270-5632

Satellite Center:

Billings Clinic
2825 8th Avenue, North
Billings, MT 59101

Appts: (406) 238-2310

Director:

Nicholas Wolter, M.D.
Fax: (406) 248-2677

Connecticut

Hartford

Cystic Fibrosis Center
Department of Pediatrics
University of Connecticut Health Center
263 Farmington Avenue
Mail Code 1827
Farmington, CT 06030

Appts: (203) 679-2647

Center Director:

Michelle Cloutier, M.D.
(203) 679-2647
Fax: (203) 679-1376

*New address and phone number
effective April 1, 1997*

Cystic Fibrosis Center
Pediatric Pulmonology Division
Connecticut Children's Medical Center
282 Washington Avenue
Hartford, CT 060630

Appts: (860) 545-9440

New Haven

Cystic Fibrosis Center
Yale University School of Medicine
333 Cedar Street, Fitkin 511
New Haven, CT 06520-8064

Appts: (203) 785-2480

Center Director:

Thomas F. Dolan Jr., M.D.
Fax: (203) 785-6337

District of Columbia

Metropolitan D.C. Cystic Fibrosis Center
   for Care, Training and Research
Children's National Medical Center
111 Michigan Avenue, N.W.
Washington, D.C. 20010-2970

Appts: (202) 884-2128

Center Director:

Robert J. Fink, M.D.
Fax: (202) 884-3461

Florida

Gainesville

Cystic Fibrosis and Pediatric Pulmonary
   Disease Center
University of Florida
P.O. Box 100296
Gainesville, FL 32610-0296

Appts: (352) 392-4458

Center Director:

Mary H. Wagner, M.D.
Fax: (352) 392-4450

Adult Program Director:

Arundhati Foster, M.D.
(352) 392-2666

Jacksonville

Nemours Children's Clinic
P.O. Box 5720
Jacksonville, FL 32247

Appts: (904) 390-3788

Center Director:

Ian Nathanson, M.D.
(904) 390-3561
Fax: (904) 390-3699

Orlando

Cystic Fibrosis Center
Orlando Regional Medical Center
85 West Miller Street, Suite 205
Orlando, Fl 32806

Appts: (407) 237-6327

Center Director:

Joseph J. Chiaro, M.D.*
(407) 237-6326
Fax: (407) 649-6986

*Preferred Mailing Address:

Arnold Palmer Hospital for Children and
   Women
85 West Miller Street, Suite 204
Orlando, FL 32806

St. Petersburg

Cystic Fibrosis Center
All Children's Hospital
880 Sixth Street South, Suite 390
St. Petersburg, FL 33731-8920

Appts: (813) 892-4146

Center Director:

Michelle Howenstine, M.D.
Fax: (813) 892-4218

Adult Program:

University of South Florida
Pulmonology Critical Care
12901 Bruce B. Downs Boulevard,
Box 33
Tampa, FL 33612

Appts: (813) 892-4146

Director:

Mark Rolfe, M.D.
(813) 972-7543

Satellite Centers:

St. Mary's Hospital, Inc.
P.O. Box 24620
901 45th Street
West Palm Beach, FL 33416-4620

Appts: (407) 881-2911

Director:

Sue Goldfinger, M.D.
Fax: (407) 882-1078

Division of Pulmonology
Miami Children's Hospital
MOB #203, 3200 S.W. 60th Court
Miami, FL 33155

Appts: (305) 662-8380

Director:

Moises Simpser, M.D.
Fax: (305) 663-8417

University of South Florida
71 Davis Boulevard, Suite 200
Department of Pediatrics
Division of Pulmonology
College of Medicine
Tampa, FL 33606

Appts: (813) 276-5520

Director:

Bruce M. Schnapf, D.O.

Outreach Clinics:

New Port Richey Specialty Care
 Clinic
5640 Main Street
New Port Richey, FL 34652

Sarasota Clinic
5881 Rand Boulevard
Sarasota, FL 34238

Tampa Clinic
12220 Bruce B. Downs Boulevard
Tampa, FL 33612

Appts: (813) 892-4146

Georgia

Atlanta

Emory University
Cystic Fibrosis Center
Department of Pediatrics
2040 Ridgewood Drive, N.E.
Atlanta, GA 30322

Appts: (404) 727-5728

Center Director:

Daniel B. Caplan, M.D.
Fax: (404) 727-4828

Augusta

Department of Pediatrics
Section of Pulmonology
Medical College of Georgia
1120 15th Street
Augusta, GA 30912

Appts: (706) 721-2635

Center Director:

Lou Guill, M.D.
(706) 721-2635
Fax: (706) 721-8512
E-mail: deptped.mquill@mail.mcg.edu

Adult Program Director

John DuPre, M.D.
(706) 721-2566
Fax: (706) 721-3069

Satellite Center:

Scottish Rite Children's Medical Center
1001 Johnson Ferry Road, N.E.
Atlanta, GA 30363

Director:

Peter H. Scott, M.D.
(404) 256-5252   Ext. 5315

Outreach Clinic:

Ware County Health Department
604 Riverside Drive
Waycross, GA 31501

Appts: (912) 283-1875

Hawaii

**See Tripler Army Medical Center
(Fort Sam Houston, Texas)**

Idaho

**See University of Utah Medical Center
(Nampa and S.E. Idaho)**

Illinois

Chicago

1. Cystic Fibrosis Center
   Children's Memorial Hospital
   Northwestern University
   2300 Children's Plaza, Box 43
   Chicago, IL 60614

   Appts: (312) 880-4382

Center Director:

Susanna A. McColley, M.D.
Fax: (312) 880-6300
E-mail: smccolley@nwu.edu

2. Wyler Children's Hospital
    Department of Pediatrics
    University of Chicago Hospitals and
        Clinics
    5841 South Maryland Avenue
    Mail Code 6057
    Chicago, IL 60637

    Appts: (312) 702-6178

Center Director:

Lucille A. Lester, M.D.
Fax: (312) 703-4041
E-mail: lalester@babies.bsd.uchicago.edu

3. Department of Pediatrics
    Loyola University Medical Center
    2160 S. First Avenue
    Maywood, IL 60153

    Appts: (708) 327-9117

Center Director:

Harold Conrad, M.D.
(708) 327-9136
Fax: (708) 327-9067

Park Ridge

Cystic Fibrosis Center
Nesset Health Center
Lutheran General Hospital
1775 Dempster Street
Park Ridge, IL 60068

Appts: (708) 318-2867
Fax: (708) 318-2903

Center Director:

Jerome R. Kraut, M.D.*
(708) 696-7700
Fax: (708) 698-6879

*Preferred Mailing Address:

1255 Milwaukee Avenue
Glenview, IL 60025

Adult Program Director:

Arvey Stone, M.D.
(708) 318-9320

Peoria

Cystic Fibrosis Center
Saint Francis Medical Center Specialty
    Clinics
Hillcrest Medical Plaza
420 N.E. Glen Oaks Avenue, Suite 201
Peoria, IL 61603

Appts: (309) 655-3889

Center Director:

Umesh C. Chatrath, M.D.*
(309) 655-4070 Ext. 3889
Fax: (309) 655-7449

*Preferred Mailing Address:

420 N.E. Glen Oak Avenue
Room #204
Peoria, IL 61603

Springfield

**See Washington University CF Center,
(St. Louis, Missouri)**

Urbana

See Washington University CF Center,
(St. Louis, Missouri)

Indiana

Indianapolis

Cystic Fibrosis and Chronic Pulmonary
  Disease Center
Riley Hospital for Children
Indiana University Medical Center
702 Barnhill Drive, Room 2750
Indianapolis, IN 46202-5225

Appts: (317) 274-7208

Center Director:

Howard Eigen, M.D.
(317) 274-3434
Fax: (317) 274-3442

Adult Program Director:

Veena Anthony, M.D.
(317) 274-7208

Satellite Centers:

Deaconess Hospital
600 Mary Street
Evansville, IN 47747

Appts: (812) 426-3217

Parkview Memorial Hospital
2200 Randallia, Ext. 4144
Ft. Wayne, IN 46805

Appts: (219) 484-6636 Ext. 41440
Fax: (219) 484-6636 Ext. 51900

Director:

Pushpom James, M.D.

South Bend

Cystic Fibrosis and Chronic Pulmonary
  Disease Clinic
St. Joseph's Medical Center
801 E. LaSalle
P.O. Box 1935
South Bend, IN 46634

Appts: (800) 206-0879

Center Director:

Edward A. Gergesha, M.D.
(219) 237-6864
Fax: (219) 239-4024

Associate Director:

James Harris, M.D.*
(219) 237-9216
Fax: (219) 239-9329

*Preferred Mailing Address:

211 North Eddy
South Bend, IN 46617

Iowa

Des Moines

Cystic Fibrosis Center
Blank Children's Hospital
1200 Pleasant Street
Des Moines, IA 50309

Appts: (515) 241-8222
Fax: (515) 241-8296

Center Director:

Veljko Zivkovich, M.D.*
(515) 244-7229
Fax: (515) 244-7233

Iowa City

Cystic Fibrosis Center
Pediatric Allergy and Pulmonary Division
Department of Pediatrics
200 Hawkins Drive
University of Iowa Hospital and Clinics
Iowa City, IA 52242-1083

Appts: (319) 356-1853

Center Codirectors:

Miles Weinberger, M.D.
Richard Ahrens, M.D.
(319) 356-3485
Fax: (319) 353-6217

Satellite Center:

McFarland Clinic
Mary Greeley Hospital
1215 Duff
Ames, IA 50010

Appts: (515) 239-4482
Fax: (515) 239-4498

Director:

Edward G. Nassif, M.D.

Kansas

Kansas City

Cystic Fibrosis Center
Kansas University Medical Center
3901 Rainbow Boulevard
Kansas City, KS 66160-7330

Appts: (913) 588-6377

Center Director:

Joseph Kanarek, M.D.
Fax: (913) 588-6319

Codirector:

Pam Shaw, M.D.
Fax: (913) 588-6319
E-mail: alieberg@kumc.edu

Wichita

Cystic Fibrosis Care and Teaching Center
Via Christi, St. Joseph Campus
3600 East Harry Street
Wichita, KS 67218

Appts: (316) 689-4707

Center Director:

Leonard Sullivan, M.D.
(316) 689-9454 or (316) 689-4709
Fax: (316) 689-5804

Kentucky

Lexington

Cystic Fibrosis Center
Department of Pediatrics
Kentucky Clinic
760 South Limestone
Lexington, KY 40536-0284

Appts: (606) 323-8023

Center Director:

Jamshed F. Kanga, M.D.
(606) 257-1226
Fax: (606) 257-7706

Louisville

Kosair Children's Fibrosis Center
233 E. Gray Street, Suite 201
Louisville, KY 40202

Appts: (502) 629-8830

Center Director:

Nemr Eid, M.D.
(502) 629-8830
Fax: (502) 629-7540

Louisiana

New Orleans

Tulane Cystic Fibrosis Center
Department of Pediatrics SL-37
Tulane University School of Medicine
1430 Tulane Avenue
New Orleans, LA 70112

Appts: (504) 587-7625

Center Director:

Scott Davis, M.D.
(504) 588-5601
Fax: (504) 588-5490

Adult Program Director:

Dean Ellithorpe, M.D.
(504) 588-2250
Fax: (504) 587-2144

Shreveport

Cystic Fibrosis and Pediatric Pulmonary
   Center
Louisiana State University Medical Center
1501 Kings Highway
P.O. Box 33932
Shreveport, LA 71130-3932

Appts: (318) 675-6094

Center Director:

Bettina C. Hilman, M.D.
Fax: (318) 675-7668

Maine

Bangor

Cystic Fibrosis Clinical Center
Eastern Maine Medical Center
489 State Street
P.O. Box 404
Bangor, ME 04402-0404

Appts: (207) 973-7559

Center Codirectors:

Erlinda Polvorosa, M.D.
Thomas Lever, M.D.
Fax: (207) 973-7674

Lewiston

Central Maine Cystic Fibrosis Center
Central Maine Medical Center
300 Main Street
Lewiston, ME 04240

Appts: (207) 795-2830

Center Director:

Fax: (207) 795-5688

Portland

Cystic Fibrosis Center
Maine Medical Center
22 Bramhall Street
Portland, ME 04102

Appts: (207) 871-2763

Center Director:

Anne Marie Cairns, D.O.*
(207) 828-8226
Fax: (207) 775-6024

Preferred Mailing Address

Maine Medical Center
Pediatric Associates
295 Forest Avenue
Portland, ME 04102

Associate Director:

Nicholas K. Fowler, M.D.*
(207) 775-4151
Fax: (207) 775-6950

Preferred Mailing Address:

Greater Portland Pediatric Associates
75B John Roberts Road
South Portland, ME 04106

Associate Director:

Jack Mann, M.D.*

Preferred Mailing Address:

884 Broadway
South Portland, ME 04106

Adult Program Director:

Edgar J. Caldwell, M.D.*
(207) 871-2489
Fax: (207) 871-4691
E-mail: caldwe.data@office.mmc.org

Maryland

Baltimore

The Johns Hopkins Hospital
Park 315, 600 N. Wolfe Street
Baltimore, MD 21287-2533

Appts: (410) 955-2795

Center Director:

Beryl J. Rosenstein, M.D.
Fax: (410) 955-1030
E-mail: brosenst@welchlink.welch.jhu.edu

Adult Program Director:

Sandra M. Walden, M.D.
(410) 955-2795
Fax: (410) 955-1030

Bethesda

Cystic Fibrosis Center
National Institute of Diabetes and
   Digestive and Kidney Diseases
National Institutes of Health
Building 10, Room 85235
Bethesda, MD 20892

Appts: (301) 496-3434

Center Director:

Milica S. Chernick, M.D.
Fax: (301) 496-9943

Massachusetts

Boston

1. Cystic Fibrosis Center
   Pulmonary Division
   Children's Hospital
   300 Longwood Avenue
   Boston, MA 02115

   Appts: (617) 355-7881

Center Director:

Mary Ellen Wohl, M.D.
Fax: (617) 355-6109

Adult Program Director:

Craig Gerard, M.D.
(617) 355-6935

2. Cystic Fibrosis Center
   Massachusetts General Hospital
   ACC 709
   15 Parkman Street
   Boston, MA 02114

   Appts: (617) 726-8707 or
            (617) 726-8708

Center Director:

Allen Lapey, M.D.
Fax: (617) 724-3948
E-mail: lapeya@al.mgh.harvard.edu

Adult Program Director:

Patricia M. Joseph, M.D.
(617) 726-3734

3. Cystic Fibrosis Center
   Tufts New England Medical Center
   Box 343
   750 Washington Street
   Boston, MA 02111

   Appts: (617) 636-5085

Center Director:

Henry L. Dorkin, M.D.
Fax: (617) 636-7760
E-mail: henry.dorkin@es.nemc.org

Springfield

Baystate Medical Center
Wesson Memorial Unit, 4th Floor
140 High Street
Springfield, MA 01199

Appts: (413) 784-2515

Center Director:

Robert S. Gerstle, M.D.
(413) 784-5066
Fax: (413) 784-5995

Worcester

University of Massachusetts Medical
   Center
Department of Pediatrics
55 Lake Avenue North
Worcester, MA 01655

Appts: (508) 856-4155

Center Director:

Robert G. Zwerdling, M.D.
(508) 856-4155
Fax: (508) 856-2609

Michigan

Ann Arbor

University of Michigan
Cystic Fibrosis Center
UMMC, D1205-0718
1500 E. Medical Center Drive
Ann Arbor, MI 48109

Appts: (313) 764-4123 (Pediatrics)
         (313) 936-5580 (Adult)

Center Director:

Samya Nasr, M.D.
Fax: (313) 436-7635

Adult Program Director:

Richard H. Simon, M.D.*
(313) 936-4570
Fax: (313) 936-7024
E-mail: rsimon@uvl.im.med.umich.edu

*Preferred Mailing Address:

3110B Taubman Center
Box 0368
Ann Arbor, MI 48109

Detroit

Children's Hospital of Michigan
Cystic Fibrosis Care, Teaching and
    Resource Center
3901 Beaubien Boulevard
Detroit, MI 48201

Appts: (313) 745-5541

Interim Director:

Ibrahim Abdulhamid, M.D.
Fax: (313) 993-2948

Adult Satellite Network:

Wayne State University
Harper Hospital
3990 John R. Street
Detroit, MI 48201

Appts: (313) 745-1735

Director:

Dana Kissner, M.D.
(313) 745-0895
Fax: (313) 993-0562

Henry Ford Hospital
2799 West Grand Boulevard
Detroit, MI 48202

Appts: (313) 876-2439

Director:

Michael Iannuzzi, M.D.
(313) 876-1394

Sinai Hospital of Detroit
Department of Medicine
6767 W. Outer Drive
Detroit, MI 48240

Appts: (313) 493-6580

Director:

Bohdan M. Pichurko, M.D.
(313) 493-6354
Fax: (313) 493-6892

Satellite Center:

Mott Children's Health Center
806 Tuuri Place
Flint, MI 48503

Appts: (810) 767-5750 Ext. 305

Director:

H. Stephen Williams, M.D., M.P.H.
Fax: (810) 768-7511

East Lansing

Michigan State University
Cystic Fibrosis Center
138 Service Road Center
East Lansing, MI 48824-1313

Appts: (517) 353-3241

Center Director:

Richard E. Honicky, M.D.*
(517) 355-4726
Fax: (517) 353-8464

*Preferred Mailing Address:

B-240 Life Sciences Building
Michigan State University
E. Lansing, MI 48824-1317

Grand Rapids

Butterworth Cystic Fibrosis Center
426 Michigan N.E.
Suite 305
Grand Rapids, MI 49503

Appts: (616) 732-8890

Center Director:

Lawrence E. Kurlandsky, M.D.*
(616) 732-3670
Fax: (616) 456-2745

*Preferred Mailing Address:

Butterworth Hospital
100 Michigan N.E.
Grand Rapids, MI 49503

Kalamazoo

Michigan State University
Kalamazoo Center for Medical Studies
1000 Oakland Drive
Kalamazoo, MI 49008

Appts: (616) 337-6430

Center Director:

Douglas N. Homnick, M.D.
Fax: (616) 337-6427
E-mail: homnick@kcms.msu.edu

Minnesota

Minneapolis

University of Minnesota
Minneapolis, MN 55455

Appts: (612) 624-0962

Center Director:

Warren J. Warwick, M.D.*
(612) 624-7175
Fax: (612) 624-0696
E-mail: warwi001@maroon.tc.umn.edu

*Preferred Mailing Address:

401 E. River Road, Room 413, Box 184
Minneapolis, MN 55455

Mississippi

Jackson

University of Mississippi Medical Center
Department of Pediatrics
2500 North State Street

Jackson, MS 39216-4505

Appts: (601) 984-5205

Center Director:

Suzanne T. Miller, M.D.
Fax: (601) 984-5982

Missouri

Columbia

Columbia Cystic Fibrosis, Pediatric
    Pulmonary and Gastrointestinal Center
University of Missouri Medical Center
Department of Child Health
One Hospital Drive
Columbia, MO 65212

Appts: (573) 882-6921

Center Director:

Peter Konig, M.D.
(573) 882-6978
Fax: (573) 882-2742

Outreach Clinics:

St. John's Regional Hospital
Medical Gardens, Suite 107
2030 S. National Avenue
Springfield, MO 65802

Appts: (573) 882-6978

Contact:

Kelly Moore, R.N., M.S.

Southeast Missouri Hospital
1701 Lacey Street
Cape Girardeau, MO 63701

Appts: (573) 651-5550

Contact:
Kelly Moore, R.N., M.S.

Kansas City

The Children's Mercy Hospital
University of Missouri, Kansas City
    School of Medicine
Pediatric Pulmonology Section
24th and Gillham Road
Kansas City, MO 64108

Appts: (816) 234-3066
Sweat Test Only: (816) 234-3230

Center Director:

Michael McCubbin, M.D.
(816) 234-3033
Fax: (816) 234-3590

St. Louis

1. Cystic Fibrosis, Pediatric Pulmonary
    and Pediatric Gastrointestinal Center
    Cardinal Glennon Memorial Hospital
    for Children
    St. Louis University School of
    Medicine
    1465 South Grand Boulevard
    St. Louis, MO 63104

Appts: (314) 577-5663

Center Director:

Anthony J. Rejent, M.D.*
(314) 268-6439
Fax: (314) 268-2798

Adult Program Director:

Mary Ellen Kleinhenz, M.D.
St. Louis University Medical Center
(314) 577-8856
Fax: (314) 577-8859

*Preferred Mailing Address:

Medical Staff Office
Cardinal Glennon Memorial Hospital
   for Children
St. Louis University School of
   Medicine
1465 South Grand Boulevard
St. Louis, MO 63104

2. Washington University School of
      Medicine
   Cystic Fibrosis Center
   One Children's Place
   St. Louis Children's Hospital
   Department of Pediatrics
   St. Louis, MO 63110

Appts: (314) 454-2694
            (314) 362-9366 (adults)
            (314) 454-6248 (sweat test
            only)
Fax: (314) 454-2515

Center Director:

George B. Mallory, Jr., M.D.
(314) 454-2694
Fax: (314) 454-2515
E-mail: mallory@al.kids.wustl.edu

Pediatric Coordinator:

Jane A. Quaute, R.N., B.S.
(314) 454-2694

Adult Program Director:

Daniel Rosenbluth, M.D.
(314) 362-6904
Fax: (314) 367-6632
E-mail: drosenbl@visar.wustl.edu

Adult Coordinator:

Sharon Muhs, B.S.N.
(314) 362-6904

Satellite Centers:

Southern Illinois University School of
   Medicine
P.O. Box 19230-MC 1311
Springfield, IL 62794-9230

Appts: (217) 782-0187 Ext. 2321
or   (217) 788-3381

Director:

Lanie E. Eagleton, M.D.
(217) 782-0187
Fax: (217) 788-5543

Coordinator:

Joni Colle, R.N., R.R.T.
Carle Clinic Association
602 W. University Avenue
Urbana, IL 61801

Appts: (217) 383-3100

Director:

Donald F. Davison, M.D.
Fax: (217) 383-4468

Montana

See Denver, Colorado

Nebraska

Omaha

Nebraska Regional Center for Cystic
   Fibrosis and Pediatric Pulmonary
   Diseases
University of Nebraska Medical Center
600 South 42nd Street
Omaha, NE 68198-5190

Appts: (402) 559-4156

Center Director:

John L. Colombo, M.D.
(402) 559-6275
Fax: (402) 559-7062

Nevada

Las Vegas

Children's Lung Specialists
2200 Rancho Drive, Suite 200
Las Vegas, NV 89102

Appts: (702) 598-4411

Center Director:

Ruben Diaz, M.D.
Fax: (702) 598-1988

New Hampshire

Hanover/Manchester

New Hampshire Cystic Fibrosis Care,
    Research and Teaching Center
Dartmouth Hitchcock Medical Center
1 Medical Center Drive
Lebanon, NH 03756

Appts: (603) 650-6244 (Lebanon) or
         (603) 695-2560 (Bedford)

Center Director:

William Boyle, Jr., M.D.
(603) 650-5541
Fax: (603) 650-8601
E-mail: william.e.boyle@hitchcock.org
        lynn.m.feenan@hitchcock.or

New Jersey

Long Branch

Cystic Fibrosis and Pediatric Pulmonary
    Center
Monmouth Medical Center
279 Third Avenue, Suite 604
Long Branch, NJ 07740

Appts: (908) 222-4474

Center Director:

Robert L. Zanni, M.D.
Fax: (908) 222-4472

Newark

New Jersey Medical School
185 South Orange Avenue
Room MSB-F534
Newark, NJ 07103-2714

Appts: (201) 982-4815

Center Director:

Nelson L. Turcios, M.D.
Fax: (201) 982-7597

Satellite Center:

Cystic Fibrosis Center
Hackensack Medical Center
30 Prospect Avenue
Hackensack, NJ 07601

Appts: (201) 996-2121

Director:

Lawrence J. Denson, M.D.
(201) 342-0922
Fax: (201) 996-2253

New Mexico

Albuquerque

University of New Mexico School of
   Medicine
Department of Pediatrics
2211 Lomas Boulevard, N.E.
Albuquerque, NM 87131

Appts: (505) 272-6633

Center Director:

Bennie C. McWilliams, M.D.
Fax: (505) 272-0329
E-mail: bmc.willi@medusa.unm.edu

New York

Albany

Pediatric Pulmonary and Cystic Fibrosis
   Center
Albany Medical College
Department of Pediatrics, A-112
47 New Scotland Avenue
Albany, NY 12208

Appts: (518) 262-6880

Center Director:

Robert A. Kaslovsky, M.D.
Fax: (518) 262-6884

Adult Program Director:

Jonathan M. Rosen, M.D.
(518) 262-5196
Fax: (518) 262-6472

Brooklyn

Long Island College Hospital
340 Henry Street
Brooklyn, NY 11201

Appts: (718) 780-1025 or
          (718) 780-1026

Center Director:

Robert Giusti, M.D.
Fax: (718) 780-2989

Outreach Clinic:

St. Vincent's Medical Center of
   Richmond
355 Bard Avenue
Staten Island, NY 10310

Buffalo

Children's Lung and Cystic Fibrosis Center
Children's Hospital of Buffalo
219 Bryant Street
Buffalo, NY 14222

Appts: (716) 878-7524

Center Director:

Drucy Borowitz, M.D.
Fax: (716) 878-7547
E-mail: dborowitz@aol.com

Adult Program Director:

Colin McMahon, M.D.

New Hyde Park

Cystic Fibrosis and Pediatric Pulmonary
   Center
Schneider Children's Hospital of Long
   Island Jewish Medical Center
Albert Einstein College of Medicine
New Hyde Park, NY 11040

Appts: (718) 470-3250

Center Director:

Jack D. Gorvoy, M.D.*
(718) 470-3305
Fax: (718) 470-9291

*Preferred Mailing Address:

Cystic Fibrosis Center
Schneider Children's Hospital of Long
   Island
L.I.J.M.C.
274-16 76th Avenue
New Hyde Park, NY 11040

Satellite Center:

Good Samaritan Hospital Medical
   Center
1000 Montauk Highway
West Islip, NY 11795

Appts: (516) 376-4191
Fax: (516) 376-4208

Director:

Louis E. Guida, Jr., M.D.

Associate Director:

Joseph S. Chiamonte, M.D.

New York City

1. Cystic Fibrosis and Pediatric
      Pulmonary Center
   Mount Sinai School of Medicine
   One Gustave L. Levy Place
   Fifth Avenue at 100th Street
   New York, NY 10029

   Appts: (212) 241-7788

Center Director:

Richard J. Bonforte, M.D.*
(212) 420-4098
Fax: (212) 420-2560

*Preferred Mailing Address:

Director of Pediatrics
Beth Israel Medical Center
First Avenue at 16th Street
New York, NY 10003

2. Pediatric Pulmonary Center, BHS 101
   Babies Hospital and Columbia
      Presbyterian Medical Center
   630 West 168th Street
   New York, NY 10032

   Appts: (212) 305-5122

Center Director:

Lynne M. Quittell, M.D.
(212) 305-6551
Fax: (212) 305-6103
E-mail: imql@columbia.edu

3. Cystic Fibrosis, Pediatric Pulmonary
      and Gastrointestinal Center
   St. Vincent's Hospital and Medical
      Center of New York
   36 Seventh Avenue, Suite 509
   New York, NY 10011

   Appts: (212) 604-8895 or
            (212) 604-8898

Center Director:

Joan DeCelie-Germana, M.D.
(212) 604-8899
Fax: (212) 604-3899

Rochester

University of Rochester Medical Center
Strong Memorial Hospital
Department of Pediatrics
601 Elmwood Avenue, Box 667
Rochester, NY 14642

Appts: (716) 275-2464

Center Director:

Karen Z. Voter, M.D.
Fax: (716) 275-8706

Satellite Center:

House of the Good Samaritan
199 Pratt Street
Watertown, NY 13601

Appts: (315) 788-2211

Director:

Ronald Perciaccante, M.D.
Fax: (315) 788-0956

Stony Brook

University Medical Center at Stony Brook
Department of Pediatrics
Health Sciences Center, 11-080
Stony Brook, NY 11794-8111

Appts: (516) 444-7726

Center Director:

Kalpana Patel, M.D.
(516) 444-2730
Fax: (516) 444-6045

Syracuse

Robert C. Schwartz Cystic Fibrosis Center
University Hospital
SUNY Health Science Center
750 East Adams Street
Syracuse, NY 13210

Appts: (315) 473-5834

Center Director:

Phillip T. Swender, M.D.
Fax: (315) 464-7564

Valhalla

The Armond V. Mascia Cystic Fibrosis
   Center
New York Medical College
Munger Pavilion, Room 106
Valhalla, NY 10595

Appts: (914) 285-7585

Center Director:

Allen Dozor, M.D.
Fax: (914) 993-4142
E-mail: pedpulm@nymc.edu

North Carolina

Chapel Hill

U.N.C. Cystic Fibrosis Center
University of North Carolina
Department of Pediatrics, CB #7220
509 Burnett-Womack Building
Chapel Hill, NC 27599

Appts: (919) 966-1055 (Pediatrics)
         (919) 966-1077 (Adults—18
         years & older)

Center Director:

Gerald W. Fernald, M.D.
(919) 966-2085
Fax: (919) 966-7299
E-mail: pedslb.pedslan@mhs.unc.edu

Adult Program:

Cystic Fibrosis/Pulmonary Research
   and Training Center
The University of North Carolina at
   Chapel Hill
CB# 7248, 7011 Thurston Bowles
   Building
Chapel Hill, NC 27599-7248

Director:

Michael Knowles, M.D.
(919) 966-1077
Fax: (919) 966-7524

Durham

Cystic Fibrosis and Pediatric Pulmonary
   Center
Duke University Medical Center
302 Bell Building
P.O. Box 2994
Durham, NC 27710

Appts: (919) 684-3364 or
             (919) 684-2289

Center Director:

Marc Majure, M.D.
Fax: (919) 684-2292

Center Codirector:

Thomas Murphy, M.D.

Adult Center Codirector:

Peter S. Kussin, M.D.
202C Bell Building, DUMC
Box 31166
Durham, NC 27710

Satellite Center:

Pediatrics Pulmonary Medicine, P.A.
16 Mills Avenue, Suite 6
Greenville, SC 29605

Director:

Jane V. Gwinn, M.D.
(803) 239-4150
Fax: (803) 239-4159

North Dakota

Bismarck

Cystic Fibrosis Center
St. Alexius Medical Center
311 North 9th Street
Bismarck, ND 58502

Appts: (701) 224-7500

Center Director:

Allan Stillerman, M.D.*
Fax: (701) 258-7015

*Preferred Mailing Address:

Heart and Lung Clinic
Morgan & Associates, M.D.'s, P.C.
311 North 9th Street
P.O. Box 2698
Bismarck, ND 58502-2698

Ohio

Akron

Lewis H. Walker, M.D. Cystic Fibrosis
Center
Children's Hospital Medical Center of
Akron
One Perkins Square
Akron, OH 44308

Appts: (216) 379-8545

Center Director:

Robert T. Stone, M.D.*
(216) 253-7753
Fax: (216) 379-8152

Preferred Mailing Address:

300 Locust Street
Suite 200
Akron, OH 44302

Cincinnati

The Children's Hospital Medical Center
Pulmonary Medicine
Department of Pediatrics
University of Cincinnati College of
Medicine
3333 Burnet Avenue
Cincinnati, OH 45229-3039

Appts: (513) 559-6771
(ask for Jeanne Weiland, R.N.)

Center Director:

Robert Wilmott, M.D.
(513) 559-6771
Fax: (513) 559-4615
E-mail: wilmott@ucbeh.san.uc.edu

Adult Program Director:

Janine Mylett, M.D.
University of Cincinnati
(513) 558-4831
Fax: (513) 558-0835

Cleveland

The Leroy Matthews Cystic Fibrosis
Center*
Rainbow Babies and Children's
Hospital/University Hospitals of
Cleveland
Case Western Reserve University School
of Medicine
2101 Adelbert Road
Cleveland, OH 44106

Appts: (216) 844-3267

Center Director:

Carl F. Doershuk, M.D.
(216) 844-3267
Fax: (216) 844-5916

Preferred Mailing Address:

The Leroy Matthews Cystic Fibrosis
Center
Rainbow Babies and Children's Hospital
2101 Adelbert Road
Cleveland, OH 44106

Columbus

Cystic Fibrosis Center
Columbus Children's Hospital
700 Children's Drive
Columbus, OH 43205-2696

Appts: (614) 722-4766

Center Director:

Karen S. McCoy, M.D.
Fax: (614) 722-4755
E-mail: mccoy%pul%chi@aloha.chi.ohio-
   state.edu

Dayton

Pediatric Pulmonary Center
The Children's Medical Center
One Children's Plaza
Dayton, OH 45404-1815

Appts: (513) 226-8376

Center Director:

William Spohn, M.D.
(513) 226-8440
Fax: (513) 463-5390
E-mail: wspohn@desire.wright.edu

Oklahoma

Oklahoma City

Children's Hospital of Oklahoma
University of Oklahoma
Health Science Center
940 N.W. 13th Street
Oklahoma City, OK 73104

Appts: (405) 271-6390

Center Director:

John E. Grunow, M.D.
(405) 271-6390
Fax: (405) 271-3017

Oregon

Portland

Cystic Fibrosis Care, Teaching and
   Research Center
Oregon Health Sciences University
UHN 56
3181 S.W. Sam Jackson Park Road
Portland, OR 97201

Appts: (503) 494-8023

Center Director:

Michael Wall, M.D.
(503) 494-8023
Fax: (503) 494-6670

Outreach Clinic:

Medford CF Clinic
Rogue Valley Hospital
Medford, OR

Pennsylvania

Harrisburg

Cystic Fibrosis Center
Kline Children's Center
Polyclinic Medical Center
2601 North 3rd Street
Harrisburg, PA 17110

Appts: (717) 782-4105

Center Director:

Christopher S. Ryder, M.D.
(717) 691-0303
Fax: (717) 691-5584

Philadelphia

1. Cystic Fibrosis Center for Care,
   Teaching and Research
   The Children's Hospital of Philadelphia
   University of Pennsylvania School of
     Medicine
   34th & Civic Center Boulevard
   Philadelphia, PA 19104-4318

   Appts: (215) 590-3749/3510
            (Mon. thru Fri. 8:30-4:30;
            evenings and weekends—ask
            for physician on call)

Center Director:

   Thomas F. Scanlin, M.D.*
   Fax: (215) 590-4298

   *Preferred Mailing Address:

   Cystic Fibrosis Center
   The Children's Hospital of Philadelphia
   Room #6125
   34th and Civic Center Boulevard
   Philadelphia, PA 19104

Adult Program:

   Department of Medicine
   Pulmonary Medicine/Critical Care
   Medicine
   Hospital of the University of
   Pennsylvania
   8035 West Gates
   3600 Spruce Street
   Philadelphia, PA 19104-4283

   Appts: (215) 662-3202

Director:

   Cynthia Robinson, M.D.
   (215) 349-5478
   Fax: (215) 349-5172

   E-mail: robinsoc@mail.med.upenn.
   edu

2. St. Christopher's Hospital for Children
   Erie Avenue at Front Street
   Philadelphia, PA 19134-1095

   Appts: (215) 427-5183

Center Director:

   Daniel V. Schidlow, M.D.
   Fax: (215) 427-4621

Adult Program:

   Pulmonary Disease and Critical Care
   Medical College of Pennsylvania
     Hospital
   3300 Henry Avenue
   Philadelphia, PA 19129

   Appts: (215) 842-7748

Director:

   Stanley Fiel, M.D.
   Fax: (215) 843-1705

Outreach Clinic:

   Mercy Hospital
   25 Church Street
   Wilkes-Barre, PA 18765

Pittsburgh

   Cystic Fibrosis Center
   Children's Hospital of Pittsburgh
   University of Pittsburgh School of
     Medicine
   One Children's Place
   3705 Fifth Avenue at DeSoto Street
   Pittsburgh, PA 15213

Appts: (412) 692-5630

Center Director:

David M. Orenstein, M.D.
Fax: (412) 692-6645

Adult Program Director:

Joel Weinberg, M.D.
(412) 621-1200
Fax: (412) 621-9958

Puerto Rico

San Juan

Cystic Fibrosis Care and Teaching Center
Pediatric Pulmonary Program
Department of Pediatrics
University of Puerto Rico Medical
   Sciences Campus
G.P.O. Box 365067
San Juan, PR 00936-5067

Appts: (809) 754-3733 or
       (809) 754-3722

Center Director:

Jose Rodriquez Santana, M.D.
Fax: (809) 763-4966

Rhode Island

Providence

Cystic Fibrosis Center
Rhode Island Hospital
CDC-APC 6th Floor
593 Eddy Street
Providence, RI 02903

Appts: (401) 444-5685

Center Director:

Mary Ann Passero, M.D.
Fax: (401) 444-6115

South Carolina

Charleston

Cystic Fibrosis Center
Medical University of South Carolina
171 Ashley Avenue
Charleston, SC 29425

Appts: (803) 792-3561

Center Director:

Hazel Moore Webb, M.D.
Fax: (803) 792-9223

Adult Program Director:

Patrick Flume, M.D.
(803) 792-9219
Fax: (803) 792-0732
E-mail: flumepa@musc.edu

South Dakota

Sioux Falls

South Dakota Cystic Fibrosis Center
Sioux Valley Hospital
1100 South Euclid Avenue
P.O. Box 5039
Sioux Falls, SD 57117-5039

Appts: (605) 333-7189

Center Director:

Rodney R. Parry, M.D.*

(605) 357-1306
Fax: (605) 357-1311

Preferred Mailing Address:

University of South Dakota
School of Medicine
1400 West 22nd Street
Sioux Falls, SD 57105-1570

Tennessee

Memphis

Memphis Cystic Fibrosis Center
Le Bonheur Children's Medical Center
University of Tennessee Center for the
    Health Sciences
50 N. Dunlap
Memphis, TN 38103-2893

Appts: (901) 572-5222

Center Director:

Robert Schoumacher, M.D.
(901) 572-5222
Fax: (901) 572-3337

Nashville

Cystic Fibrosis Care Teaching and
    Research Center
Vanderbilt University Medical Center
S-0119 MCN
Nashville, TN 37232-2586

Appts: (615) 343-7617

Center Director:

Preston W. Campbell, M.D.
(615) 343-7617
Fax: (615) 343-1763

Satellite Centers:

East Tennessee Children's Hospital
2018 Clinch Avenue
Knoxville, TN 37920

Appts: (615) 541-8336

Director:

Don Ellenburg, M.D.
(615) 525-2640
Fax: (615) 525-9536

Codirector:

John Rogers, M.D.
(615) 541-8583
Fax: (615) 541-8629

T.C. Thompson Children's Hospital
910 Blackford Street
Chattanooga, TN 37403

Appts: (615) 778-6505

Director:

Joel Ledbetter, M.D.
(615) 778-6501
Fax: (615) 778-6215

Texas

Dallas

Cystic Fibrosis Care, Teaching and
 Research Center
Children's Medical Center
1935 Motor Street, Room 316
Dallas, TX 75235

Appts: (214) 640-2361 or
 (214) 640-2362

Center Director:

Claude Prestidge, M.D.
Fax: (214) 640-2563

Adult Program:

St. Paul Medical Center
5939 Harry Hines Boulevard
Dallas, TX 75235

Director:

Randall Rosenblatt, M.D.
(214) 879-6555
Fax: (214) 879-6312

Satellite Centers:

Permian Basin Allergy Center
Allergy Alliances
606B North Kent Street
Midland, TX 79701

Appts: (915) 561-8183

Director:

John D. Bray, M.D.
(915) 686-8659

Fax: (915) 684-7003

Scott & White Clinic
2401 South 31st Street
Temple, TX 76508

Appts: (817) 724-4950

Director:

James F. Daniel, M.D.
(817) 724-2708
Fax: (817) 724-5857

Tulsa Ambulatory Pediatric Center
2815 South Sheridan Road
Tulsa, OK 74129

Appts: (918) 838-4820
Fax: (918) 838-4729

Director:

John C. Kramer, M.D.*
(918) 749-6458
Fax: (918) 749-3869

Preferred Mailing Address:

1980 Utica Square
Suite 251
Tulsa, OK 74114-1611

The University of Texas
Health Center at Tyler
P.O. Box 2003
Tyler, TX 75710

Appts: (903) 877-7220

Director:

Robert B. Klein, M.D.

(903) 834-2541

Fort Sam Houston

Tri-Services Military CF Center
Pulmonary/Critical Care Medicine
  Department
Wilford Hall USAF Medical Center
200 Berquest Drive, Suite 1
59 Medical Wing/PSMP
Lackland AFB, TX 78236-5300

Appts: (210) 670-7347

Center Codirector:

Dr. Stephen Inscore, LTC, MC, USA
Fax: (210) 760-6180

Center Codirector:

Dr. Jan Westerman, MAJ., MC, USAF*
(210) 670-5235
Fax: (210) 670-6180

Satellite Centers:

Naval Hospital San Diego
Department of Pediatrics
San Diego, CA 92134

Appts: (619) 532-6896

Director:

B. Gaston, CDR
E-mail: suredjb@aol.com

Tripler Army Medical Center
Department of Pediatrics
Tripler AMC, HI 96859

Appts: (808) 433-6407

Director:

Dr. Charles Callahan, MAJ, MC
Fax: (808) 433-4837

National Naval Medical Center
Pediatric Clinic, Building 9, Room 123
8901 Wisconsin Avenue
Bethesda, MD 20889-5000

Appts: (301) 295-4902 or
         (301) 295-4903

Director:

Dr. Donna Perry, CAPT, MC, USN
Fax: (301) 295-6173

Clinic Coordinator:

Jane A. Dean, R. N.
(301) 295-4929

USAF Medical Center Keesler
81st MDOS/SGOCC
301 Fisher Street, Room 1A132
Keesler AFB, MS 39534-2519

Appts: (601) 377-6620

Director:

Dr. James Woodward, MAJ., USAF
Fax: (601) 377-6304

William Beaumont Army Medical
  Center
Department of Pediatrics
El Paso, TX 79920-5001

Appts: (915) 569-2000

Director:

Dr. Larry Tremper, LTC, MC, USA
Fax: (915) 569-1396

Portsmouth Naval Medical Center
620 John Paul Jones Circle
Portsmouth, VA 23321

Appts: (804) 398-7558 (DSN 564)

Director:

John Pfaff, CDR, MC, USNR
Fax: (804) 398-5964

Madigan Army Medical Center
Department of Pediatrics
Pediatric Pulmonary Medicine
Tacoma, WA 98431

Appts: (206) 968-1980 or
         (206) 968-3333

Director:

Dr. Donald Moffitt, COL, MC, USA
Fax: (206) 968-0384

Fort Worth

Cystic Fibrosis Center
Cook-Ft. Worth Children's Medical Center
801 Seventh Avenue
Fort Worth, TX 76104

Appts: (817) 885-4202

Center Codirector:

James C. Cunningham, M.D.
Fax: (817) 885-1090

Center Codirector:

Nancy Dambro, M.D.

Outreach Clinic:

Texas Tech University Health Sciences
 Center
1400 Coulter
Amarillo, TX 79106

Appts: (806) 354-5613
         (800) 237-0167

Codirectors:

James C. Cunningham, M.D.
Maynard Dyson, MD

Houston

Cystic Fibrosis Center
Pulmonology Section
Department of Pediatrics
Baylor College of Medicine
One Baylor Plaza
Houston, TX 77030

Appts: (713) 770-3013

Center Director:

Peter W. Hiatt, M.D.*
(713) 770-3300
Fax: (713) 770-3308

*Preferred Mailing Address:

Clinical Care Center
Texas Children's Hospital
6621 Fannin, MC3-2571
Houston, TX 77030

Satellite Center:

Seton Medical Center
1201 West 38th Street
Austin, TX 78705

Appts: (512) 454-3387

Director:

Allan L. Frank, M.D.*
(512) 454-3387

Preferred Mailing Address:

Capital Pediatric Group Associates
1100 West 39½ Street
Austin, TX 78756

San Antonio

Cystic Fibrosis–Chronic Lung Disease
  Center
Santa Rosa Children's Hospital
519 West Houston Street
P.O. Box 7330, Station A
San Antonio, TX 78207

Appts: (210) 228-2058 or
         (210) 228-2201

Center Director:

Ricardo Pinero, M.D.*
(210) 271-0321
Fax: (210) 271-0880

Preferred Mailing Address:

343 W. Houston Street, Suite #906
San Antonio, TX 78205

Utah

Salt Lake City

Intermountain Cystic Fibrosis Center
Department of Pediatrics
University of Utah Medical Center
50 North Medical Drive
Salt Lake City, UT 84132

Appts: (801) 588-2621 (pediatrics)
         (801) 581-2410 (adults)

Center Codirector:

Dennis Nielson, M.D., Ph.D.
(801) 581-2410
Fax: (801) 581-4920

Center Codirector (Adult Program):

Bruce C. Marshall, M.D.
(801) 581-7806
Fax: (801) 585-3355

Satellite Centers:

Mercy Medical Center
1512 12th Avenue Road
Nampa, ID 83651

Appts: (208) 463-3190

Director:

Eugene M. Brown, M.D.*
(208) 463-3000
Fax: (208) 465-4825

Preferred Mailing Address:

215 East Hawaii
Nampa, ID 83686

537 S. 12th Avenue
P.O. Box 4730
Pocatello, ID 83201

Appts: (208) 232-1443

Director:

Don McInturff, M.D.
Fax: (208) 233-1434

890 Oxford Avenue
Idaho Falls, ID 83401

Appts: (208) 523-3060

Director:

George H. Groberg, M.D.

Vermont

Burlington

Cystic Fibrosis and Pediatric Pulmonary
  Center
One Kennedy Drive
South Burlington, VT 05403

Appts: (802) 862-5529

Center Director:

Donald R. Swartz, M.D.
Fax: (802) 863-9633

Virginia

Charlottesville

Cystic Fibrosis Care, Teaching and
  Research Center
University of Virginia School of Medicine
Charlottesville, VA 22908

Appts: (804) 924-2250

Center Director:

Robert F. Selden, Jr., M.D.*
(804) 924-5935 or

(804) 924-2250
Fax: (804) 924-0390

*Preferred Mailing Address:

University of Virginia Medical Center
Department of Pediatrics
P.O. Box 386
Charlottesville, VA 22908

Norfolk

Eastern Virginia Medical School
Children's Hospital of the King's
  Daughters
601 Children's Lane
Norfolk, VA 23507

Appts: (804) 668-7132

Center Director:

Thomas Rubio, M.D.
(804) 668-7238
Fax: (804) 668-9767

Adult Program Director:

Ignacio Ripoll, M.D.

Richmond

Cystic Fibrosis Program
Medical College of Virginia
Box 980271
Richmond, VA 23298

Appts: (804) 786-9445

Center Director:

David A. Draper, M.D.
(804) 828-9612 or

(804) 828-9613
Fax: (804) 371-5481

Washington

Seattle

Pulmonary Disease and Cystic Fibrosis
    Center
Children's Hospital and Medical Center
P.O. Box C5371
4800 Sand Point Way, N.E.
Seattle, WA 98105

Appts: (206) 526-2024

Center Director:

Bonnie W. Ramsey, M.D.
Fax: (206) 528-2639
E-mail: bramsey@u.washington.edu

Adult Program:

Cystic Fibrosis Clinic
Division of Pulmonary and Critical
    Care Medicine
University of Washington Medical Center
Box 356522
Seattle, WA 98195

Appts: (206) 548-4615

Clinic Coordinator:

Gwen McDonald, R.N., M.S.
(206) 548-8446
Fax: (206) 548-2105
E-mail: gwen@u.washington.edu

Director:

Moira Aitken, M.D.
(206) 543-3166
Fax: (206) 685-8673
E-mail: moira@u.washington.edu

Satellite Centers:

Anchorage Cystic Fibrosis Clinic
Providence Hospital
3200 Providence Drive
P.O. Box 196604
Anchorage, AK 99508

Appts: (907) 561-5440

Director:

Dion Roberts, M.D.*

**Preferred Mailing Address:*

4001 Date Street, Suite 210
Anchorage, AK 99508

Mary Bridge Children's Health Center
311 South Street
Tacoma, WA 98405

Appts: (206) 552-1415
Fax: (206) 383-5320

Codirectors:

Lawrence A. Larson, D.O.
David Ricker, M.D.

Deaconess Medical Center
West 800 Fifth Avenue
P.O. Box 248
Spokane, WA 99210-0248

Appts: (509) 458-7300
Fax: (509) 459-8796

Director:

Michael M. McCarthy, M.D.
(509) 455-6739
Fax: (509) 624-7973

West Virginia

Morgantown

Mountain State Cystic Fibrosis Center
Robert C. Byrd Health Science Center
West Virginia University School of
   Medicine
P.O. Box 9214
Morgantown, WV 26506

Appts: (304) 293-1841

Center Director:

Stephan C. Aronoff, M.D.
Fax: (304) 293-4341

Wisconsin

Madison

University of Wisconsin
Cystic Fibrosis/Pediatric Pulmonary
   Center
Clinical Sciences Center - H6/380
600 Highland Avenue
Madison, WI 53792-4108

Appts: (608) 263-8555

Center Director:

Michael J. Rock, M.D.
Fax: (608) 263-0440
E-mail: mjrock@facstaff.wisc.edu

Adult Program:

University of Wisconsin
Adult Cystic Fibrosis Program
Clinical Sciences Center-E5/369
600 Highland Avenue
Madison, WI 53792

Appts: (608) 263-7203

Adult Program Director:

Guillermo A. doPico, M.D.
(608) 263-3612
Fax: (608) 263-3104

Adult Nurse Coordinator:

Lorna Will, R.N., M.A.
(608) 263-8937
Fax: (608) 263-1987

Milwaukee

Children's Hospital of Wisconsin,
   MS #777A
Medical College of Wisconsin
Cystic Fibrosis Clinic
9000 West Wisconsin Avenue
Milwaukee, WI 53201

Appts: (414) 266-6730

Center Director:

Mark Splaingard, M.D.
(414) 266-6730

Adult Program Director:

Julie A. Biller, M.D.
(414) 266-6730

CHAPTERS

Alabama Chapter

502 Montgomery Highway, Suite 101
Vestavia Hills, AL 35216

(205) 823-9113
(800) 523-2357 (in Alabama)
Fax: (205) 823-8970

Executive Director:

Ms. Robin Reed

Arizona Chapter

2345 East Thomas Road, Suite 420
Phoenix, AZ 85016

(602) 224-0068 (Phoenix)
(520) 884-9441 (Tucson)
Fax: (602) 224-0432

Executive Director:

Ms. Kelly Swanson

Arkansas Chapter

7101 W. 12th Street, Suite 401
Little Rock, AR 72204

(501) 664-1200
Fax: (501) 663-6711

Executive Director:

Southern California/Utah Chapter (Excluding San Diego and Imperial Counties)

2150 Towne Centre Place, Suite 120
Anaheim, CA 92806

(714) 938-1393
Fax: (714) 938-1462

Executive Director:

Ms. Helen Johnson

Los Angeles Office

1950 Sawtelle Boulevard, Suite 328
Los Angeles, CA 90025

(310) 479-8585
Fax: (310) 473-7307

Director of Special Projects:

Ms. Laura Squair

Hacienda Heights Office

2440 South Hacienda Boulevard
Hacienda Heights, CA 91746

(818) 855-2896
Fax: (818) 961-2404

Director of Development:

Ms. Mary Schraeger

Utah Office

4848 South Highland Drive, Suite 653
Salt Lake City, UT 84117

(801) 322-2226
Fax: (714) 938-1462

Director of Development:

Mr. Gary Green

Northern California Chapter

417 Montgomery Street, Suite 404
San Francisco, CA 94104

(415) 677-0155
Fax: (415) 677-0156

Executive Director:

Ms. Geraldine M. Dooley

Southern California Chapter
(San Diego/Imperial Counties)

2320 Fifth Avenue, Suite A
San Diego, CA 92101

(619) 234-5880
Fax: (619) 234-4803

Executive Director:

Ms. Kae Meyer

Colorado Chapter

1755 Blake Street
Denver, CO 80202

(303) 296-6610
Fax: (303) 296-6923

Executive Director:

Ms. Penny Barnow

Pikes Peak Office

118 North Tejon Street, #205H
Colorado Springs, CO 80903

(719) 444-8966

Director of Special Events:

Ms. Debby Fowler

Connecticut Chapter

185 Silas Deane Highway
Wethersfield, CT 06109-1219

(203) 257-6907
(800) 841-2828 (in CT)
Fax: (203) 257-6903

Executive Director:

Mr. Gregory L. Hollinger

Delaware: See Delaware Valley
Chapter (Pennsylvania)

Metropolitan Washington, D.C.,
Chapter

6931 Arlington Road, Suite 200
Bethesda, MD 20814

(301) 657-8444
Fax: (301) 652-9571

Executive Director:

Ms. Regina Schewe

Florida Chapter

Two Prospect Park Business Center
3443 N. W. 55th Street, Building 7
Ft. Lauderdale, FL 33309

(954) 739-5006
Fax: (954) 739-2890

Executive Director:

Ms. Christina Landshut

Orlando Regional Office

378 Whooping Loop, Suite 1272
Altamonte Springs, FL 32701

(407) 339-8334

Director of Development:

Ms. Kerry Huffman

Palm Beach Regional Office

319 Belvedere Road, Suite 7
West Palm Beach, FL 33405

(407) 655-9577
Fax: (407) 655-9750

Executive Director:

Ms. Marie Cook

Tampa Regional Office

1211 N. Westshore Boulevard
Suite 602
Tampa, FL 33607

(813) 286-0266
Fax: (813) 289-4472

Director of Development:

Ms. Randy Harris

Georgia Chapter

2250 North Druid Hills Road, NE
Suite 275
Atlanta, GA 30329

(404) 325-6973
(800) 476-4483
Fax: (404) 325-7921

Executive Director:

Ms. Maureen A. Fraser

Hawaii: See Southern California Chapter

Idaho: See Oregon/Idaho/Montana

Greater Illinois Chapter

150 North Michigan Avenue, 4th Floor
Chicago, IL 60601

(312) 236-4491
(800) 824-5064 (in Illinois)
Fax: (312) 236-2797

Executive Director:

Mr. Chuck Saponaro

Indiana Chapter

50 South Meridian Street, Suite 505
Indianapolis, IN 46204

(317) 631-4115
(800) 622-4826 (in Indiana)
Fax: (317) 631-4410

Executive Director:

Ms. Suzanne McKeever Collins

Iowa Chapter

2600 72nd Street, Suite M
Des Moines, IA 50322

(515) 252-1530
(800) 798-5151
Fax: (515) 252-7684

Executive Director:

Ms. Yvonne M. Putze

Heart of America Chapter

5750 W. 95th Street, Suite 214
Overland Park, KS 66207

(913) 648-2323
Fax: (913) 648-2171

Executive Director:

Ms. Pamela Gale

Kentucky/West Virginia Chapter

1941 Bishop Lane, Suite 507
Louisville, KY 40218

(502) 452-6353
Fax: (502) 456-2936

Executive Director:

Ms. Mary Lee Stevens

Louisiana Chapter

4621 W. Napolean Avenue, Suite 207
Metairie, LA 70001

(504) 455-5194
(800) 257-4166
Fax: (504) 889-2592

Executive Director:

Ms. Renee Ganucheau

Baton Rouge Regional Office

1200 South Acadian Thruway, Suite 214
Baton Rouge, LA 70806

(504) 389-9993
Fax: (504) 387-4573

Director of Development:

Ms. Nancy Wertz

Maine: See Northern New England Chapter (New Hampshire)

Maryland Chapter

10616 Beaver Dam Road, S-1
Hunt Valley, MD 21030

(410) 771-9000
Fax: (410) 771-3208

Executive Director:

Ms. Josephine Schaeffer

Massachusetts Chapter

220 North Main Street, Suite 104
Natick, MA 01760

(508) 655-6000
(800) 966-0444
Fax: (508) 653-6942

Executive Director:

Mr. John F. Cox

Greater Michigan Chapter— Eastern Region

2118 Marshall Court
Saginaw, MI 48602-3368

(517) 790-2233
(800) 986-7169 (in Michigan)
Fax: (517) 790-1050

Executive Director:

Ms. Carolyn Cameron

Genesee Valley Regional Office

3553 S. Dort Highway
Flint, MI 48507-2047

(810) 743-5160
(800) 968-6796 (in Michigan)
Fax: (810) 743-6130

Director of Development:

Ms. Kelly McFarlan

Greater Michigan Chapter— Western Region

404 McKay Tower
146 Monroe Center Street, N.W.
Grand Rapids, MI 49503

(616) 451-4225
(800) 968-1050 (in Michigan)
Fax: (616) 451-8615

Executive Director:

Ms. Cindy Sharp

Metro Detroit Chapter

1133 E. Maple Road, Suite 201
Troy, MI 48083-2853

(810) 524-2873
Fax: (810) 524-4755

Executive Director:

Ms. Patricia Cavitt

Washtenaw County Chapter

1430 Kearney Road
Ann Arbor, MI 48104

(313) 662-4635

Minnesota Chapter

Century Plaza
1111 3rd Avenue, South, Suite 370
Minneapolis, MN 55404

(612) 338-0885
Fax: (612) 338-1601

Executive Director:

Ms. Linda L. Mahoney

Mississippi Chapter

4800 McWillie Circle, Suite B-6
Jackson, MS 39206

(601) 981-3100
Fax: (601) 981-0609

Executive Director:

Ms. Renda McGowan

Gateway Chapter

200 South Hanley, Suite 620
St. Louis, MO 63105

(314) 721-2490
Fax: (314) 721-2809

Executive Director:

Mr. L. Ashton Chase

Montana: See Oregon/Idaho/Montana Chapter

Nebraska Chapter

10838 Old Mill Road, Suite 6
Omaha, NE 68154

(402) 330-6164
Fax: (402) 330-8458

Executive Director:

Ms. Susan Simon

Nevada Chapter

1516 East Tropecana, Suite A-5
Las Vegas, NV 89119

(702) 597-0435
Fax: (702) 597-0668

Executive Director:

Ms. Regale Komzak

Northern New England Chapter

136 Harvey Road, Building A
Londonderry, NH 03053

(603) 669-8682
(800) 757-0203
Fax: (603) 669-9729

Greater New Jersey Chapter

1710 Route 10, Suite 225
Parsippany, NJ 07054

(201) 605-2525
Fax: (201) 605-2929

Executive Director:

Mr. Richard J. McCourt

New Mexico Chapter

4004 Carlisle, N.E., Suite B
Albuquerque, NM 87107

(505) 883-1455
Fax: (505) 883-3998

Executive Director:

Ms. Jennifer Threet

Central New York Chapter

110 Marlborough Road
Syracuse, NY 13206

(315) 463-7965
(800) 962-6578
Fax: (315) 463-8221

Executive Director:

Ms. Michele E. Argentieri

Greater New York Chapter

60 East 42nd Street, Suite 1563
New York, NY 10165

(212) 986-8783
Fax: (212) 697-4282

Executive Director:

Ms. Doris Tulcin

Long Island Office

265 Post Avenue, Suite 115
Westbury, NY 11590-2237

(516) 876-0580
Fax: (516) 876-0585

Associate Executive Director:

Ms. Yolan J. Wolf

Hudson Valley Branch

c/o Carol Hosdale
95 Croton Lake Road
Katonah, NY 10536

(914) 232-5401

Brooklyn Branch

c/o Gerald Balsam
2765 W. 5th Street
Brooklyn, NY 11224

(718) 996-1324

Northeastern New York Chapter

50 Colvin Avenue
Albany, NY 12206

(518) 489-2677
Fax: (518) 489-2751

Executive Director:

Ms. Linda Traylor

Rochester Chapter

307 Exchange Boulevard
Rochester, NY 14608

(716) 546-5890
Fax: (716) 546-3903

Executive Director:

Ms. Kelly Powers

Western New York Chapter

4213 N. Buffalo Road
Orchard Park, NY 14127

(716) 662-3710
Fax: (716) 662-4080

Executive Director:

Ms. Barbara Almeter

Carolinas Chapter

P.O. Box 31572
Raleigh, NC 27622

For deliveries:
3716 National Drive, Suite 111
Raleigh, NC 27612

(919) 782-5530
(800) 822-9941
Fax: (919) 782-5831

Executive Director:

Ms. Nancy Mallory

Charlotte Office

301 E. 7th Street, Suite 202
Charlotte, NC 28202

(704) 344-0329
(800) 336-0329
Fax: (704) 344-1864

Carolinas Telemarketing Center

P.O. Box 639
Wilson, NC 27894

For deliveries:
1704 South Tarboro Street, Suite 200
Wilson, NC 27893

(919) 291-7190
(800) 682-6858
Fax: (919) 291-3482

Director of Telemarketing:

Mr. Bruce Joyner

North Dakota - Please Contact:

Foundation Office

6931 Arlington Road
Bethesda, MD 20814

Field Manager:

Ms. Marcia Ritchie

(301) 951-4422
(800) FIGHT CF
Fax: (301) 951-6378

Central Ohio Chapter

6555 Busch Boulevard, Suite #108
Columbus, OH 43229

(614) 846-2440
Fax: (614) 846-2472

Executive Director:

Mr. Dave Anderson

Greater Cincinnati Chapter

2011 Madison Road
Cincinnati, OH 45208

(513) 533-9300
Fax: (513) 533-9301

Executive Director:

Ms. Susan Berliant

Rainbow Chapter

5755 Granger Road, Suite 630
Independence, OH 44131

(216) 485-8700
Fax: (216) 485-8711

Executive Director:

Ms. Sara Weiss

Sooner Chapter

2642 East 21st Street, Suite 100
Tulsa, OK 74114

(918) 744-6354
Fax: (918) 744-0806

Executive Director:

Ms. JoAnn Winn

Oregon/Idaho/Montana Chapter

4445 S.W. Barbur Boulevard
Suite C-101
Portland, OR 97201

(503) 226-3435
(800) 448-8404 (Oregon, Idaho,
   Washington)
Fax: (503) 226-4165

Executive Director:

Ms. Mary Miller

Central Pennsylvania Chapter

55 South Progress Avenue
Harrisburg, PA 17109

(717) 671-4000
Fax: (717) 671-4007

Executive Director:

Ms. Norma Frame

Delaware Valley Chapter

1601 Market Street, Suite 2310
Philadelphia, PA 19103

(215) 587-2800
Fax: (215) 587-9530

Executive Director:

Ms. Patricia Fulvio

Northeastern Pennsylvania Chapter

1541 Alta Drive, Suite 102
Whitehall, PA 18052

(610) 820-0206
(800) 552-2199 (in Pennsylvania)
Fax: (610) 820-9367

Executive Director:

Ms. Kathleen Houlihan

Western Pennsylvania Chapter

119 Federal Street, Room 509
Pittsburgh, PA 15212

(412) 321-4422
Fax: (412) 321-9305

Executive Director:

Ms. Mary Pat Root

Rhode Island Chapter

Office Commons 95
335 Centerville Road, Building 5
Warwick, RI 02886

(401) 739-6900
Fax: (401) 738-0054

South Carolina: See Carolinas Chapter (North Carolina)

South Dakota - Please Contact:

Foundation Office

6931 Arlington Road
Bethesda, MD 20814

Field Manager:

Ms. Marcia Ritchie

(301) 951-4422
(800) FIGHT CF
Fax: (301) 951-6378

Tennessee Chapter

3814 Cleghorn Avenue
Nashville, TN 37215

(615) 297-3582
Fax: (615) 385-1032

Executive Director:

Ms. Belinda Dinwiddie

Memphis Branch

3475 Central Avenue
Memphis, TN 38111-4407

(901) 452-2151 Ext. 120

Director of Special Events:

Ms. Catheryn Gay

Lone Star Chapter

8620 North New Braunfels, Suite 110
San Antonio, TX 78217

(210) 829-7267
Fax: (210) 829-4204

Executive Director:

Ms. Marti Alpard

Northeast Texas Chapter

2929 Carlisle, Suite 230
Dallas, TX 75204-1058

(214) 871-2222 or
Metro (214) 263-7299
Fax: (214) 969-7439

Executive Director:

Ms. Sila N. Foote

Texas Gulf Coast Chapter

3730 Kirby Drive, Suite 810
Houston, TX 77098

(713) 523-9044
Fax: (713) 523-9684

Executive Director:

Ms. Sissy Boyd

Utah: See Southern California/Utah Chapter

Vermont: See Northern New England Chapter (New Hampshire)

Virginia Chapter

2720 Enterprise Parkway, Suite 107
Richmond, VA 23294

(804) 527-1500
Fax: (804) 527-0016

Executive Director:

Ms. Deborah Golden

Hampton Roads Office

1423 North Great Neck Road
Suite 204
Virginia Beach, VA 23454

(804) 481-1383
(800) 572-3213
Fax: (804) 481-5919

Washington Chapter

100 West Harrison
North Tower, Suite 510
Seattle, WA 98119

(206) 282-4770
(800) 647-7774 (in Washington)
Fax: (206) 283-8359

Executive Director:

Ms. Dottie Moore

West Virginia: See Kentucky/ West Virginia Chapter

Wisconsin Chapter

2421 North Mayfair Road
Suite 320
Milwaukee, WI 53226

(414) 778-4820
(800) 472-7720 (in Wisconsin)
Fax: (414) 778-4824

Executive Director:

Ms. Lisa Weisman

Wyoming: See Colorado Chapter

APPENDIX G

Cystic Fibrosis Care Centers Worldwide

ARGENTINA

Hospital de Ninos Recardo Gutierrez
(Unidad 3)
Sanchez de Bustamante 1399
1425 Buenos Aires
Tel: 962-9212/9229/9232

Instituto Nacional de Genetica Medica
Dpto. Genetica Experimental
Av. Las Heras 2670 - 4o. Piso
1425 Buenos Aires
Tel: 801-2326
802-0011 to 0018 (Ext. 112)

Hospital de Pediatria (Dr. Pedro de
Elizalde)
Av. Montes de Oca 40
1270 Buenos Aires
Tel: 28-0056

Hospital de Pediatria (Juan P. Garrahan)
Combate de los Pozos 1881
1245 Buenos Aires
Tel: 941-6809/8486/6012/6191

Hospital de Ninos Sor Maria Ludovica
Calle 14 entre 65 y 66
1900 La Plata
Tel: 021-210448

Hospital de Ninos (Dr. Carlos Rezzonico)
Corrientes 643
5000 Cordoba

Dr. Otmar Bertero

Belgrano 3071 - ler piso
3000 Santa Fe
Tel: 042-32484

Institute del Nino
Entre Rios 1647
2000 Rosario

Hospital de Neuquen
Buenos Aires 353
8400 Neuquen

Hospital Emilio Civit
Labertador S/N - Parque Gral. San Martin
5300 Mendoza

AUSTRALIA
Victoria

Professor Haydn Walters
Dept. of Respiratory Medicine
The Alfred Hospital
Cystic Fibrosis Adult Clinic
Commercial Road
Prahran, Victoria 3181
Tel: 61 3 276 3476
Fax: 61 3 521 2365

Dr. Anthony Olinsky
Department of Thoracic Medicine
Royal Children's Hospital
Flemington Road
Parkville, Victoria 3052
Tel: 61 3 345 5522
Fax: 61 3 349 1289

South Australia

Dr. Mark Holmes, Consultant
The Royal Adelaide Hospital
Cystic Fibrosis Adult Clinic
The Chest Clinic
275 North Terrace
Adelaide, South Australia 5000
Tel: 61 8 223 0230
Fax: 61 8 223 4761

Dr. James Martin—Consultant
Pulmonary Department
Women's and Children's Hospital
King William Road
North Adelaide, South Australia 5006
Tel: 61 8 204 7000
Fax: 61 8 204 7459

Tasmania

Dr. Ian Stewart
Royal Hobart Hospital
48 Liverpool Street
Hobart, Tasmania 7000
Tel: 61 02 38 8308
Fax: 61 02 312 043

(Not a formal clinic)
Dr. J. Markos
Launceston General Hospital
Charles Street
Launceston, Tasmania 7250
Tel: 61 03 32 7111
Fax: 61 03 327 577

Queensland

Dr. P. Francis, Dr. A. Isles
Royal Children's Hospital
Heston Road
Herston, Queensland 4006
Tel: 61 7 253 8111
Fax: 61 7 257 1768

Dr. B. Masters, Dr. I. Robertson,
  Dr. M. Harris
Mater Children's Hospital
Raymond Terrace
South Brisbane, Queensland 4101
Tel: 61 7 840 8270
Fax: 61 7 844 8873

Dr. P. Zimmerman, Dr. R. Nolan, Dr. W.
  Oliver
Prince Charles Hospital
Rode Rd
Chermside, Queensland 4032
Tel: 61 7 350 8111
Fax: 61 7 359 5756

Dr. D. McEvoy, Dr. I. Brown, Dr. S.
  Morrison
Royal Brisbane Hospital
Herston, Queensland 4006
Tel: 61 7 253 8111
Fax: 61 7 257 1765

Dr. D. Lindsay, Dr. D. Price
Southport General Hospital
Southport, Queensland 4215

Dr. P. Roper, Dr. H. Mercer
Rockhampton Base Hospital
Rockhampton, Queensland 4700

Dr. J. Williams
Bundaberg Hospital
Bundaberg, Queensland 4670

Dr. M. Williams
Mackay Base Hospital
Mackay, Queensland 4740

Dr. P. Ryan
Townsville General Hospital
Townsville, Queensland 4810

Dr. R. Messer
Cairns Base Hospital
Cairns, Queensland 4870

New South Wales

Dr. Peter Bye
Royal Prince Alfred Hospital
Cystic Fibrosis Adult Clinic
Brown Street Outpatients
Page Chest Pavilion
Missenden Road
Camperdown, New South Wales 2050
Tel: 61 2 516 6111
Fax: 61 2 550 5865

Dr. Peter Cooper
Westmead Hospital (Adults & Children)
Hawkesbury Road
Westmead, New South Wales 2145
Tel: 61 2 633 6333
Fax: 61 2 633 4984

Dr. John Morton
The Prince of Wales Hospital
Cystic Fibrosis Clinic (Adults & Children)
High Street
Randwick, New South Wales 2031
Tel: 61 2 399 0111
Fax: 61 2 399 5414

Dr. John Brown
Royal Alexandra Hospital for Children
Pyrmont Bridge Road
Camperdown, New South Wales 2050
Tel: 61 2 519 0466
Fax: 61 2 519 3662

Dr. Richard Henry
John Hunter Hospital
Lookout Road
New Lambton Heights
New South Wales 2305
Tel: 61 49 213 000
Fax: 61 49 213 599

Dr. J. Pendergast
Gosford District Hospital
Cystic Fibrosis Clinic
Holden Street
Gosford, New South Wales 2250
Tel: 61 43 202 111
Fax: 61 43 202 804

Australian Capital Territory

Dr. M. Hurwitz
Woden Valley Hospital (Adult patients
  only)
Yamba Drive
Garran ACT 2605
Tel: 61 6 244 2154 (Physio Dept.)
Fax: 61 6 285 3127

Dr. C.S. May (Adult patients only)
Calvary Hospital
Cnr Haydon Drive & Belconnen Way
Bruce ACT 2617
Tel: 61 6 201 6111
Fax: 61 6 253 1907
Note: Children attend private pediatricians

Western Australia

Professor Lou Landau
University Department of Pediatrics
Princess Margaret Hospital for Children
  (Children's Clinic)
GPO Box D184
Perth WA 6001
Tel: 61 9 340 8222
Fax: 61 9 388 2097

Dr. Gerard Ryan
Sir Charles Gairdner Hospital (Adult
  Clinic)
Verdun Street
Nedlands WA 6009
Tel: 61 9 389 3333
Fax: 61 9 389 3606

Other Centers in Western Australia (not formal clinics)

Dr. John Hobday
Dr. Jacqueline Scurlock
Princess Margaret Hospital for Children
GPO Box D184
Perth WA 6001
Tel: 61 9 340 8222
Fax: 61 9 340 8111

AUSTRIA

University Children's Hospital, CF-Clinic
Director: Prof. Dr. M. Zach
Auenbruggerplatz 36
A-8036 Graz
Tel: 0316/385-2367

University Children's Hospital, CF-Clinic
Director: Dr. Ellemunter
Anichstrasse 35
A-6020 Innsbruck
Tel: 0512/504-0, -2001, -2008

Children's Hospital, CF-Clinic
Director: Dr. I. Huttegger, Dr. S. Riedler
Mullner Haupstrasse 48
A-5020 Salzburg
Tel: 0662/4482

University Children's Hospital, CF-Clinic
Director: Prof Dr. M. Gotz
Wahringer Gurtel 18-20
A-1090 Wien (Vienna)
Tel: 40400/3232

Prim. Dr. Franz Eitelberger
Krankenhaus der Barmherzigen Schestern
 Wels
Grieskirchner Strasse 42
4600 Wels
Tel: 07242/415-0

BELGIUM

Docteur Baran
Antoine Depage
Tel: 02/538 61 40

Hopital Erasme
route de Lennik 808
1070 Bruxelles
Tel: 02/526 39 85
 02/526 36 93

Docteur Bertrand
Clinique St. Vincent
rue Francois Lefevre 207

4000 Rocourt
Tel: 041/46 62 65
 041/46 62 66

Docteur Lebeque
U.C.L. Saint-Luc
avenue Hyppocrate 10
1200 Bruxelles
Tel: 02/764 11 11

Docteur Leclercq
Centre Hospitalier
Regional de la Citadelle
bld.du 12e de Ligne 1
4000 Liege
Tel: 041/25.61.11

Docteur Casimir
Hopital Universitaire d'enfants
Reine Fabiola
Place Van Gehuchten 4
1020 Bruxelles
Tel: 02/477 21 11

Docteur Dab
Azvub
Laarbeeklaan 101
1090 Jette
Tel: 02/477 60 61

Dokter Debaets
A.Z. - De Pintelaan 9000 Gent
Tel: 091/22 57 41

Dokter Deboeck
U.Z. Gasthuisberg
 Herestraat 49 3999 Leuven
Tel: 016/21 21 11

Professor Eggermont
U.Z. Gasthuisberg
 Herestraat 49 3000 Leuven
Tel: 016/21 21 11

Dokter van Schil
St. Vincentiusziekenhuis
 St. Vincentiusstraat 2000 Antwerpen
Tel: 03/218 60 00

Dokter H. Franckx
Zeepreventorium
  Koninklijke Baan 8420 de Haan
Tel: 059/23 39 11

Dokter Schuddinck
Preventorium St. Jozef
  Reebergenlaan 4 2240 Zandhoven
(Pulderbos)
Tel: 03/484 36

BRAZIL

Dr. Fernando de Abreu e Silva
Setor de Pneumologia Pediatrica
Hospital de Clinicas de Porto Alegre
Rua Ramiro Barcellos no 2350
Porto Alegre RS 90210
Fax: 51 227 4082

Dr. Daurinda Higa
Instituto Fernandes Figueira
Av. Rui Barbosa no 716 - Botafogo
Rio de Janeiro 22250

Dr. Neiva Damasceno
Departamento de Pediatria
Santa Casa de Misericordia de Sao Paulo
Rua Jose de Magalhaes no 20 - Vila
  Clementino
Sao Paulo

Dr. Tatiana Rozov
Instituto de Crianca
Av. Dr. Eneas de Carvalho Aguiar no 647
Pinheiros
Sao Paulo 05403

Dr. Antonio Fernando Ribeiro
Departamento de Pediatria
Faculdade de Ciencias Medicas
Caixa Postal 6111
Campinas 13083

Dr. Francisco Caldeira Reis
Departamento de Pediatria
Hospital das Clinicas de Belo Horizonte

Rua Ceara no 161 grupo 103/106
Belo Horizonte 30150

Dr. Nelson Rosario Filho
Departamento de Pediatria
Rua General Carneiro no 181
Curitiba 80000

Dr. Murilo Carlos Amorin de Brito
Instituto Materno Infantil de Pernambuco
Rua dos Coelhos no 300 - Boa Vista
Recife 50070

Dr. Lairton Valentin
Clinica Curumim
Rua Blumenau 321
Joinville 89200

Dr. Norberto Ludwig
Hospital Infantil Joana de Gusmao
Rua Rui Barbosa no 152
Agronomica
Florianopolis 88025

Dr. Maria Angelica Santana
Hospital Carlos Otavio Mangabeira
Largo do Paul Miudo

BULGARIA

Dr. Anni Kufardjieva
Pediatric Clinic
University Alexander Hospital
St. G. Sofiisky Str 1
Sofia 1431
Bulgaria

CANADA

British Columbia

B.C. Children's Hospital
4480 Oak Street
Vancouver, British Columbia
V6H 3V4

Director: Dr. A.G.F. Davidson
Nurse Coordinator: Maureen O'Loane
Clinic: 604/875-2146
Fax: 604/875-2292
Emergency: 604/875-2345
Office: 604/875-2142
Office Fax: 604/875-2349

University Hospital
Shaughnessy Site
4500 Oak Street
Vancouver, British Columbia
V6H 3N1
Director: Dr. E.M. Nakielna
Clinic Coordinator: Janet Hopkins
Clinic: 604/875-2146
Fax: 604/875-2643
Emergency: 604/875-2222
Office: 604/874-9212
Fax: 604/875-2643

Victoria General Hospital
35 Helmcken Road
Victoria, British Columbia
V8Z 6R5
Director (Pediatric): Dr. S. Kent
Nurse Coordinator: Susanne Laughren
Clinic: 604/727-4187
Fax: 604/727-4391
Attn: Local 5100
Emergency/Main: 604/727-4212
Office: 604/727-4189
Office Fax: 604/727-4221
Director (Adult): Dr. I. Waters
Office: 604/727-4212
Nurse Coordinator: Sharon Wiltse

Alberta

Alberta Children's Hospital
1820 Richmond Road S.W.
Calgary, Alberta
T2T 5C7
Director: Dr. I. Mitchell
Nurse Coordinator: Kay Jamieson

Clinic: 403/229-7319
Fax: 403/229-7221

Emergency/Main: 403/229-7211
Office: 403/229-7818
Office Fax: 403/229-7221

Foothills Hospital
University of Calgary Medical Clinic
3350 Hospital Drive N.W.
Calgary, Alberta
T2N 4N1
Director: Dr. H.R. Rabin
Nurse Coordinator: Christine Hegi
Clinic: 403/229-7319
Fax: 403/229-7221
Emergency/Main: 403/229-7211
Office: 403/220-5951
Office Fax: 403/270-2772

University of Alberta Hospitals
112 Street and 84th Avenue
8th Floor, Room #113D
Edmonton, Alberta
T6G 2B7
Director: Dr. P. Zuberbuhler
Nurse Coordinator: Inez Brown
Clinic: 403/492-6745
Fax: 403/426-2223
Emergency/Main: 403/492-8822
Office: 403/423-6911 x.235
Office Fax: 403/426-2223

Saskatchewan

Plains Health Centre
4500 Wascana Parkway
Regina, Saskatchewan
S4S 5W9
Director: Dr. G. White
Nurse Coordinator: Ms. Gerry Thompson
Clinic: 306/584-6314
Fax: 306/584-6334
Emergency: 306/584-6330
Main: 306/584-6211
Office: 306/584-6314
Office Fax: 306/584-6334

Regina General Hospital
1440-14th Avenue
Regina, Saskatchewan

S4P OW5
Director: Dr. B. Holmes
Nurse Coordinator: Marlene Hall
Clinic: 306/359-4289
Fax: 306/359-4723
Emergency: 306/359-4444
Office: 306/352-7633
Office Fax: 306/359-4723

University Hospital—Pediatric Clinic
Saskatoon, Saskatchewan
S7N OXO
Director: Dr. B.F. Habbick
Nurse Coordinator: Shirley Patola
Clinic: 306/966-8108
Fax: 306/975-3767
Emergency/Main: 306/244-2323
Office: 306/966-7930
Office Fax: 306-966-8799

University Hospital - Adult Clinic
Saskatoon, Saskatchewan
S7N OXO
Director: Dr. D. Cotton
Nurse Coordinator: Shirley Patola
Clinic: 306/966-8108
Fax: 306/975-3767
Emergency/Main: 306/244-2323
Office: 306/966-8694
Office Fax: 306/966-8694

Manitoba

Children's Hospital
840 Sherbrooke Street
Winnipeg, Manitoba
R3A 1S1
Director: Dr. V. Chernick
Nurse Coordinator: Roberta Woodgate
Clinic: 204/787-2401
Fax: 204/788-6489
Emergency: 204/787-2306
Main: 204/787-2993
Office: 204/788-6670
Office Fax: 204/788-6489

Ontario

Children's Hospital at Chedoke-McMaster
Department of Pediatrics
1200 Main Street West, Room 3F30
Hamilton, Ontario
L8N 3Z5
Director: Dr. W.M. Wilson
Nurse Coordinator: Rosamund Hennessey
Clinic: 416/521-5011
Fax: 416/521-1703
Emergency: 416/521-2100
Office: 416/521-2100 x5617
Page: 416/521-5030
Office Fax: 416/521-1703
(attn: June, x5617)

Children's Hospital of Eastern Ontario
401 Smyth Road
Ottawa, Ontario
K1H 8L1
Director: Dr. N. MacDonald
Nurse Coordinator: Anne Smith
Clinic: 613/737-2214
Fax: 613/738-3216
Emergency: 613/737-2328
Main: 613/737-7600
Office: 613/737-2651
Office Fax: 613/738-4832

Children's Hospital of Western Ontario
800 Commissioners Road East
London, Ontario
N6A 4G5
Director: Dr. E.R. Ecclestone
Nurse Coordinator: Elizabeth Hunter
Clinic: 519/685-8500
Emergency: 519/685-8142
Main: 519/685-8500
Office: 519/685-8221
Office Fax: 519/685-8156

Hotel Dieu Hospital
166 Brock Street
Kingston, Ontario
K7L 5G2
Director: Dr. D.W. Geiger
Nurse Coordinator: Jo-Ann Koster

Clinic: 613/544-1365
Fax: 613/544-9897
Emergency/Main: 613/544-3310
Office: 613/544-2266
Fax: 613/544-9897

Hotel Dieu of St. Joseph Hospital
1030 Ouellette Avenue
Windsor, Ontario
N9A 1E1
Director: Dr. E. Varga
Nurse Coordinator: Dagmar Ray
Clinic: 519/973-4444 x247
Fax: 519/973-1516
Emergency: 519/973-4444
Office: 519/258-4354
Office Fax: 519/258-9918

Kitchener-Waterloo Hospital
835 King Street West
Kitchener, Ontario
N2G 1G3
Co-Director: Dr. Kuldip Malhotra*
Co-Director: Dr. Mary Jackson**
Nurse Coordinator: Wendy Down
Clinic: 519/749-4204
Fax: 519/749-2376
Emergency/Main: 519/742-3611
*Office: 519/744-2691
Fax: 519/749-4204 (must call first)
**Office: 519/741-8660
Fax: 519/741-5772

Laurentian Hospital
41 chemin du Lac Ramsey
Sudbury, Ontario
P3E 5J1
Director: Dr. V.J. Kumar
Nurse Coordinator: Charlene Piche
Clinic: 705/522-2200 x3264
Fax: 705/523-7017
Emergency: 705/522-2200
Office: 705/674-1499
Office Fax: 705/671-2471

The Hospital for Sick Children
555 University Avenue
Toronto, Ontario

M5G 1X8
Director: Dr. H. Levison
Nurse Coordinator: Louise Taylor
Clinic: 416/813-5826
Fax: 416/813-7505
Emergency/Main: 416/813-1500
Office: 416/813-6167
Office Fax: 416/813-6246

The Wellesley Hospital
160 Wellesley Street East
Toronto, Ontario
M4Y 1J3
Director: Dr. E. Tullis
Nurse Coordinator: Susan Carpenter
Clinic: 416/926-7053
Fax: 416/926-4921
Emergency: 416/926-7037
Main: 416/966-6600
Office: 416/926-7745
Office Fax: 416/926-4921

The Rehabilitation Centre
505 Smyth Road
Ottawa, Ontario
K1H 8M2
Director: Dr. R.E. Dales
Nurse Coordinator: Therese Corbin
Clinic: 613/737-7350 x619
Fax: 613/737-8470
Emergency/Main: 613/737-7350
Office: 613/737-8198
Office Fax: 613/737-8141

Quebec

Centre Hospitalier Regional de l'Outaouais
116, boul. Lionel Emond
Hull, Quebec
J8Y 1W7
Directeur: Dr. G. Cote
Infirm. Coordonnatrice: Denise Levesque
Clinic: 819/595-6053
Emergency: 819/771-8367
Office: 819/595-6000
Office Fax: 819/595-1582

Centre Hospitalier Regional de Rimouski
150, ave. Rouleau
Rimouski, Quebec
G5L 5T1
Directeur: Dr. J. Boucher
Infirmiere Coordonnatrice: Denise
    Michaud
Clinic: 418/724-8561
Emergency: 418/724-4221
Office: 418/724-4221

Centre Hospitalier de l'Universite Laval
2705, boul. Sir Wilfred Laurier
STE-Foy, Quebec
G1V 4G2
Co-Directors: Dr. P. Bigonesse, Dr. G.
    Rivard
Directeur De La Clinique Pour Adultes:
    Dr. M. Ruel
Infirmiere Coordonnatrice: Anne-Marie
    Robert
Clinic: 418/654-2272
Emergency: 418/656-4141
Office: 418/656-4141 x7510
Office Fax: 418/654-2771

Centre Hospitalier Universitaire de
    Sherbrooke
3001 12e ave. n.
Sherbrooke, Quebec
J1H 5N4
Directeur: Dr. J. Lippe
Infirm. Coordonnatrice: Marguerite Plante
Clinic: 819/563-5555 x4638
Emergency/Main: 819/563-5555
Office: 819/563-6232
Office Fax: 819/822-2673

Hopital de Chicoutimi, Inc.
C.P. 5006
Chicoutimi, Quebec
67H 5H6
Directeur: Dr. G. Aubin
Infirmiere Coordonnatrice: Simone Aubin
Clinic: 418/696-9978
Emergency/Main: 418/696-9978
Office: 418/549-1034
Office Fax: 418/696-4673

Hopital Ste-Justine
3175, chemin Ste-Catherine
Montreal, Quebec
H3T 1C5
Directeur: Dr. A. Lamarre
Infirm. Coordonnatrice: Diane Dupont
Clinic: 514/345-4724
Fax: 514/345-4769
Emergency: 514/345-4611
Office: 514/345-4654
Office Fax: 514/345-4804

Hotel-Dieu de Montreal
Service de Pneumologie
3840, rue St-Urbain
Montreal, Quebec
H2W 1T8
Directeur: Dr. A. Jeanneret
Inf. Coordonnatrice: Marie-Claire
    Michoud
Clinic: 514/843-2670
Fax: 514/843-9486
Emergency/Main: 514/843-2670
Office: 514/843-2670
Office Fax: 514/843-2708

Montreal Chest Hospital
3650 St-Urbain Street
Montreal, Quebec
H2X 2P4
Director: Dr. E. Matouk
Nurse Coordinator: Leticia De La Calzada
Clinic: 514/849-5201 x280
Fax: 514/982-6840
Emergency/Main: 514/849-5201
Office: 514/345-3104
Office Fax: 514/849-6075
(Attn: Research Department)

Montreal Children's Hospital
2300 Tupper Street
Montreal, Quebec
H3H 1P3
Director: Dr. N. Sweezey
Nurse Coordinator: Jackie Townshend
Clinic: 514/934-4400 x2643
Emergency/Main: 514/934-4400
Office: 514/934-4442
Office Fax: 514/934-4477

New Brunswick

Saint John Regional Hospital
P.O. Box 2100
Saint John, New Brunswick
E2L 4L2
Director: Dr. D.N. Garey
Nurse Coordinator: Diana Peacock
Clinic: 506/648-6793
Emergency/Main: 506/648-6000
Fax: 506/648-6282
Office: 506/634-1016

Nova Scotia

I.W. Killam Hospital for Children
5850 University Avenue
Halifax, Nova Scotia
B3J 3G9
Director: Dr. D. Hughes
Nurse Coordinator: Paula Barrett
Clinic: 902/428-8111
Fax: 902/422-9229
Emergency: 902/428-8050
Main: 902/428-8111
Office: 902/428-8219
Office Fax: 902/422-9229

Victoria General Hospital
1278 Tower Road
Halifax, Nova Scotia
B3H 2Y9
Director: Dr. R.T. Michael
Nurse Coordinator: Joanne Brown-
  Bonomo
Clinic: 902/428-4194
Fax: 902/428-5561
Emergency: 902/428-2110
Office: 902/422-1708

Newfoundland

The Dr. Charles A. Janeway Child Health
  Centre
710 Newfoundland Drive
St. John's, Newfoundland
A1A 1R8

Director: Dr. D. Vaze
CoDirector: Dr. R. Morris
Nurse Coordinator: Elizabeth Sheppard
Clinic: 709/778-4389
Fax: 709/722-9605
Main: 709/778-4222
Office: 709/778-4222
Office: 709/778-4150
Office Fax: 709/722-9605

COSTA RICA

Cystic Fibrosis Center
Hospital Nacional de Ninos
San Jose, Costa Rica
Director: Reina Gonzalez, M.D.
Apdo. 337-1200
San Jose, Costa Rica
Tel: Hospital (506) 22-01-22, ext. 313
Fax: Hospital (506) 55-49-07

CUBA

Dr. Tomas Perez
Servicio de Respiratorio
Hospital "J.M. Miranda"
Ave. 26 de Julio y 1a
Reparto Escambray
Cividad de Villa Clara
Santa Clara Prov. CP: 50100
Cuba
Tel: 72129, 72013

Dr. Luis Climent
Hospital Pediatr. Provincial "P. Gonzalez"
Calle 39 #3602
Cividad de Cienfuegos CP: 55100
Prov. Cienfuegos
Cuba
Tel: 7129

Dr. Guillermo Ramirez
Hospital Pediatr. Provincial de Holguin
Ave Libertadores #91
Cividad Holguin CP: 80100
Provincia Holguin
Cuba
Tel: 45012

Dra. Concepcion Estrada
Hosp. Infantil de Matanzas
Sta. Isabel el America y Compostela
Cividad de Matanzas CP: 40100
Matanzas
Cuba
Tel: 7012 ext. 52

Dr. Guillermo Amaro Ivonet
Hospital Pediatr. Sur de Santiago; 24 de
    Febrero 402
Cividad de Santiago de Cuba CP: 90100
Provincia de Santiago de Cuba
Cuba
Tel: 6556

Dr. Fidel Rodriquez
Servicio de Respiratorio
Hospital "Calixto Garcia"
Municipio Plaza CP: 10400
Cividad de La Habana
Cuba
Tel: 329501-07

Dra. Juana Maria Rodriguez
Servicio de Afecciones Respiratorias
Hosp. Pediatr. Pedro Borras
F entre 27y29 CP: 10400
Muicipio Plaza
Cividad de La Habana
Cuba
Tel: 32-6533

Dr. Roberto Razon
Servicio de Apecciones Respiratorias
Hospital Pediatrico "William Soler" Ave de
    Vento
Municipio de Alta habana CP: 10800
Cividad de La Habana
Cuba
Tel: 443621

Dra. Gladys Abreu
Servicio de Apecciones Respiratorias
Hospital Pediatr. de Centro Habana
Municipio de Centro-Habana
Cividad de La Habana
Cuba
Tel: 704556, 703292

Dr. Manuel Rojo Concepcion
Hospital Pediatrico "J.M. Marquez"
Ave. 31 esq. 76 CP: 11400
Municipio de Marianao
Cividad de la Habana
Cuba
Tel: 20 2860
Fax: Buro FAX H.P.J.M.M.
    53-7-338212
    53-7-338213

CZECHOSLOVAKIA

Dr. A. Kolek
Pediatric Department
University Hospital
I.P. Pavloa 6,
775 20 Olomouc Czechoslovakia
Tel: 4268 474 1111

Dr. Holcikova
Pediatric Department
Cernopolni 9
662 63 Brno Czechoslovakia
Tel: 425-5165

Dr. Lenka Toukalkova
Pediatric Department
Bata Hospital
Havlickovo n. 600
760 01 Zlin Czechoslovakia
Tel: 42967 25 102

Dr. H. Vanicek
Pediatric Department
University Hospital
500 36, Hradec Kralove Czechoslovakia
Tel: 4249 39 05

Dr. Helena Honomichlova
Pediatric Department
University Hospital
Dr. E. Benese 13
305 99 Plzen Czechoslovakia
Tel: 4219 2162

Dr. Ivana Tumova
Department, TRN, ILF
Masaryk Hospital
401 13 Usti nad Labem - Bukov
    Czechoslovakia
Tel: 4247 42 241

Dr. I. Sekyrova
Pediatric Department ILF,
B. Nemcove 54
370 87 Ceske Budejovice Czechoslovakia
Tel: 4238 821911

Dr. Hubova
Pediatric Department ILF,
Syllabove 19
703 86 Ostrava Czechoslovakia
Tel: 4269 449 117

Dr. Vera Vavrova
2nd Pediatric Department,
University Hospital Motol
V uvalu 84
150 18 Praha 5-Motol
Czechoslovakia
Tel: 422 5295 2269
Fax: 422 5295 2220

DENMARK

Dr. Christian Koch, M.D. Ph.D.
Chairman
Cystic Fibrosis Center - Copenhagen
Dept. of Pediatrics GGK-5002
University Hospital (Rigshospitalct)
Blegdamsvej 9
DK-2100 Copenhagen
Tel: (+45) 3545 3545, ext. 4822, or 4832,
    or 5006
Fax: (+45) 3536 8717

Professor P.O. Schiotz, Ph.D.
Chairman
Danish Cystic Fibrosis Center - Aarhus
Dept. of Pediatrics A
University Hospital (Kommunehospitalet)
DK-8000 Aarhus

Tel: (+45) 8612 5555, ext. 2043 or 2014
Fax: (+45) 8615 9377

ESTONIA

Dr. Katrin Ounap
Medical Genetics Centre
Tartu University Children's Hospital
EE2400 Tartu, Estonia
Tel: 7 01434 34986
Fax: 7 01434 32119

Maris Teder
Tartu University
Inst. Gen & Mol Path,
34 Veski Street,
EE2400 Tartu,
Estonia
Tel: 7 01434 35169
Fax: 7 01434 35430

FINLAND

Dr Erkki Savilahti
University of Helsinki Children's Hospital
Stenbackinkatu 11
00290 Helsinki
Finland

FRANCE

Hauet Normandie

M. le Dr. Lashinat
Hopital des Feugrais
7 rue Petou
BP 346
76503 Elbeuf
Tel: 35.87.35.35

M. le Dr. Le Luyer
Hopital General Du Havre
55bis rue Gustave Flaubert
76083 Le Havre
Tel: 35.55.25.25

M. le Dr. Mouterde
Hopital Charles Nicoles
1 rue de Germont
76031 Rouen Cedex
Tel: 38.08.81.81

Langeudoc Roussillon

M. le Dr. Ariole
Institut St. Pierre
34250 Palavas les flots
Tel: 67.07.75.00

M. le Dr. Rodiere
Centre Medico-Churugical
Guy de Chauliac
2 avenue Bertin Sans
34090 Montpellier
Tel: 67.63.90.50

M. le Pr. Rieu
Hopital St. Charles
300 rue Auguste Broussonnet
34000 Montpellier
Tel: 67.33.67.33

Basse Normandie

M. le Pr. Duhamel
Hopital Clemenceau
avenue Georges Clemenceau
14033 Caen Cedex
Tel: 31.44.81.12

M. le Dr. Guillot
Hopital Robert Bisson
4 rue Roger Aini
BP223
14107 Lisieux Cedex
Tel: 31.31.17.76

Picardie

M. le Dr. Pautard
Mme le Dr. Lenaerts
Centre Hospitalier Universitaire

Place Victor Pauchet
80054 Amiens Cedex
Tel: 22.66.80.00

Nord

M. le Dr. Druon
Institut A. Calmette
62176 Camiers
Tel: 21.84.91.44

M. le Pr. Farriaux
Hopital C. Huriez
Place de Verdun
59037 Lille Cedex
Tel: 20.44.44.27

M. le Dr. Loeville
Hopital General de Dunrerque
130 avenue Louis Herbeaux
BP6-367
59385 Dunkerque Cedex 01
Tel: 28.29.59.00

Paca

M. le Dr. Albertini
Hopital de Cimiez
4 avenue Victoria
BP179-06003 Nice
Tel: 92.03.44.44

M. le Dr. Chazalette
Hopital Renee Sabran
Bd Edouard Herriot
Giens 83406 Hyeres
Tel: 94.58.92.00

Mme le Dr. Lafferre
Les Cadrans Solaires
BP 86 - 11 route de St. Paul
06140 Vence
Tel: 93.24.55.00

M. le Dr. Sarles
Hopital de la Timone
Pediatric et Genetique
13005 Marseille Cedex 5
Tel: 91.38.60.00

M. le Dr. Theveniau
Hopital D'zix en Provence
avenue des Tamaris
3616 Aix en Provence Cedex 1
Tel: 42.33.50.00

Auvergne

M. le. Pr. Labbe
Hotel Dieu
Pavillion Hacquart
Bd Leon Malfreyt - BP 69
63003 Clermont Ferrand cedex 1
Tel: 73.31.60.60

Rhone-Alpes

M. le Pr. Bellon
M. le Pr. Vital Durand
Centre Hospitalier Lyon Sud
J. Courmont Ste Eugenie
165 Chemin du Grant Revoyet
69310 Pierre Benite
Tel: 78.50.95.15

M. le Dr. Clavel
Centre Medical Climatique
Bellevue
26220 Dieutefit
Tel: 75.46.35.35

M. le Dr. Gout
Chru de Grenoble
BP217
38043 Grenoble Cedex 9
Tel: 76.76.76.76

Bordeaux Aquitaine

Mme le Dr. Ceccato
Hopital Pellegrin—Tripode
Place Amelie Raba Leon

33076 Bordeaux Cedex
Tel: 56.79.56.79

M. le Dr. Domblides
Hopital Xavier Arnozan
avenue Haut Leveque
33604 Pessac
Tel: 56.55.65.65

M. le Dr. Contraires
Hopital de Bayonne
Service de Pediatrie
13 rue de l'Interne J. Loeb
64100 Bayonne
Tel: 59.44.35.35

Pays de Loire

Mme le Dr. David
Chru
5 allee de l'Ile Gloriette
Immeuble Deurbroucq
BP 1005
44035 Nantes Cedex 01
Tel: 40.08.42.42

M. le Dr. Ginies
Chru d'Angers
1 avenue de l'Hotel Dieu
49033 Angers Cedex 01
Tel: 41.35.36.37

M. le Dr. Picherot
Chg de St. Nazaire
BP 414
44606 St. Nazaire Cedex
Tel: 40.90.60.60

Bretagne

M. le Dr. Journel
Hopital P. Chubert
Bd General Guillaudot
BP 555
56017 Vannes Cedex
Tel: 97.01.41.41

M. le Dr. Lefur
Hopital Augustin Morvan
5 avenue Foch
29609 Brest Cedex
Tel: 98.22.33.33

M. le Dr. Rault
Centre Helio Marin
Presquile de Perharldy
29684 Roscoff Cedex
Tel: 98.29.39.39

M. le Pr. Roussey
Hopital de Pontchaillou
rue Henri le Guilloux
35033 Rennes Cedex
Tel: 99.28.43.21

Lorraine

M. le Pr. Vidailhet
Mme le Dr. Derelle
Hopital d'Enfants de Brabios
5 allee du Morvan
54511 Vandoeuvre les Nancy
Tel: 83.15.30.30

Champagne-Ardennes

M. le Pr. Pennaforte
Chru de Reims
23 rue des Moulins
51092 Reims Cedex
Tel: 26.78.78.78
Ile de France Est
M. le Dr. Steinschneider

Centre Hospitalier General
BP 218
6/8 rue St. Fiacre
77108 Meaux Cedex
Tel: 64.33.49.35

Ile de France Ouest

Mme le Pr. Caubarrere
M. le Dr. Stern
Hopital Foch
40 rue worth
BP36
92151 Suresnes
Tel: 46.25.20.00

M. le Dr. Feigelson
Cabinet Medical
153 rue de saussure
75017 Paris
Tel: 42.67.12.15

M. le Dr. Foucaud
Hopital A. Mignot
177 rue de Versailles
78157 Le Chesnay
Tel: 39.63.91.33

Mme le Dr. Hubert
Hopital Cochin
27 rue du Fg St. Jacques
75674 Paris Cedex 14
Tel: 42.34.12.12

M. le Pr. Lenior
M. le Pr. Scheinman
Hopital Necker
Enfants Malades
149 rue de Sevres
75015 Paris
Tel: 42.73.80.00

M. le Pr. Navarro
Hopital Robert Debre
48 Bd Serurier
75019 Paris
Tel: 40.03.20.00

M. le Pr. Tournier
Mme le Dr. Sardet
Hopital Trousseau
26 av. du Dr. Netter
75571 Paris 12eme
Tel: 43.46.13.90

Bourgogne

M. le Pr. Nivelon
Hopital d'Enfants
2 Bd Marechal de Lattre de
Tassigny - BP 1542
21000 Dijon
Tel: 80.29.30.31

Midi-Pyrenees

M. le Pr. Dutau
M. le Pr. Ghisolfi
Hopital de Purpan
Place du Dr. Baylac
31052 Toulouse Cedex
Tel: 61.77.82.33

M. le Dr. Sablayrolles
Cabinet Medical
Groupe de Pneumologie
2 rue Ozenne
31000 Toulouse
Tel: 61.52.64.36

Poitou-Charentes

M. le Dr. Massicot
Centre Helio Marin
19 Bd Felix Faure
17370 St. Trojan
Tel: 46.76.00.09

Franche-Comte

M. le Pr. Noir
Hopital de Besancon
Chru
2 Place St. Jacques
25030 Besancon Cedex
Tel: 81.66.81.66

Centre

M. le Dr. Feron
Hopital d'Orleans

1 rue Pte. Madelcine
45032 Orleans Cedex
Tel: 38.51.44.44

M. le Pr. Grenier
Hopital Gatien de Clocheville
40 Bd Beranger
37044 Tours Cedex
Tel: 47.47.47.47

Limousin

Dr. Gautry
Hopital General de Brive
Pediatrie
BP 432
19312 Brive la Gaillarde Cedex
Tel: 55.92.60.00

M. Pr. de Lumley
Chru Dupuytren
Pediatrie I
2 Avenue Alexis Carrel
87042 Limoges
Tel: 55.05.61.23

GERMANY

CF-Ambulanz
Krankenhaus Zehlendorf
Zum Heckeshorn 30-33
1000 Berlin 39

CF-Ambulanz
Kreiskrankenhaus Nauen, Betriebsstatte
   Staaken/Kinderabt.
Chefarzt Dr. Med. K.-D. Stettnich
Schulstrasse 13
1000 Berlin 20
Tel: 030/3634011
Fax: 030/3634016

CF-Ambulanz
Altonaer Kinderkrankenhaus
Bleickenallee 38
2000 Hamburg 50

CF-Ambulanz
Universitäts-Kinderklinik
Hamburg
Dr. med. M. Ballmann
Martinstrasse 52
2000 Hamburg 20
Tel: 040/4717-3710
Fax: 040/4717-5108

CF-Ambulanz
der Universitätskinderklinik
Dr. med. A. Claass
PD Dr. M. Krawinkel
Schwanenweg 20
2300 Kiel 1
Tel: 0431/597-1622
Fax: 0431/597-1831

CF-Ambulanz
Klinik fur Padiatrie der
Med. Universitat Lubeck
Dr. F.K. Testmeyer, Dr. S. Jonas
Kahlhorstrasse 31-35
2400 Lübeck 1
Tel: 0451/50025-67 o. 55
Fax: 0451/5006222

CF-Ambulanz
Kinderdlinik "Links der Weser"
Dr. Classen
Prof. Bachmann
Senator-Wessling-Strasse 1
2800 Bremen 61
Tel: 0421/879-0 o. 322
Fax: 0421/879599

CF-Ambulanz
Prof. Hess-Kinderklinik
Zentralkrankenhaus
OA Dr. med. Wolfram Wiebicke
St. Jurgen-Strasse
2800 Bremen 1
Tel: 0421/497-5410
Fax: 0421/497-3311

Kinderabteilung
St. Marienhospital
Dr. H. Koch

Marienstrasse 6
2848 Vechta
Tel: 04441/14222
Fax: 04441/81194

CF-Ambulanz
Reinhard-Nieter-Krankenhaus
Kinderklinik
Friedrich-Paffrath-Strasse 100
2940 Wilhelmshaven
Tel: 04421/89-0

CF-Ambulanz
MHH Hannover
Kinderklinik
Prof. Dr. med. H. von der Hardt
Postfach 61 01 80
3000 Hannover 61
Tel: 0511/532/3251
Fax: 0511/532-6125

CF-Ambulanz
der Inneren Medizin der MHH
Frau Dr. C. Smaczny
Postfach 61 01 80
3000 Hannover 61
Tel: 0511/532-325
Fax: 0511/532-6125

CF-Ambulanz
Allgemeines Krankenhaus
Kinderklinik
Prof. Dr. H. Jacobi
Siemensplatz 4
3100 Celle
Tel: 05141/308260
Fax: 05141/308558

CF-Ambulanz
Universtäts-Kinderklinik
Dr. Jutta Domagk
Robert-Koch-Strasse 40
3400 Göttingen
Tel: 0551-396239
Fax: 0551-396252

CF-Ambulanz
Kinderklinik der Städtischen
Kliniken Kassel
Prof. Dr. H. Wehinger
Mönchebergstrabe 41
3500 Kasse
Tel: 0561/9803365
Fax: 0561/9806971

CF-Ambulanz
Zentrum für Kinderheilkunde d.
 Universität Marburg
Deutschhausstrasse 2
3550 Marburg

CF-Ambulanz
Universitäts-Kinderklinik
Dusseldorf
Dr. Ballauf, Dr. Calaminus
Moorenstrasse 5
4000 Düsseldorf 1
Tel: 0211/311-8297
Fax: 0211/311-6266

CF-Ambulanz
Städt. Krankenanstalten Krefeld
Kinderklinik
OA Muhlenberg, R. Meisen
Lutherplzatz 40
4150 Krefeld 1
Tel: 02151/3223-10 o.49

CF-Ambulanz
Universitäts-Kinderklinik Essen
Drs. Ratjon, Wiesemann, Kuster
Prof. Stephan
Hufelandstrasse 55
4300 Essen 1
Tel: 0201/72333-55 o.50

CF-Ambulanz
Clemenshospital
Kinder-und Jugendabteilung
Dr. med. J. Uekotter
Duesbergweg 124
4400 Münster
Tel: 0251-9762601
Fax: 0251-9762002

CF-Ambulanz
Kinderklinik der Universitat
Dr. med. Hans Georg Koch
Dr. med. Anne Schulze-Everding
Albert-Schweitzer-Strasse 33
4400 Münster
Tel: 0251/837750
Fax: 0251/838045

CF-Ambulanz
Kinderhospital Osnabruck
OA Dr. med. Rudiger Szczepaiski
Iburger Strasse 187
4500 Osnabrück
Tel: 0541/5602-0 o.114
Fax: 0541/5602110

CF-Ambulanz
Kinderklinik der Universitat
zu Koln
OA Dr. Ernst Reitschel
Joseph-Stelzmann-Strasse 9
5000 Köln 41
Tel: 0221/478-361 o.358
Fax: 0221/4784689

CF-Ambulanz
Klinikum der Stadt Koln
Kinderkrankenhaus-Koln-Riehl
Dr. V. Soditt, Dr. R. Grolik
Amsterdamer Strasse 59
5000 Koln 60
Tel: 0221/7774-1
Fax: 0221/7774576

CF-Ambulanz
Dr. Jachertz/Dr. Tinschmann
Gemeinschaftspraxis
Hauptstrase 19-21
5020 Frechen

CF-Ambulanz
Med. Fakultät d. RWTH Aachen
Kinkerklinik
Pauwelstrasse
5100 Aachen

CF-Ambulanz
Johanniter-Kinderklinik

OA Dr. Gerhard Koch
Arnold-Janssen-Strasse 29
5205 Sankt Augustin 1
Tel: 02241/249303
Fax: 02241/204578

CF-Ambulanz
Zentrum fur Kinderheilkunde
der Universitat Bonn
OA Dr. K.M. Keller
Adenauerallee 119
5300 Bonn 1
Tel: 0228/287-3355
Fax: 0228/287-3314

CF-Ambulanz
Kreiskrankenhaus Mechernich
Dr. med. Jorg Schriever
Stiftsweg 18
5353 Mechernich
Tel: 02443/17-1401
Fax: 02243/17-1005

CF-Ambulanz
Mutterhaus der Borromaerinnen
Padiatrische Abteilung
Dr. Wolfgang Rauh, Dr. St. Bratz
Feldstrasse 16
5500 Trier
Tel: 0651/711-2656
Fax: 0651/7112587

CF-Ambulanz
Zentrum der Kinderheilkunde
Abt. Allgemeine Pädiatrie 1
Dr. H.-G. Posselt, Dr. Hummel
Theodor-Stern-Kai 7
6000 Frankfurt 70
Tel: 069/6301-5034
Fax: 069/6301-5229

CF-Ambulanz
Universitäts-Kinderklinik
Prof. Dr. H. Lindemann
Feulgenstrasse 12
6300 Gieben
Tel: 0641/702-4405

CF-Ambulanz
Kinder u. Kinderpoliklinik
d. J. Gutenberg-Uni/Allergologie
u. Pneumologie/Prof. Dr. Dorsch
Langenbeckstrasse 1
6500 Mainz
Tel: 06131-172602
Fax: 06131-222332

CF-Ambulanz
Universitätsklinik
Kinder-und Jugendmedizin Amb.
Prof. Dr. G. Dockter, Dr. S. Lipfert
6650 Homburg
Tel: 06841/164047
Fax: 06841-164011

CF-Ambulanz
Kinderklinik St. Anna Stift
Prof. Dr. med. H. Chr. Dominick
OA Dr. med. C. Ehringhaus
Karolina-Burger-Strasse 51
6700 Ludwigshafen
Tel: 0621/5702269
Fax: 0621/5702221

CF-Ambulanz
Klinikum der Stadt Mannheim
Kinderklinik Haus 2
Priv. Doz. Dr. med. M. Teufel
Grenadierstrasse 1
6800 Mannheim 1
Tel: 0621/383-2243 o. 2410
Fax: 0621/3833829

CF-Ambulanz
Olgaspital Stuttgart
Herrn Dr. V. Zenkl
Bismarckstrasse 8
7000 Stuttgart 1
Tel: 0711/99224-30 o. 31

CF-Ambulanz
Kinderklinik Heilbronn
Dr. med. Norbert Geier
Am Gesundbrunnen
7100 Heilbronn
Tel: 07131/493702

CF-Ambulanz
Kinderklinik fur Kinder u. Jugendliche
Frau Dr. med. Kathrin Schmidt
Frau Dr. med. Susanne Luxenhofer
Hirschlandstrasse 97
7300 Esslingen
Tel: 0711/3103-3510
Fax: 0711/3103-726

CF-Ambulanz
Universitäts-Kinderklinik
Prof. Dr. M. Stern, Dr. M. Reuter
Rümelinstrasse 23
7400 Tubingen
Tel: 07071/293781
Fax: 07071/294713

CF-Ambulanz
Kinderklinik Karlsruhe
Dr. Angelika Loesch
Karl-Wilhelm-Strasse 1
7500 Karlsruhe 1
Tel: 0721/797-670
Fax: 0721/607485

CF-Ambulanz
Kinderklinik des Stadtischen
Krankenhauses Pforzheim
Prof. Dr. Diethelm Kaiser
Kanzlerstrasse 2-6
7530 Pforzheim
Tel: 07231/601401
Fax: 07231/601901

CF-Ambulanz
Kinderklinik KKH Offenburg
Dr. J. Hautz
Ebertplatz 12
7600 Offenburg
Tel: 0781/4722790

CF-Ambulanz
Universitäts-Kinderklinik Ulm
Dr. Anna Wolf, Dr. M. Rank
Pritzwitzstrasse 43
7900 Ulm
Tel: 0731/5027791

CF-Ambulanz
Med. Uni-Klinik, Innere Med. II
OA Dr. med. S. Wieshammer
Robert-Koch-Strasse 8
7900 Ulm

CF-Ambulanz
Kinderkrankenhaus St. Nikolaus
OA Dr. Gerdaliese Wolfle
Nikolausstrasse 10
7980 Ravensburg
Tel: 0751/873285
Fax: 0751/873202

CF-Ambulanz
Dr. von Haunersches Kinderspital
Prof. Dr. Harms
Dr. Bertele-Harms
Lindwurmstrasse 4
8000 Munchen 2
Tel: 089/5160-3138
Fax: 089/5160-4725

CF-Ambulanz
der Kinder-u. Kinderpoliklinik
der Techn. Uni am KKH Schwabing
OA Dr. B. Hilz u. Dr. R. Franz
Kolner Platz 1
8000 Munchen 40
Tel: 089/3068-632
Fax: 089/3007464

CF-Ambulanz
Kinderpoliklinik der
Universitat Munchen
Prof. Dr. Reinhardt
Pettenkoferstrasse 81
8000 Munchen 2

CF-Ambulanz
Klinik mit Poliklinik fur Kinder
und Jugendliche der Universitat
Akad. Dir. Dr. med. B. Bowing
Loschgestrasse 15
8520 Erlangen
Tel: 09131-853134
Fax: 09131-853113

CF-Ambulanz
Kinderklinik der Universitat
Wurzburg
Josef-Schneider-Strasse 2
8700 Wurzburg

CF-Ambulanz
Bezirkskrankenhaus Brandenburg
Kinderklinik
Hochstrasse 29
0-1000 Bradenburg

CF-Ambulanz
Stadtisches Klinikum Berlin-Buch
III. Kinderklinik
Karower Strasse 11
0-1115 Berlin

CF-Ambulanz
Krankenhaus Berlin-Lichtenberg
Ortl. Bereich Kinderkl. Lindhof
Dr. Generlich, OA Dr. B. Leucht
Gotelindestrasse 2-20
0-1130 Berlin
Tel: 030/5554-0 o. 291
Fax: 030/5554-100

CF-Ambulanz
Klinikum Frankfurt/Oder
Dr. med. Harald Ronitz
Seelower Kehre 3/4
0-1200 Frankfurt/Oder
Tel: 0335/63080
Fax: 0335/42031

CF-Ambulanz
Bezirkskrankenhaus Potsdam
Herrn OA Dr. med. Opitz
Leninallee 114-117
0-1560 Potsdam

CF-Ambulanz
Ruppiner Krankenhaus
Chefarzt Dr. Kalz
Fehrbelliner Strasse 38
0-1950 Neuruppin
Tel: 03391/393701
Fax: 03391/3745

CF-Ambulanz
Klinikum Neubrandenburg
Kinderklinik
Prov.-Doz. Dr. F.J. Heydolph
Dr.-Salvador-Allende-Str. 30
0-2000 Neubrandenburg
Tel: 0395/75-0 o. 2917

CF-Ambulanz
Klinik fur Kinderheilkunde der
Ernst-Moritz-Arndt-Uniersitat
Prof. Dr. S. Wiersbitzky
Soldtmannstrasse 15
0-2200 Greifswald
Tel: 03834/7533
Fax: 03834/75329

CF-Ambulanz
Universitats-Kinderklinik
Frau Dr. med. K. Breuel
Rembrandstrasse 16/17
0-2500 Rostock
Tel: 0381/396891
Fax: 0381/39874

CF-Ambulanz
Kinderklinik des Klinikums
Schwerin
Dr. med. Joachim Venzmer
Wismarsche Strasse 397
0-2758 Schwerin
Tel: 0385/892694

CF-Ambulanz
Kinderklinik der Medizinischen
Akademie Magdeburg
Frau Dr. med. Ursula Klaer
Wiener Strasse
0-3014 Magdeburg
Tel: 677303
Fax: 677267

CF-Ambulanz
Martin-Luther-Univers./Klinikum
Krollwitz/Klinik fur Kinderheil-
  kunde/Frau Dr. med. S. Bromme
Postfach 63
0-4010 Halle
Tel: 672500 o. 672053

Cf-Ambulanz
Kinderklinik der Medizinische
Akademie Erfurt
OA Dr. med. habil. G. Weinmann
Am Schwemmbach 32 a
0-5083 Erfurt
Tel: 0361-39131
Fax: 0361-31478

CF-Ambulanz
Bezirkskrankenhaus Suhl
Kinderklinik
Albert-Schweitzer-Strasse 3
0-6013 Suhl

CF-Ambulanz
Thurinen-Klinik
"Georgius Agricola"
OA Dr. med. S. Mattes
Rainweg 54
0-6800 Saalfeld
Tel: 03671/827500

CF-Ambulanz
Universitats-Kinderklinik
Dr. L. Vogt, Dr. E. Janitzky
Kochstrasse 2
0-6900 Jena
Tel: 03641/8850
Fax: 03641/885470

CF-Ambulanz
Bezirkskrankenhaus fur
Lungenkrankheiten
Nikolai-Rumjanzew-Strasse 100
0-7031 Leipzig

CF-Ambulanz
Uni-Kinderpoliklinik Leipzig
Frau Dr. med. T. Leitz
Ostrasse 21-23
0-7050 Leipzig
Tel: 0341/6820341
Fax: 0341/603004

CF-Ambulanz
Dr. med. Gisa Schubert
Kinderarztpraxis

Leipziger Strasse 46
0-7500 Cottbus
Tel: 0355/421440

CF-Ambulanz
Klinik u. Poliklinik f. Kinderheilkunde
Med. Akademie "Carl Gustav Carus"
Dr. J. Henker
Fetscherstrasse 74
0-8019 Dresden
Tel: 0351-4582287
Fax: 0351-4584311

CF-Ambulanz
Bezirkskrankenhaus
Neucoswiger Strasse 21
0-8270 Coswig

CF-Ambulanz
Kinderklinik der Stadtischen
Kliniken Chemnitz
Doz. Dr. Klaus Dietel
Dresdner Strasse 178
0-9075 Chemnitz
Tel: 0371/47060
Fax: 0371/41166

CF-Ambulanz
Kinderklinik des Klinikums Aue
Dr. med. Gunter Frey
Schneeberger Strasse 98
0-9400 Aue
Tel: 03771/22302

CF-Ambulanz
Stadtisches Klinikum
"Heinrich Braun," Kinderklinik
OA Dr. med. Werner Wende
Karl-Keil-Strasse 35
0-9547 Zwickau
Tel: 0375/512409
Fax: 0375/529551

CF-Ambulanz
der Kinderklinik des Vogtland-klinikums
    Plauen
OA Dr. med. Karin Thoss
Rontgenstrasse 2

0-9900 Plauen
Tel: 03741/493237
Fax: 03741/494499

GREECE

Children's Hospital "Aghia Sophia"
Goudi, Athens 11527
CF Center
Director: G. Adam, M.D.
Tel: 01-7771811 (ext. 8018)

General Hospital "Kentriko"
Ethnikis Amynas 41
Thessaloniki
CF Center
Dr. Sonta Noussia-Arvanitaki
Tel: 031-211222 (ext. 200)

HUNGARY

Klara Holics M.D.
Hem Pal Hospital for Children
CF Center
H-1089 Budapest
Ulloi ut. 86
Tel: (36-1) 133000-718/332
Fax: (36-1) 1334-553

Szabadsigheyl Gyermekgyogyintezet
1121 Budapest, Mironhegyi ut 6.
Tel: 1-564-922

Somogy megyei Tanacs Tudogyogyintezete
7257 Mosdos
Tel: 82-77-055

SOTE I. sz. Gyermekklinika
1083 Budapest, Bokay j. u. 53
Tel: 1-343-186

SOTE II. sz. Gyermekkiinika
1094 Budapest, Tuzolto u. 7-9
Tel: 1-331-380

Heim Pal Gyermekkorhaz
1089 Budapest, Olloi ut 86
Tel: 260-072

DOTE Gyermekklinika
4012 Debrecen, Nagyerdei krt. 98
Tel: 52-12-594

POTE Gyermekklinika
7623 Pecs, Jozsef A. u. 7
Tel: 72-10-144

SZOTE Gyermekklinika
6725 Szeged, Koranyl fasor 14-15
Tel: 62-23-133

Mogyei Korhaz-Rendelointezet
  Gyermekegeszsegugyi Kozpont
3501 Miskolc, Szentpeteri kapu 76
Tel: 46-18-681

Megyei Korhaz-Rendalointezet Korhaz II,
  Gyermekosztaly
4431 Sostogyogyfurd 8
Tel: 42-13-422

Megyei Korhaz-Rendelointezet
9023 Gyor, Magyar u.8
Tel: 96-18-244

Orszagos Koranyi Tbe es Pulmonologial
  Intezet, II. Bel. Oszt.
1529 Budapest, Pineho ut 1.
Tel: 1-767-511

IRELAND

Professor Edward Tempany
Our Lady's Hospital for Sick Children
  (Pediatric)
Crumlin, Dublin 12
Tel: 01-558111

Professor M. FitzGerald
St. Vincent's Hospital (Adult Clinic)
Elm Park
Dublin 4
Tel: 01-2694533

Drs. Brendan Watson, T. O'Halloran & C.
  Bredin
(Adult Clinic)
Regional Hospital
Wilton, Cork.
Tel: 021-546400

Dr. N. O'Brien
The Children's Hospital
Temple Street
Dublin 1
Tel: 01-748763

Dr. Brian Denham
National Children's Hospital
Harcourt Street
Dublin 2
Tel: 01-752355

Dr. J. Cosgrove
Ardkeen Hospital
Waterford
Tel: 051-75429

Dr. F. Leahy
St. Catherine's Hospital
Tralee, Co. Kerry
Tel: 066-26222

Professor G. Loftus
Regional Hospital
Merlin Park, Galway
Tel: 091-57631

Dr. Mahony
Regional Hospital
Dooradoyle, Limerick
Tel: 061-28111

Dr. B. McDonagh
General Hospital
Sligo
Tel: 071-42161

Dr. D. O'Kane
General Hospital
Castlebar, Co. Mayo
Tel: 094-22196

Dr. C. Ryan
General Hospital
Letterkenny, Co. Donegal
Tel: 074-22022

Drs. A. Murphy & Joseph O'Sullivan
Our Lady of Lourdes Hospital
Drogheda, Co. Louth
Tel: 041-37601

ISRAEL

Sheba Medical Center
Tel Hashomer
Ramat Gan
Tel: 03-5303030

Beilinson Hospital
Petah Tikva
Tel: 03-9377377

Hadassah Medical Center
Ein Karem
Jerusalem
Tel: 02-427427

Soroka Hospital
Beer Sheba
Tel: 057-400111

Hacarmel Hospital
Haifa
Tel: 04-250211

Kaplan Hospital
Rehovot
Tel: 08-441211

ITALY

Servizio presso Divisione Pediatrics
Ospedale di Bolzano
Alto Adige
Responsabile: Dr. ssa Lydia Pescolderung
Tel: 0471/908111

Servizio presso Divisione Pediatrica
Ospedale di Livorno
Toscana
Responsabile: Dr. ssa Maria Vittoria Perez
Tel: 0586/418111

Servizio presso Divisione Pediatrica
Ospedale di Cerignola (Foggia)
Puglia Nord
Responsabile: Dr. Luigi Ratclif
Tel: 0885/24386

Servizio presso Divisione Pediatrica
Ospedale di S. Giovanni Rotondo
Puglia Nord
Responsabile: Dr. Germano Pio Ercolino
Tel: 0882-853721-853621

Servizio presso Divisione Pediatrica
Ospedale di Acquaviva delle Fonti (Bari)
Basilicata
Responsibile: Dr. Nicola D'Andrea
Tel: 080/760374

Servizio presso Divisione Pediatrica
Ospedale di Soverato (Catanzaro)
Calabria
Responsabile: Dr. Pasquale Alcaro
Tel: 0967/539111

Servizio presso Divisione Pediatrica
Ospedale di Guilianova (Teramo)
Abruzzo e Molise
Responsabile: Dr. Paolo Moreti
Tel: 085/8619270

Centro Fibrosi Cistica - Divisione di
    Pediatria e Neonatologia
Ospedale del Bambini "G. Salesi" ULSS n.
    12
Ancona
Responsabile: Prof. Giuseppe Caramia
Tel: 071/5962351
Fax: 071/5962354

Servizio di Prevenzione e Cura della
    Mucoviscidosi
Clinica Pediatrica II - Policlinico - Piazza
    Giulio Cesare

Bari
Responsible: Prof. Nicola Rigillo
Tel: 080/5227527
Fax: 080/278911

Divisione di Pediatria
Ospedale G. Brotzu - ULSS n.21 -
    Regione Sardegna -
Via Peretti
Cagliari
Responsabile: Prof. Mario Silvetti
Tel: 070/539551

Centro Regionale Toscano per la Fibrosi
    Cistica
Dipartimento di Pediatria - Ospedale
    Meyer
Via L. Giordano, 13
Firenze
Responsabile: Prof. ssa Lore Marianelli
Tel: 055/5662474

Centro per la Fibrosi Cistica
Divisione di Pediatria e Patologia
    Neonatale - Ospedale "M. Bufalini"
    ULSS 39
Cesena (Forli)
Responsabile: Prof. Giancarlo Biasini
Tel: 0547/352837-302322

Centro Regionale per le Malattle
    Endocrine e Metaboliche dell'Eta
    Evolutiva
Sez. Fibrosi Cistica
Clinica Pediatrica I - Instituto
    "G. Gaslini"
Via Largo Gerolamo Gaslini, 5
Genova
Responsabile: Prof. Cesare Romano
Tel: 010/387496(Direttore)
    5636366(Reparto)5636367(Laboratorio)
Fax: 010/3776590

Instituto Clinica Pediatrica
Policlinico Universitario
Messina
Responsible: Prof. Giuseppe Magazzu
Tel: 090/2935007
Fax: 090/2935007

Centro per la Prevenzione, Diagnosi e
Terapia della Fibrosi Cistica
Instituto Policattedra di Pediatria - Via
della Commenda, 9
Milano
Responsabile: Prof. ssa Annamaria Giunta
Tel: 02/5511043-57992456
Fax: 02/5452051

Centro Regionale di Diagnosi, Cura e
Ricerca per la Mucoviscidosi
Cattedra di Pediatria - Dipartimento di
Pediatria II Facolta
di Medicina e Chirurgla - Via Pansini, 5
Napoli
Tel: 081/7463273-7463500

Centro per la Fibrosi Cistica
Cattedra di Clinica Pediatrica dell
Universite - Via Giustiniani, 3
Padova
Responsabile: Prof. Franco Zacchello
Tel: 049/8211111

Servizio per la Diagnosi e Cura della
Fibrosi Cistica
IV Divisione Ospedale del Bambini "G.
De Cristina" - Plazza Porta Montalto
Palermo
Responsabile: Prof. Vincenzo Balsamo
Tel: 091/6666074
Fax: 091/6666226

Centro per la Fibrosi Cistica
Centro di fisiopatologia respiratoria
Infantile dell Universita - Via Gramsci
14
Parma
Responsabile: Prof. ssa Augusta Battistini
Tel: 0521/991198-290461

Servizio supporto Fibrosi Cistica e
Fisloterapia
Ospedale "Calai" - Divisione di Pediatria -
Gualdo Tadino (Pg)
Perugia
Responnnsible: Dott. Angelo Cosimi

Tel: 075/9109301

Servizio Fibrosi Cistic e Fisioterapia
Insitituo Clinica Pediatrica Policlinico
"Umberto I" - Viale Regina Elena, 324
Roma
Responsiabile: Prof Mariano Antonelli
Tel: 06/497891 Int. 289
Fax: 06/4454898

Centro di Diagnosi e Terapla della Fibrosi
Cistica
Divisione Pediatrica di Gastroenterologia
Ospedale Bambino Gesu Piazza S.
Onofrio, 4
Roma
Responsibile: Dott Massimo Castro
Tel: 06/65192333-329

Centro Dipartimentale Clinico-
Ospedaliero per la Fibrosi Cistica
Ospedale Infantile Regina Margherita -
Plazza Polonia, 94
Torino
Responsabile: Prof. ssa Nicoletta Ansaldi
Prof. Domenico Castello

Servizio per la Cura della Fibrosi Cistica
Istituto di Clinica Pediatrica - IIa Divisione
Pediatrica - Via dell'Istria, 65
Trieste
Responsabile: Dott. Dino Faragune
Tel: 040/7787397

Verona
Centro Regionale Veneto di Ricerca,
Prevenzione, Riabilitazione
ed Insegnamento per la Fibrosi Cistica
Ospedale Civile Magglore - Piazzale
Stefani, 1
Responsabile: Prof. Gianni Mastella
Tel: 045/932370 - 8301200
Fax: 045/8301200

KAZAKHSTAN

Dr. Munira Bayjanova
Research Institute for Pediatrics of
   Kazakhstan
pr. Al-Faraby, 146, 480123 Alma-Ata,
   Kazakhstan

MEXICO

Dr. Rodolfo Boites
No. Releccion 311
Cd. Obregon 85000 Sonora
Mexico
Tel: 324-84

Dr. Jose Luis Lezana
Asociacion Mexicana de Fibrosis Quistica,
Altavista 21, CP 01000
Mexico, DF
Tel: 548-3021/548-4256

Dr. Carlos Nesbitt
Calle de la llave 1419, CP 31020
Chihuahua, Chih.
Tel: 15-1355

Dr. Lorenzo Perez Fernandez
Instituto Nacional de Pediatria
Neumologia y Cirugia de Torax
Insurgentes Sur 3700 C, CP 04530
Mexico DF
Tel: 606-0002

Dr. Sergioi A. Castaneda R.
Hospital de Pediatria CMO
Isla Salina 2302, CP 44950
Tel: 16-8864/16-9469

NETHERLANDS

Dr. Roos, Dr. Breed, Dr. Griffioen
Academisch Medisch Centrum (AMC)
Emma Kinderziekenhuis
Meibergdreef 9
1105 NL Amsterdam
Tel: 020-5669111

Dr. Bakker
Dr. Heijerman
Ziekenhuis Leijenburg
afd. Longziekten
Leyweg 75
2545 CH Den Haag
Tel: 070-3592000

Dr. Dijkman
Academ. Ziekenhuis Leiden
afd. Longziekten
Rijnsburgerweg 10
2333 AA Leiden
Tel: 071-26950/269111

Dr. Schilte
Medisch Centrum Alkmaar
Wilhelminalaan 12
1815 JD Alkmaar
Tel: 072-145454

Dr. de Jongste
Sophia Kinderziekenhuis
Gordelweg 160
3038 GE Rotterdam
Tel: 010-4656566

Dr. vd Laag
Wilhelmina Kinderziekenhuis
Nieuwe Gracht 137
3512 LK Utrecht
Tel: 030-320911

Dr. Gerritsen
Academisch Ziekenhuis Groningen
Oostersingel 59
9713 EZ Groningen
Tel: 050-619111

NEW ZEALAND

Dr. Pli Pattemore
Department of Paediatrics
Christchurch Hospital
Private Bag
Christchurch, New Zealand

Dr. Christopher Hewitt
Dunedin Hospital
Private Bag
Dunedin, New Zealand

Dr. John Gillies
Paediatrician
Waikato Hospital
Private Bag
Hamilton, New Zealand

Dr. Archie Kerr
Paediatrician
Hutt Hospital
Private Bag
Lower Hutt, New Zealand

NORWAY

Helge Michalsen, M.D.
Dept. of Pediatrics
Aker University Hospital
N-0514 Oslo 5
Tel: 02-89 40 00

Ole Chr. Haanas, M.D.
Dept. of Internal Medicine
Aker University Hospital
N-0514 Oslo 5
Tel: 02-89 40 00

Dag Skyberg, M.D.
Dept. of Pediatrics
Aust-Agder Sentralsykehus
N-4800 Arendal
Tel: 041-24600

Gjermund Fluge, M.D.
Dept. of Pediatrics
Ph.D.
Haukeland Hospital
N-5016 Haukeland Sykehus
Tel: 05-29 80 60

Sigurd Borsting, M.D.
Dept. of Pediatrics
Innherred sykehus
N-7600 Levanger
Tel: 076-81-900

Bjorn Nilsen, M.D.
Dept. of Pediatrics
Nordland Sentralsykehus
N-8000 Bodo
Tel: 081-20 040

POLAND

Dr. Anna Nowakowska
Institut of Mother and Child
Clinics Pediatrics
ul. Kasprzaka 17 A
01-211 Warszawa

Dr. Leszek Olchowik
Institut of Mother and Child
Clinics Pediatrics
ul. Kasprzaka 17A
01-211 Warszawa

Prof. Jerzy Socha
Child Health Centre
Al. Dzieci Polskich 20
04-736 Warszawa

Dr. Jerzy Zebrak
Institut of Mother and Child
Rabka Branch
ul. Polna 3
34-700 Rabka

Dr. Ewa Kopytko
Institut of Mother and Child
Rabka Branch
ul. Polna 3
34-700 Rabka

Prof. Wojciech Cichy
Medical Academy in Poznan
ul. Szpitalna 27/23
60-572 Poznan

Prof. M. Prochorow
Pomeranian Medical Academy
ul. Unii Lubelskiej 1
71-344 Szczecin

Dr. Teresa Malaczynska
Specjalistyczny Zespol Opieki
Zdrowotnej nad Matka i Dzieckiem
ul. Polanki 119
80-308 Gdansk-Oliwa

Prof. A. Balcar-Boron
Medical Academy in Bydgoszcz
ul. Chodkiewicza 44
85-667 Bydgoszcz

Dr. Krystyna Sawielajc
Medical Academy in Bydgoszcz
ul. Chodkiewicza 44
85-667 Bydgoszcz

Prof. F. Iwanczak
ul. M.C. Sklodowskiej 50/52
50-376 Wroclaw

Dr. Tadeusz Latos
Specjalistyczny Zespol Gruzlicy
i Chorob Pluc Dzieci
ul. Mysliwska 17
58-450 Karpacz

Dr. M. Kaczmarski
Medical Academy in Bialystok
ul. M.C. Sklodowskiej 26
19-950 Bialystok

PORTUGAL

Dr. Luiz Marques Pinto
Unidade de Pneumologia
Servico de Pediatria
Hospital de Santa Maria
Av. Egas Moniz
1600 Lisboa
Tel: 802131 (extensao 46)

Dr. Mario Diniz Esteves
Servico de Pediatria

Hospital de D. Estefania
Rua Jacinto Marto
1100 Lisboa
Tel: 3561954

Dra. Maria Lurdes Chieira
Hospital Pediatrico
3000 Coimbra
Tel: 3929788 (extensao 395)

Dr. Lourenco Gomes
Servico de Pediatria
Hospital Pediatrico Maria Pia
4000 Porto
Tel: (2) 699861

Dr. Amil Dias
Servico de Pediatria
Hospital de S. Joao
4000 Porto
Tel: (2) 487151

ROMANIA

Professor dr. loan Popa
Institutul De Medicina Timisoara
SEF Clinica II Pediatrie
Spital Bega Bv Dr. V Babes 12
1900 Timosoara, Romania
Tel: (40-96) 18.29.46

RUSSIA

Prof. V. Baranov
Chief of Centre of Prenatal Diagnostic
Institute of Obstetrics and Gynecology
Mendeleevskaya line 3
St. Petersburg, 199034
Russia
Tel: 218-04-87

Prof. N. Kapranov (Children)
Russian CF Centre
Moskvozeshie 1
Moscow, Russia
Tel: 936-93-33

Prof. T. Guembitskaia (adults, children)
Dr. Jelenina L. (Children)
Institute of Pulmonology
12 Roentgen st.
St. Petersburg 197089
Russia
Tel: 238-48-31
Fax: 812/315-17-01

Dr. A. Orlov (Children)
44th Children's City Hospital
2 Zemledelcheskaya st.
St. Petersburg, 194156
Russia
Tel: 245-69-98

Prof. A. Bogdanova (Children)
Children's Hospital
6 Komsomola st.
St. Petersburg, 195009
Russia
Tel: 542-53-62

Pr. Sergei M. Gavalov, M.D.
Novosibirsk Medical Institute
Chief, Pediatrics Dept.
Zolotodolinskays st., 36/1
Novosibirsk 630090
Russia

Pr. Ludmila Matveeva, M.D.
Tomsk Medical Institute
Chief, Pediatrics Dept.
Lenin av., 15b, app. 3
Tomsk 634028
Russia

Dr. Alla Neretina
Voronezh Medical Institute
Chief, Pediatrics Dept.
Lenin squir, 5, app. 41
Voronezh 394018
Russia

Dr. V. Pavlov (Children)
Dr. L. Belenko (Adults)
Ekaterinburg Medical Institute

Dept. of Pediatrics
Beloretchenskaya str., 34/2, app. 79
Ekaterinburg 620102
Russia

SAUDI ARABIA

Professor Hisham Nazer
King Faisal Specialist Hospital
P.O. Box 3354
Riyadh 11211
Kingdom of Saudi Arabia
Tel: 4647272 Ext. 1942/7761
Fax: 4414839 or 4424493

SIBERIA

Lilia V. Belenko
Pulmonary Department
Central City Clinic 2
North Side-Street 2
620035 Ekaterinburg
Siberia
Tel: /3432/ 51 33 47

Professor Vladimir I. Shilko
Assistant professor Gennady V. Pavlov
Chair of Children's Diseases
Ekaterinburg State Medical Institute
Repin Street 3
620219 Ekaterinburg
Siberia
Tel: /3432/ 44 51 64

REPUBLIC OF SLOVAKIA

Dr. Hana Kayserova
Pediatric Dept. 1VZ
Derer Hospital
Limbova uL
833 05 Bratislava
Slovakia
Tel: 427 37 4649

SOUTH AFRICA

Prof M Bowie
Cape Town CF Clinic
Department of Paediatrics and Child
  Health
Red Cross Children's Hospital
Rondenbosch
7700
Tel: (021) 658 5325
Fax: (021) 689 1287

Dr Dave Richard
Johannesburg CF Clinic
Department Paediatrics
Johannesburg General Hospital
Johannesburg 2000
Tel: (011) 488 3282
Fax: (011) 643 1612

Dr S Naude
Pretoria CF Clinic
Department of Paediatrics
H F Verwoerd Hospital
Pretoria
0001
Tel: (012) 21 3211
Fax: (012) 26 2401

Dr J Egner
Durban CF Clinic
Department of Paediatrics
Addington Hospital
P O Box 977
Durban
4000
Tel: (031) 322 1111
Fax: (031) 368 3300

Dr C Househam
Bloemfontein CF Clinic
Department Paediatrics
University of the Orange Free State
P O Box 339
Bloemfontein
9300
Tel: (051) 405 3181
Fax: (051) 47 3222

SPAIN

Hospital Generall Nuetra Senora del
  Perpetuo Socorro (Badajoz)
Carretera de Valverde s/n
06080 Badajoz
Medico encargado: Antonio Serrano

Hospital Infantil Valle de Hebron
Paseo del Valle de Hebron s/n
08023 Barcelona
Medico encargado: Nicholas Cobos
  Barroso

Hospital de San Juan de Dios
Carretera de Esplugas s/n
08034
Medico encargado: Luis Amat Ballarin

Hospital Infantil de Cruces
Plaza de Barrios Cruces s/n
48903 Bilbao
Medico encargado: Carlos Vazquez

Hospital Infantil Reina Sofia
Avenida Menendez Pidal, 1
14004 Cordoba
Medico encargado: Francisco Sanchez
  Ruiz

Hospital Infantil Teresa Herrera
C/Las Jubias de Arriba
15006 La Coruna
Medico encargado: Leopoldo Garcia
  Alonso

Hospital Materno Infantil
Avenida Maritima del Sur s/n
35016 Las Palmas de Gran Canaria
Medico encargado: Luis Pena

Hospital Infalntil La Paz
Paseo de la Castellana, 261
28046 Madrid
Medico encargado: Maria del Carmen
  Antelo

Hospital del Nino Jesus
Avenida Menendez Pelayo, 65
28009 Madrid
Medico encargado: Maria Dolores Garcia
    Novo

Hospital Infantil 12 de Octubre
Carretera de Andalucia, Km 5.400
28041 Madrid
Medico encargado: Javier Manzanarez

Hospital Ramon y Cajal
Carretera de Colmenar Km 9.100
28034 Madrid
Medico encargado: Hector Escobar Castro

Hospital Infantil Carlos Haya
Avenida Carlos Haya s/n
29010 Malaga
Medico encargado: Francisco Perez Frias
    & Carlos Sierrea Salinas

Hospital Virgen de la Arreixaca
Carretera Madrid - Cartagena
30120 El Palmar - Murcia
Medico encargado: Jose Maria Nadal

Hospital Nuestra Senora de Covadonga
C6 Celestino Villamil s/n
33006 Oviedo
Medico encargado: Carlos Bousono

Hospital Son Dureta
C/ Andrea Doria, 55
07014 Palma de Mallorca
Medico encargado: Juana Roma Pena

Hospital Clinico Universitario
Avenida del doctor Fedriani, s/n
41009 Sevilla
Medico encargado: Federico Arguelles

Hospital Infantil Virgen del Rocio
Avenida Manuel Siurot s/n
41013 Sevilla
Medico encargado: Federico Arguelles

Hospital Infantil Virgen del Rocio
Avenida Manuel Siurot s/n

41013 Sevilla
Medico encargado: Francisco Dapena

Hospital Infantil Virgen de la Candelaria
Carretera Rosario s/n
41013 Santa Cruz de Tenerife
Medico encargado: Amado Zurita

Hospital Infantil La Fe
Avenida Campanar, s/n
46009 Valencia
Medico encargado: Juan Ferrer Calvete

Hospital Clinico Universitario
Avenida Ramon y Cajal, 7
47005 Valladolid
Medico encargado: Margarita Alonso
    Franch

Hospital Miguel Servet
Paseo Isabel la Catolica s/n
50009 Zaragoza
Medico encargado: Soleadad Heredia
    Gonzalez

SWEDEN

Lena Hjelte
Pediatric Clinic
University Hospital
141 986 Huddinge
Tel: 08-7461000
Fax: 08-7741317

Ragnhild Kornfalt
Pediatric Clinic
University Hospital
221 85 Lund
Tel: 046-171000
Fax: 046-145459

Birgitta Strandvik
Pediatric Clinic
University Hospital
416 85 Goteborg
Tel: 031-374000
Fax: 031-217023

SWITZERLAND

PD Dr. M. Rutishauser
Universitäts-Kinderklinik
Römergasse
4058 Basel
Tel: 061-6912626

Prof Dr. Richard Kraemer
Universitäts-Kinderklinik
Inselspital
Freiburgstrasse
3010 Bern
Tel: 031-642711

Drs Dominique Belli, Thierry Rochat and
PD Dr Susanne Suter
Hôspital Cantonal Universitaire de Genève
Clinique De Pédiatrie
30, Bd de la Cluse
1211 Genève 4
Tel: 022-226396

Dr Michel Roulet
Centre Hospitalier Universitaire
Vaudois CHUV
Av. de Beaumont 21
1011 Lausanne
Tel: 021-411111

Prof. Dr. D.H. Shmerling
Universitäts-Kinderklinik
Steinwiesstrasse 75
8032 Zürich
Tel: 01-2597111

Dr Felix H. Sennhauser
Ostschweiz Kinderspital St. Gallen
Claudiusstrasse 6
9006 St. Gallen
Tel: 071-263161

PD Dr. H.P. Gnehm
Kinderklinik
Kantonsspital Aargau
Bucherstrasse
5000 Aarau
Tel: 064-214141

Dr. Peter Kilcher
Kinderklinik
Kantonsspital Luzern
Spitalstrasse
6004 Luzern
Tel: 041-253151

Dr. Martin Schöni
Alpine Kinderklinik
"Pro Juventute"
Scalettastrasse 5
76270 Davos Platz
Tel: 83-36131

UKRAINE

Prof. T. Buzhievskaya
Head, Dept. of Medical Genetics
Kiev State Institute for Postgraduate
   Medical Studies
Dorogoshittskaya str., 9, Kiev, 252112
Ukraine

UNITED KINGDOM

Royal Victoria Hospital
Queen Victoria Road
Newcastle upon Tyne
NE1 4LP
Dr. R. Nelson (Children)
Dr. A. Brewis (Adults)
Tel: 091 232 5131

South Cleveland Hospital
Marton Road
Middlesbrough
Cleveland
TS4 3BW
Dr. G. Wyatt (Children)
Tel: 0642 824877

St. James's University Hospital
Beckett Street
Leeds
LS9 7TF
Dr. J. Littlewood (Children)
Dr. R. Page (Adults)
Tel: 0532 433144

Seacroft Hospital
York Road
Leeds
LS14 6UH
Dr. S.P. Conway (Adults)
Tel: 0532 648164

Nottingham City Hospital
Hucknall Road
Nottingham
NG5 1PB
Dr. J. Hiller (Children)
Dr A. Knox (Adults)
Tel: 0602 691169

Children's Hospital
Western Bank
Sheffield
S10 2TH
Dr. C. Taylor (Children)
Tel: 0742 761111

Leicester Royal Infirmary
Leicester
LE2 7LX
Dr. C. O'Callaghan (Children)
Tel: 0533 523268/9

Peterborough District Hospital
Thorpe Road
Peterborough PE3 6DA
Dr. J. Kuzemko (Children)
Tel: 0733 67451

The Brompton Hospital
Fulham Road
London
SW3 6HP
Dr. A. Bush (Children)
Dr. M. Hodson (Adults)
Dr. D. Geddes (Adults)
Tel: 071 352 8121

The Hospital for Sick Children
Great Ormond Street
London
WC1N 3JH

Dr. R. Dinwiddie (Children)
Tel: 071 405 9200

Queen Elizabeth Hospital for Children
Hackney Road
Behnal Green
London E2 9JX
Tel: 071 739 8422

King's College Hospital
Denmark Hill
London
SE5 9RS
Dr. J. Price (Children)
Dr. D. Hutchison (Adults)
Tel: 071 274 6222

Lewisham Hospital
High Street
Lewisham
London
SE13 6LH
Dr. C.E. Daman Willems (Children)
Dr. J. Stroobant (Children)
Dr. P. Rees (Adults)
Tel: 081 690 4311

Southampton General Hospital
Tremona Road
Southampton
SO9 4XY
Dr. C. Rolles (Children)
Prof. J. Warner (Children)
Dr. G. Sterling (Adults)
Tel: 0703 777222

John Radcliffe Hospital
Headington
Oxford
OX3 9DU
Dr. A. Thompson (Children)
Tel: 0865 64711

Royal Devon and Exeter Hospital
Barrack Road
Exeter
EX2 5DW
Dr. J. Tripp (Children)

Dr. A. Ferguson (Adults)
Tel: 0392 411611

Royal Hospital for Sick Children
St. Michael's Hill
Bristol
BS2 8BJ
Dr. F. Carswell (Children)
Tel: 0272 215411

City General Hospital
Newcastle Road
Stoke-on-Trent
ST4 6QC
Dr. C. Campbell (Children)
Dr. C. Pantin (Adults)
Tel: 0782 621133

Children's Hospital
Ladywood Middleway
Birmingham
B16 8ET
Dr. P. Welle (Children)
Tel: 021 454 4851

East Birmingham Hospital
Bordesley Green
Birmingham
B9 5ST
Dr. D. Stableforth (Adults)
Tel: 021 766 6611

Alder Hey Children's Hospital
Eaton Road
Liverpool
L12 2AP
Dr. D. Heaf (Children)
Tel: 051 228 2024

Booth Hall Children's Hospital
Charlestown Road
Manchester
M27 1HA
Prof. T. David (Children)
Tel: 061 795 7000

Royal Manchester Children's Hospital
Hospital Road
Pendlebury

Manchester
M27 1HA
Dr. M. Super (Children)
Dr. G. Hambleton (Children)
Tel: 061 794 4696

Monsall Hospital
Newton Heath
Manchester
M10 8WR
Dr. K. Webb (Adults)
Tel: 061 205 2393

Royal Gwent Hospital
Newport
Gwent
NPT 2UB
Dr. S. Magwire (Children)
Dr. I. Petherham (Adults)
Tel: 0633 252244

University Hospital of Wales
Heath Park
Cardiff
South Glamorgan
CF4 4XW
Dr. M. Goodchild (Children)
Tel: 0222 755944

Llandough Hospital
Llandough
Penarth
South Glamorgan
CF6 1XX
Prof. D. Shale (Adults)
Dr. I. Campbell (Adults)
Tel: 0222 708601

Aberdeen City Hospital
Urquhart Road
Aberdeen
AB2 1NJ
Dr. J. Friend (Adults)
Tel: 0224 681818

Royal Aberdeen Children's Hospital
Cornhill Road
Aberdeen
AB9 2ZG

Prof. P. Helms (Children)
Prof. G. Russell (Children)
Tel: 0224 681818

Ninewells Hospital Medical School
Dundee
DD1 9SY
Prof. R.E. Olver (Children)
Tel: 0382 60111

Royal Hospital for Sick Children
Sciennes Road
Edinburgh
EH9 1LF
Dr. T. Marshall (Children)
Tel: 031 667 1991

Western General Hospital
Crewe Road
Edinburgh
EH4 2XU
Dr. A. Greening (Adults)
Tel: 031 332 2525

Western Infirmary
Dumbarton Road
Glasgow
G11 6NT
Dr. B. Stack (Adults)
Tel: 0382 60111

Royal Hospital for Sick Children
Yorkhill
Glasgow
G38SJ
Dr. J. Paton (Children)
Dr. J. Evans (Children)
Tel: 041 339 8888

Royal Belfast Hospital for Sick Children
Falls Road
Belfast
BT12 4BE
Dr. A. Redmond (Children)
Tel: 0232 240503

URUGUAY

Drs. Stella Cabeza de Latourrette
Costa Rica 2061
Montevideo
Tel: 603842 (Private)
Tel: 795512 (Policlinica)
Fax: 816728 (International 598-2-816728)

Dra. Liria Martinez
Departamento de Neumologia Pediatrica
(Respiratory Unit)
Catedra B y C
Hospital Pereyra Rossell
Bulevar Artigas s,n
Montevideo
Tel: 773651 (Private)

Dra. Virginia Mendez
Amsterdam 1496
Montevideo
Tel: 695359 (Private)

Dr. Sergio Orsi
Ellauri 419 piso 7
Montevideo
Tel: 703193 (Private)

VENEZUELA

Josefa Vegas M.D.
Susana Raffally
Nutrition Departament
Centro Medico
de Caracas
Plaza El Estanque C.P.
1011 San Bernandino
Caracas-Venezuela
Tel: 9858-2-5099228
Fax: 9858-2-5641930

Ana Judith Chacon M.D.
O.R.L. Department
Hospital Vargas
Caracus-Venezuela
Fax: 9858-2-5641930

Georgette Daoud M.D.
Gastroenterology Division
Hospital General Miguel
Perez Carreno
Caracus-Venezuela
Fax: 9858-2-2631516

Hans Romer M.D.
Gastroenterology Department
The Children's Hospital
"J.M. de los Rios"
Caracas-Venezuela
Tel: 9858-2-5748375
Fax: 9858-2-2631560

Isaac Tueti M.D.
Fundacardin Hospital
Dr. Carlos Arvelo
Caracas-Venezuela
Fax: 9858-2-263-15-60

Luis Quisber M.D.
Venezuelan Central University
Pediatric Clinic
University Hospital of Caracas
Caracas-Venezuela
Tel: 9858-2-2633338
Fax: 9858-2-2631519

Beatriz Carrasquel M.D.
Teolinde Morales M.D.
O.R.L. Departament
The Children's Hospital J.M.
de los Rios Av. Vollmer
C.P. 1011 San Bernandino
Caracas-Venezuela
Tel: 9858-2-9743511
Fax: 9858-2-2631560

Gustavo Medrano
Pulmonary Phisicology Lab.
Chest Division
University Hospital of Caracas
Venezuela
Tel: 9858-2-6067695
Fax: 9858-2-2631560

Alida Pascualone M.D.
Pediatric Surgeon and
Departament of Pediatric Surgery
Transplant Surgeon
The Children's Hospital
J.M. de los Rios
Caracas-Venezuela
Tel: 9858-2-2631560
Fax: 9858-2-518823

Jorge Prieto M.D.
Cardiopulmonary Division
The Children's Hospital
J.M. de los Rios
Caracas-Venezuela
Tel: 9858-2-2631560
Fax: 9858-2-5710082

Eduardo Mezza
Pulmonary Division
Central Hospital of Valencia
Valencia Edo. Carabobo
Venezuela
Tel: 9858-041-312283
Fax: 9858-2-2631519

Guillermo Isturiz M.D.
Tuberculosis Departament and Respiratory
   Diseases
The Algodonal Hospital
Caracas-Venezuela
Tel: 9858-2-494258
Fax: 9858-2-2631519

Bebella Nieto M.D.
Clinica Razzetti, Barquisimeto Estado
Lara
Venezuela
Tel: 9858-2-319077 Ext. 415 or 417
Fax: 9858-2-2631560

Oscar Machado M.D.
The Luis Gomez Lopez Hospital
Barquisimeto Edo. Lara
Venezuela
Fax: 9858-2-263-15-60

Evila Davila M.D.
Pediatric Clinic
University Hospital Los Andes
Merida, Venezuela
Fax: 9858-2-2631560

YUGOSLAVIA

Faculty of Medicine
The Pediatrical Clinic
ul. Vodnjanska bb
91000 Skopje, Yugoslavia
Tel: 38-91 226-111, ext. 2761

APPENDIX H

Cystic Fibrosis Associations Worldwide

ARGENTINA

Mrs. M.L. Saporiti de Endler
Assoc. Argentina de Lucha Contra La
Enfermedad
Fibroquistica del Pancreas
Mansilla 2814
3o piso Depto. 14 Capital
1425 Buenos Aires, Argentina
Tel: (54)962-6313

AUSTRALIA

Mrs. Helen Griffiths
President ACFA
P.O. Box 746
Petersham New South Wales
2049, Australia
Tel: (02) 564 3089
Fax: (02) 564 3080

AUSTRIA

Mr. Wolfgang Dangl
Osterreichische Gesellschaft zur Bekämp-
fung der Cystic Fibrose
Obere Augartenstrasse 26-2
A-1020 Wien, Austria
Tel/Fax: 0043/1/332.6376

BELGIUM

M. Marcel De Paepe
Assoc. Belge de Lutte contre la

Muscoviscidose
Place Georges Brugmann 29
B.1060 Brussels, Belgium
Tel: (32)2 347 30 64
Fax: (32)2 347 35 06

BRAZIL

Associacao Brasileira de Ass. a
Mucoviscidose
Hospital de Clinicas de P. Alegre, C.P. #5082
90041 Porto Alegre-RS, Brazil
Tel/Fax: 55-512-274082

BULGARIA

Cystic Fibrosis Assoc. of Bulgaria
Research Institute of Pediatrics
Medical Academy
D. Nesterov str.II
1606 Sofia, Bulgaria
Tel: (359)51-70-85

CANADA

Mrs. Cathleen Morrison
Canadian Cystic Fibrosis Foundation
Suite 601
2221 Yonge Street
Toronto, Ontario, Canada M4S 2B4
Tel: (416)485-9149
Fax: (416)485-0960

CHILE

Mr. Patricio Lira
Corp. para la Fibrosis Quistica del Pancreas
La Canada 6505 (i)
La Reina, Santiago, Chile

COLOMBIA

Dr. Jorge Palacios
Calle 20N 4N45 202
Cali, Colombia
Tel: 61-2300

COSTA RICA

Associacion Costarricense
de Fibrosis Quistica
Dra. Reina Gonzalez Pineda
Apdo. 337, Zona 9, Pavas
San Jose, Costa Rica
Fax: (506)55-49-07

CUBA

Dr. Manuel Rojo Concepcion
Comision Cubana de Fibrosis Quistica
Hospital Pediatrico J.M. Marquez
Ave. 31 esq.a 76, CP 11400
Municipio Marianao,
Ciudad Habana, Cuba
Tel: 53-7-202860
Fax: 53-7-338212-3

CZECHOSLOVAKIA

Mrs. Helena Holubova
Bitouska 1226/7
Praha 4 140 00 Czechoslovakia
Tel/Fax: 42.242.1381

DENMARK

Mrs. Hanne Wendel Tybkjaer
Danish Cystic Fibrosis Association
Hyrdebakken 246
DK-8800 Viborg, Denmark
Tel: (45)8667 4422
Fax: (45)8667 6666

EL SALVADOR

Fundaccion para la Fibrosis
Quistica de El Salvador (Fiqes)
Res. Bethania, Pje., 4
No. 14-e, Santa Tecla, El Salvador
Tel: 503-210-915

ESTONIA

Institute of General & Molecular
Pathologyult
Attn: Dr. Maris Teder de Tartu University
Mucoviscidose
Veski 34, EE2400 Tartu Estonia
Tel: 7.01434.35169
Fax: 7.01434.35430

FINLAND

Keuhkovammaliitto r.y.
PL35
SF-00621 Helsinki, Finland

FRANCE

Monsieur Herve Garrault
Association Francaise de Lutte contra la Mucoviscidose
76, rue Bobillot
75013 Paris, France
Tel: 33.1.40.78.91.91
Fax: 33.1.45.80.86.44

GERMANY

Mr. Michael Hartje
Deutsche Gesellschaft zur Bekampfung der
Mukoviszidose e.V
Bendenweg 101
D-5300 Bonn 1, Germany
Tel: (0228) 66 10 26
Fax: (0228) 66 92 64

GREECE

Mrs. Z. Papavassilopoulou
Hellenic Cystic Fibrosis Assoc.
Angelou Sikelaniou 8
Neo Psychico
Athens 15452, Greece
Tel: (30)1.64.31.883

HUNGARY

Mr. Denes Baan
Hungarian CF Families
H-1134 Budapest, Dozsa Gyorgy ut 150,
Hungary

ICELAND

Mr. Hordur Bergsteinsson
Cystic Fibrosis Assoc. of Iceland
Barnaspitali Hringsins
Landspitalinn v/Baronsstig
101 Reyjavik, Iceland
Tel: (354)1 601000
Fax: (354)1 601519

IRELAND

Mrs. Bridie Maguire
Cystic Fibrosis Assoc. of Ireland
CF House
24 Lower Rathmines Road
Dublin 6, Ireland

Tel: 353-1-962433
Fax: 353-1-962201

ISRAEL

Mr. Ami Kolumbus
Israel Cystic Fibrosis Assoc.
5 Benymini Street
Tel Aviv, Israel
Tel: 972 2 86.0965
Fax: 972 2 632 312

ITALY

Mr. Vittoriano Faganelli
Lega Italiana Delle Assiazioni per la Lotta
contra la Fibrosi Cistic
c/o Ospedale Civile Maggiore
Piazzali A. Stefani 1
37126 Verona, Italy
Tel: (45)8344060
Fax: (45)8348125

MEXICO

Dr. Jose Luis Lezana
Asociacion Mexicana de Fibrosis Quistica,
AC
Altavista # 21 CP.01000
Col. San Angel, Mexico D.F.
Tel: (52)5 548-3021
Fax: (52)5 548-4256

NETHERLANDS

Mr. Hank van Lier
Nederlandse Cystic Fibrosis Stichting
N.C.F.S.
Lt. Gen. van Heutszlaan 6
3743 JN Baarn, Netherlands
Tel: (31)2 154 18 408
Fax: (31)2 154 21 616

NEW ZEALAND

Mr. Bruce Dunstan
Cystic Fibrosis Assoc. of New Zealand
187 Cashel St, P.O. Box 22776
Christchurch 1, New Zealand
Tel: (03)3651-122
Fax: (03)3668-535

NORWAY

Ms. Reidun Jahnsen
Norsk Forening For Cystic Fibrose
  (NFCF)
Postboks 114, Kjelsas
0411 Oslo 4, Norway

PAKISTAN

Research Director
Attn: Dr. T. Akhtar
PMRC, Research Centre
Khyber Medical College
Peshawar, Pakistan

POLAND

Mr. Stanislav Sitko
Polish Society Against Cystic Fibrosis
os. Tysiaclecia 62/64
Krakow, Poland
Tel: (0-187)760-60 w 331
Fax: (0-187)76-069

PORTUGAL

Dr. Luiz Marques Pinto
Associacao Portuguesa de Fibrose Quistica
Hospital de Santa Maria
Av. Egas Moniz
1900 Lisboa, Portugal
Tel: 802131 (ext.46)

ROMANIA

Professor dr. Ioan Popa
Romanian CF Association
Str. Iancu Vacarescu Nr.8
ap. 16 - 1900 Timisoara, Romania
Tel/Fax: (040-96)11.52.86

RUSSIA

Dr. Tatiana E. Gembitzkaya
Dept. of Therapy of Lung Diseases
All-Union Research Institute
197089 Leningrad
Roentgen str. 12, Russia

SAUDI ARABIA

Dre Hisham Nazer, FRCP
Prof. of Pediatrics
King Faisal Specialist
Hosp. & Research Centre
P.O. Box 3354
Riyadh 11211, Saudi Arabia
Tel: 464-7272 ext. 7761/1942
Fax: 442-4493

SOUTH AFRICA

Mr. Alain Woolf
National CF Assoc.
25 Hope Road
Orange Grove 2192, South Africa
Tel: 27 7 728 4096

SPAIN

Mr. Andres Casanova
Federacion Espanola de
Fibrosis Quistica
c/Lladro y malli - 10
46007 Valencia, Spain
Tel/Fax: 34-6-380 08 75

SWEDEN

Mrs. Birgitta Hellquist
Swedish Cystic Fibrosis Association
Box 1827
751 48 Uppsala, Sweden
Tel: (46) 18 151 622
Fax: (46) 18 127 074

SWITZERLAND

Mrs. Regula Salm-Muller
Schweizerische Gesellschaft fur Cystische
Fibrose (Mucoviscidose)
Bellevuestrasse 166
3095 Spiegel/Bern, Switzerland
Tel: (41) 31.972.28.28

TURKEY

Dr. Ayhan Gocmen
Professor of Pediatrics
Institute of Child Health
Hacettepe University
Hacettepe/Ankara Turkey

UNITED KINGDOM

Cystic Fibrosis Research Trust
5 Blyth Road, Bromley
Kent BR1 3RS, England U.K.
Tel: (44)0-81 464-7211
Fax: (44)0-81 313-0472

UNITED STATES

Robert J. Beall, Ph.D.
Cystic Fibrosis Foundation
6931 Arlington Road
Bethesda, Maryland 20814
Tel: (301) 951-4422
Fax: (301) 951-6378

URUGUAY

Mr. Enrique Silver
Asociacion de Fibrosis Quistica del Uruguay
Francisco Rodrigo 2975, aptdo 4
11, 600 Montevideo, Uruguay
Tel: (598) 2 81-6728
Fax: (598) 2 907161

VENEZUELA

Mrs. Lisbeth Abad
Fibrosis Quistica de Venezuela
Avenida Jose Felix Sosa
Torre Britanica Piso 2
Oficinas EFG Altamire si
Caracas, Venezuela
Tel: 58 2 263 3338
Fax: 58 2 564 1930
     58 2 263 1519

INTERNATIONAL

Aisha Ramos
Secretary, ICF(M)A
Avda. Campanar, 106-3o-6.a
46015 Valencia, Spain
Tel: (34-6)346 14 14 (office hours:
     0830–1330)
Fax: (34-6) 349 40 47
Tel: (34-6) 369 94 64 (home)
E-Mail: aramos.fq@vlc.sevicom.es.

APPENDIX I

Bibliography

General

Davis P B (editor). *Cystic Fibrosis.* Marcel Dekker, Inc., New York, 1993. Also an excellent text.
Hodson M E, Geddes D M (editors). *Cystic Fibrosis.* Chapman & Hall Medical, London, 1995. A comprehensive text on cystic fibrosis; an excellent resource.
Welsh MJ, Smith AE. Cystic Fibrosis. *Scientific American,* December 1995, 52–59. Very good overview, including good pictures.
Welsh, MJ, Tsui L-C, Boat TF, Beaudet AL. Cystic fibrosis, in *Metabolic and Molecular Basis of Inherited Disease.* Edited by Scriver CR, Beaudet AL, Sly WS, Valle D. McGraw-Hill, 1994.

Of Historical Interest

Andersen D H. "Cystic fibrosis of the pancreas and its relation to celiac disease; a clinical and pathologic study." *American Journal of Diseases of Children,* 1938; **356:**344–395. The earliest description of cystic fibrosis as a single entity.
di Sant'Agnese P A, Darling R C, Perera G A, Shea E. "Abnormal electrolyte composition of sweat in cystic fibrosis of the pancreas: Clinical significance and relationship of the disease." *Pediatrics* 1953; **12:**549–563. Original description of the high salt content in CF sweat.
Doershuk C F, Matthews L W, Tucker A S, et al. "A five-year clinical evaluation of a therapeutic program for patients with cystic fibrosis." *Journal of Pediatrics,* 1964; **65:**677–693. The first paper to show the benefit of a comprehensive treatment program for patients with CF.
Drumm M L, Pope H A, Cliff W H, et al. "Correction of the cystic fibrosis defect in vitro by retrovirus-mediated gene transfer." *Cell* 1990; **62:**1227–1233.
Gibson L E, Cooke, R E. "A test for concentration of electrolytes in sweat in cystic fibrosis of the pancreas utilizing pilocarpine by iontophoresis." *Pediatrics* 1959; **23:**545–549. Landmark report detailing a laboratory method for collection and analysis of CF sweat.
Knowles M, Gatzy J, Boucher R. "Increased bioelectric potential difference across respiratory epithelia in cystic fibrosis." *New England Journal of Medicine,* 1981; **305:**1489–1495. The first of the papers to elucidate the problem of electrolyte transport across mucous membranes in CF.
Quinton P M, Bijman J. "Higher bioelectric potentials due to decreased chloride absorption in the sweat glands of patients with cystic fibrosis." *New England Journal of Medicine,* 1983; **308:**1185–1189. Initial publication demonstrating that the problem in the nose and respiratory tree also existed in sweat glands, and that it was primarily a problem with chloride not being able to pass through mucous membranes.
Rich D P, Anderson M P, Gregory R J, et al. "Expression of cystic fibrosis transmembrane conductance regulator corrects defective chloride channel regulation in cystic fibrosis airway epithelial cell." *Nature* 1990; **347:**358–363. This paper and the Drumm et al. paper listed above appeared almost simultaneously and showed that the CF cell defect could be cured in the laboratory with gene transfer.

Romens J M, Iannuzzi M C, Kerem B-S, et al. "Identification of the cystic fibrosis gene: chromosome walking and jumping." *Science* 1989; **245**:1059–1065. Landmark paper announcing discovery and cloning of CF gene by Drs. Lap-Chee Tsui, Francis Collins, and Jack Riordan (and their colleagues), from Toronto and Michigan.

For Classroom Teachers

Young, A. *Cystic Fibrosis in the Classroom.* Distributed via Scandipharm. Superb introduction to CF for teachers who have a child with CF in their classes.

Subject Index

A

Abdominal pain, 91–92
  appendicitis, 92
  constipation, 92
  coughing, 92
  DIOS, 91. *See also* Distal intestinal
    obstruction syndrome
  gallstone, 91
  gastroenteritis, 92
  gynecologic problem, 92
  intussusception, 85–86, 91
  lactose intolerance, 92
  meconium ileus equivalent. *See* Distal
    intestinal obstruction syndrome
  pancreatitis, 82, 91
  psychologic stress, 92
  stomach flu, 92
  ulcer, 91
  urinary tract infection, 92
Abortion, 236
Absolute contraindications, lung transplantation, 144
Accelerase, 90, 311
Accessory muscles of respiration, 24
Accurbron, 311
Acetylcysteine, 41, 311, 318
Acid reflux. *See* Gastroesophageal
  reflux
Actifed, 311
Actigall. *See* Ursodeoxycholic acid
Actin, 31
Active cycle of breathing technique,
  39–40, 333
"Active" status, on transplant list, 150–151
Activity, for hospitalized child, 126
Acute rejection, lung transplant, 162
Acyclovir, 312

ADA (Americans with Disabilities Act),
  255–256
ADEK, 312
Adolescence, 180–181. *See also* Teenagers
  concerns about dying, 265
Adrenalin, 312, 316
Adults
  attitudes and outlook, 244
  CF patients as, 243–244
  communicating with other CF adults,
    259–260
  concerns about dying, 265
  cystic fibrosis and adulthood, 243–260
  death, 258–259
  education, 253–255
  employment, 255–256
  gastrointestinal system in, 245–247
  health and disability insurance for,
    251–253
  health issues in, 249–250
  marriage and family, 256–258
  medical care issues, 250–251
  psychological issues, 258
  reproductive system in, 247–249
  respiratory system in, 244
Aerobic exercise, 188
  college students, 254
Aerobid, 312
Aerolate Jr. and Sr., 312
Aerosol, 41–42, 48–49, 289
  antibiotics, 48–49
  bronchodilator medication, 41–42
  hospital treatments, 129
Aerosol machine, 42, 42f
Afrin, 312
Aides. *See* Patient care assistants
Air embolism, 137

Air hunger, 262
Air sac, 20, 22
Airplane travel, 184
Airway, 20–21, 21f, 289
    bacteria in, as lung transplant contra-
        indication, 145–146
    infection of, causes, 6–7
    narrowing following lung transplan-
        tation, 164, 166
    reducing inflammation in, 43–44
    research areas, 272–275
        fluid composition, 273–274
        infection, 272–273
        inflammation, 274
        mucus-thinning agents, 274–275
Airway clearance, techniques, 321–334.
    See also specific techniques
Airway fluid composition, research into,
    273–274
Airway inflammation, 29–31
    clinical research, 274
    reducing, 43–44
Airway obstruction, treatment, 38–44. *See
    also* Mucus-thinning agents
Albumin, low blood levels, 104–105
Albuterol, 42, 298, 312, 320
    exercise-induced asthma, 191
    prior to running, 191
Alcohol, 254
Aldactone, 305, 312
Allerest, 312
Allergic bronchopulmonary aspergillosis, 36
Allergy, medication, 304
    allergy shot, 304
Alpha-1-antitrypsin, future treatments
    with, 278
Altitude, 184
    oxygen effects, 61
Aluminum carbonate gel, 312
Aluminum hydroxide gel, 311
Alupent. *See* Metaproterenol sulfate
Alveolus, 20, 21–22, 289
Amantadine hydrochloride, 46, 312
Amcill. *See* Ampicillin
Americans with Disabilities Act, 255–256
Amikacin sulfate (Amikin), 296, 312
Amiloride, 9
    future treatments with, 278

    sodium channel blocker, 4
Aminodur, 312
Aminoglycosides, 295–296
Aminophylline, 299, 312
Amnesia, retrograde, 170
Amniocentesis, 213
Amoxicillin, 294, 312, 317, 319
Amoxicillin/clavulanate potassium, 195,
    312
Amoxil. *See* Amoxicillin
Amphojel, 312
Amphotericin, 312
Ampicillin, 294, 312, 318
Amylase, 76, 77
Anabolic steroid, 309
Anaerobic exercise, 187
Anastomosis, 289
Ancef. *See* Cefazolin sodium
Androgen, 309
Anemia, iron-deficiency, 105–106
Anger, 218
Anorexia, 289
Anorexia of malnutrition, 104
Antacids, 82, 306–307
Anterior-inferior transthoracic incision,
    lung transplantation, 152
Anthropometrics, 102
Anti-acid medication, 82, 306–307
Antibiotics, 44–45
    aerosol, 48–49
    bronchus, 44–45
    intravenous treatments. *See* Intravenous
        (IV) treatments
    lungs, 293–294
    oral, 44–45, 48
    resistance, 74
    side effects, 294
    therapeutic considerations, 49–52
    treatment, 2
Antibloating medication, 309
Anticoagulants, 289
    in lung transplantation, 153
Anticonstipation medicine, 307–309
Antihistamine, 304
Antiinfective treatment, future, 278
Anti-inflammatory treatment, 231–232
    future, 278
    in hospital, 129

Antilymphocyte antibodies, organ transplants, 157
Antilymphocyte drugs, 310–311
Antimetabolites, 310–311
  organ transplants, 157
Antireflux drugs, 307
Antirejection drugs, 142–143, 310–311
Antithymocyte globulin, 311
  transplant rejection therapy, 162, 165
Apical pleurectomy, 58
Appendicitis, 92
  abdominal pain, 92
Appetite
  caloric intake, 104
  malabsorption of food and, 103
Appetite stimulant, 309–310
AquaMephyton, 312
Aquasol A, 312
Aquasol E, 107, 312
Asbron, 312
Ascites, 90
  treatment, 91
Aspergillus fumigatus, 36
Aspirin, 44, 65
Assisted ventilation, 34
Asthma, 31–32
  antiinflammatory inhalers, 231–232
  bronchodilator medications, 41–42
  causes, 32
  chest pain, 63
  exercise-induced, 191
  medicine, 298–299
  pain, 63
  reactive airways, 69
  tests, 69–70
    bronchial provocation test, 70
    inhalation challenge test, 70
  tightness, 63
  treatment, 41–42
Atelectasis, 59–61, 289
  treatment, 59–61
  x-ray, 59, 60
ATG. *See* Antithymocyte globulin
Atgam, 312
Atrovent, 312
Atuss, 312
Augmentin, 294, 312
Autogenic drainage, 40, 334

  in teenage years, 227, 228
Autopsy, 267
Avazyme, 77, 312
Azactam, 298, 312
Azlocillin, 295, 312
Azmacort, 312
Azothioprine, 311, 312
  organ transplants, 158
  side effects, 160
Aztreonam, 298, 312

B
b.i.d., defined, 289
Bacteria, 35–36, 72–74. *See also specific organisms*
  growth in lung, 226
  infection control for hospitalized child, 126–127
  lung transplant contraindication, 144–145
  protection against, 26–27
  resistance, 74
Bactrim, 295, 312
Bactrim DS, 312
BAL. *See* Bronchoalveolar lavage
Basaljel, 312
Baseline, 289
Basic research. *See* Research, basic scientific
Beclomethasone dipropionate (Beclovent, Beconase), 300, 312, 320
Beepen-VK, 312
Benadryl, 312
Beta-agonist, 298–299
Betapen-VK, 313
Bethanechol, 89
Biaxin. *See* Clarithromycin
Bicarbonate, 289
Bicillin, 313
Bicycling, 199–200
  clothes, 200
  equipment, 199
  preparing bicycle, 200
  safety, 200
  starting, 200
Bile duct, blocked, 90–91
Bile salts, 77, 90
Bilezyme, 313

Biliary cirrhosis, 90
Biliary fibrosis, 90
Bilogen, 313
Biopsy, 289
  liver, 177
  open lung, 172
  transbronchial, posttransplant, 162, 168, 169–170, 171–172
Birth control, 241, 248–249
Bisacodyl, 313
Blebs, 58
Bleeding
  as central line complication, 137
  in chest, following lung transplantation, 161
Blood, 1
  in mucus, 52. See also Hemoptysis
Blood clots, following lung transplantation, 161–162
Blood gas, 289
  test, 70
Blood glucose, 82–83
Blood tests, in hospital, 130
Body box, 69
Body image, 237–238
Body temperature, CFTR function and, 9
Bone problem, 64–65
Boost Liquid, 118t
Bottle feeding, 109, 257
Bowel movement, pancreatic insufficiency, 79–80
Bowel stimulant, 308
Brain, 1
Bran, 313
"BRAT" diet, 104
Breast feeding, 109, 257
Breath, shortness of, 57
  assessing need for treatment, 230
Breathing control, 22–23, 40, 333
  carbon dioxide, 22–23
  oxygen, 22–23
Breathing tests, in teenage years, 230–231
Brethine. See Terbutaline sulfate
Bricanyl. See Terbutaline sulfate
Bristagen. See Gentamicin
Bristamycin, 313
Brompheniramine maleate, 315
Bronchial artery embolization,

  hemoptysis, 54
  disadvantages, 54
Bronchial blockage, minimizing in teenage years, 227–229
Bronchial cells, healthy, fluid secretion from, 3–4
Bronchial infection. See Pulmonary exacerbation
Bronchial provocation test, 70
Bronchial tree, 20
Bronchial tube, 1, 20. See also Bronchus
  adult, 244–245
Bronchiectasis, 30
Bronchiole, 20–21, 289
  cartilage, 20
  dilation, 30
  infection, 29–31
  inflammation, 29–31
  muscle, 21
  pneumothorax, 56
Bronchiolectasis, 30
Bronchiolitis, 29, 34
  infant, 34
Bronchitis, 29, 34
Bronchoalveolar lavage, 168, 169, 289
  complications, 171
Bronchobid Duracaps, 313
Bronchodilator, 298–299
  for exercise-induced asthma, 191
  oral, 41–42
  prior to running, 191
Broncholate Capsules, 177, 313
Bronchoscope, 289
Bronchoscopy, 60, 290
  complications, 170–172
  hemoptysis, 54
  posttransplant, 162, 169
    biopsy via. See Transbronchial biopsy
    lavage via. See Bronchoalveolar lavage
Bronchospasm, 32, 69
Bronchus, 20–21, 290
  antibiotics, 44–45
  cartilage, 20
  dilation, 30
  inflammation, 29–31, 30f
  muscle, 21
  pneumothorax, 56

reducing infection
  preventing bacterial infection, 45–56
  viral infections, 46–47
reducing infection between CF patients,
  45–46
Brondecon, 313
Brondelate. *See* Brondecon
Bronitin Mist, 313
Bronkaid, 313
Bronkaid Mist, 313
Bronkodyl, 313
Bronkolixir, 313
Bronkometer, 313
Bronkosol, 313
Bronkotabs, 313
Broviac catheter, 134, 135
"Buddy system," 198
Burkholderia cepacia, 35, 36, 45
  infection control for hospitalized child,
    126, 127
  as lung transplant contraindication, 146,
    148, 151
BVRs. *See* Vocational rehabilitation
  programs

C
Calcium-dependent chloride channel, 3
Calories Plus Liquid, 118t
Carbenicillin, 295, 313
Carbohydrate, 76, 109, 110t–111t
Carbon dioxide, 20
  breathing control, 22–23
  death, 262
  gas delivery, 21–22
  gas transfer, 21–22
  high levels, 22, 61, 261–262
  respiratory failure, 22, 61
Carbon monoxide, 20
Cardiopulmonary bypass, 290
  in lung transplantation, 153
Cardiovascular system, 20, 290
Care issues. *See* Medical care; Medical
  issues
Career opportunities, 242
Carnation Breakfast Liquid, 118t
Carotene, 105
Carrier, 10–11, 17, 204, 214–215, 214t
  carrier test, 214–215

risk of being carrier, 214–215, 214t
Ceclor, 313
Cefaclor, 297, 313
Cefadroxil, 313
Cefadyl, 313
Cefamandole, 313
Cefataxime, 297
Cefazolin sodium, 312, 313, 317
Cefobid, 313
Cefoperozone, 313
Cefotaxime, 314
Cefoxitin, 314
Cefprozil, 314
Ceftazidime, 297, 314, 316
Ceftin, 314
Cefulac, 308, 314
Cefuroxime, 314
Cefzil, 314
Celbenin, 314
Cell growth, 8–9
Cell membranes, salt and water movement
  across
  in CF, 4–5
  normal, 2–4
Cenalax, 314
Centers, cystic fibrosis treatment, 345–427
  United States, 345–390
  worldwide, 391–427
Central lines, 134–137, 290
  care of, 136–137
  complications, 137
  equipment, 135
  location, 136–137
  placement, 135, 136–137
  types, 134–135
Cephalexin, 297, 314, 317
Cephaloglycin, 314
Cephaloridine, 297, 314
Cephalosporin, 296–297, 314
Cephalothin sodium, 297, 314, 317
Cephapirin sodium, 314
Cephradine, 314
Cerose, 314
Cervix, 98, 234
Cerylin, 314
CF gene, 1–2, 209–211
  basic scientific research, 270
  discovery, 2

CF gene *(contd.)*
  survival, 9–11
CF Roundtable newsletter, 260
CFTR protein, 2–3
  basic scientific research, 271
  cell growth and, 8–9
  as a chloride channel and regulator of
      sodium transport, 2–5
  gene therapy trials, 275
  in healthy cells, 7
  mutations, 7–8
Check in, hospital admission, 123–124
Checkup, 179
Chemical pleurodesis, 58
Chemical sclerosing, 58
Chest pain, 57, 63–64
  asthma, 63
  esophagus, 63
  pulmonary exacerbation, 63
Chest physical therapy, 38–40, 179
  college students, 254
  drawbacks, 38
  equipment, 38–39
  in hospital, 129
  posttransplant, 172
  procedure, 38–40
  in teenage years, 227–228
Chest PT. *See* Chest physical therapy
Chest tube, 57, 58–59
Chest X-ray, 71–72, 73
  increased markings, 71
  overinflation, 72
  pneumothorax, 71
  sternal bowing, 72
Chicken pox, 46
Child development specialists, hospital-
      based, 132
Child-life workers, hospital-based, 132
Children, CF patients having, 256
Chlor-Trimeton, 314
Chloramphenicol, 296, 314
Chloride, 1, 3–4, 93–97
CFTR protein, 4–5
  heat training, 193–194
Chloride block, 94
Chloromycetin, 314
Choledyl, 314
Cholera, 10

Chorionic villus sampling, 213
Chromosome, 21
Chronic rejection, lung transplant, 162
Chronulac, 308
Chymex test, 80
Chymotrypsin, 77, 312
Cigarette smoke, 24, 25, 32, 37, 88, 182,
      238, 254
Cilia, 25, 25f, 290
Cimetidine, 82, 89, 306, 314, 320
Cipro, 314
Ciprofloxacin, 314
Cirrhosis.. *See* Liver cirrhosis
Cisapride, 89, 307, 314
Citrotein, 80
Claforan, 314
"Clamshell" approach, lung transplanta-
      tion, 152
Clarithromycin, 313, 314
Cleocin, 314
Clindamycin, 314
Clinic. *See* Cystic fibrosis clinic
Clinical research. *See* Research, clinical
      studies
Clothing, for hospitalized child, 126
Clotrimazole, 314
Clotting test, 108
Cloxacillin sodium, 295, 314, 320
Cloxapen, 314
Clubbed finger, 64–65, 290
  testing for CF, as indication for, 14
  treatment, 65
Clubbing. *See* Clubbed finger
CMV infection. *See* Cytomegalovirus
      infection
Co-Pyronil, 314
Co-trimoxazole, 314
Co-Tylenol, 314
COBRA, 251–252
Cod liver oil, 314
Codeine, 314
Coffee, 314
Colace, 309, 314
Cold, 32–33
  causes, 32–33
  cold virus, 32–33
  infant, 181
  prevention, 33

symptoms, 33
Cold weather, running in, 191, 198
Colipase, 77
Colistin sulfate, 314
Collapsed lung, 55–59, 232
College, leaving home for, 253–254
Colon
 fibrosis of, 82, 86
 role in digestion, 77
Colonization, 34
 vs. infection, 34
Coly-Mycin S, 314
Communication
 between adult CF patients, 259–260
 friends, 222
 grandparents, 222
 newsletters, 260
 spouse, 222–223
Comprehensive Omnibus Budget
  Reconciliation Act, 251–252
Comprehensive treatment program, 2–3
Concentrators, oxygen, 139
Conduction, CFTR mutations, 8
Confusion, 218
Constipation, 92
 abdominal pain, 92
Consultants, hospital-based, 132
Contac, 314
Contraindications
 to liver transplantation, 175
 to lung transplantation, 144–145
Cor pulmonale, 62–63
 treatment, 63
Coricidin, 315
Corticosteroids, 299–300. *See also*
  Steroids
 organ transplants, 156
Costs, transplantation, 166
Cotazym, 315
Cotazym-B, 90, 315
Cotazym-S, 315
Cough, 24–25
 abdominal pain, 92
 assessing need for treatment, 230
 defined, 24
 as sign of pulmonary exacerbation, 47
 steps, 24–25
Cough medicine, 303

Cough reflex, 163
Cough suppressant, 303
Cow milk, 105
Crackles, lung, 230
Creon, 315
Criticare, 315
Cromolyn, 44, 232, 300, 315, 317
Cross-country skiing, 194–195
Culture, 72–74
CVS. *See* Chorionic villus sampling
Cyclacillin, 315
Cyclapen, 315
Cyclosporine, 142, 310
 organ transplants, 158
 side effects, 160
Cyst, 290
Cystic fibrosis
 associations (worldwide), 429–433
 basic defect, xvii–xviii
 care centers, xviii–xix, 345–427
  United States, 345–390
  worldwide, 391–427
 causes, xv–xvi
 complications, 52
 defined, xv
 diagnosis
  emotional reaction to, 218
  importance of making, 13–14
  indications, 14
  tests confirming, 15–17
  unusual cases, 18
 education of family and friends,
  220–221
 epidemiology, xv–xvi
 gene. *See* CF gene
 genetic causes, 203–216
 historical aspects, xvi–xvii, 343
 information sources, xviii–xix
 life span, xvi–xvii
 organs affected, xv
 organs not affected, xv
 prenatal testing, 213–214
 prognosis, xvi–xvii
 research. *See* Research
 risk of being carrier, 214–215, 214t
 risk of inheriting, 204–206, 205f, 206t
  sibling, 205–206, 214
 tests, 65–74

Cystic fibrosis *(contd.)*
  transmembrane conductance regulator.
    See CFTR protein
Cystic fibrosis clinic
  financial and logistical issues, 223
  visit preparation, 223
  visit schedule, 223
Cystic Fibrosis Foundation, xviii–xix,
    281–287
  Care Center Program, 285
  clinical research, 284–285
  Consumer Affairs program, 286
  fellowships, 283–284
  field services, 282
  future directions, 286–287
  individual research grants, 282–283
  local chapters, 281–282, 380–390
  medical/scientific programs, 282–284
  mission, 281
  NIH partnership, 285–286
  organization, 281–286
  peer review, 284
  Public Policy program, 286
  research centers, 282
Cystic fibrosis gene. *See* CF gene
Cystic fibrosis tissue, basic scientific
    research, 272
Cystic fibrosis transmembrane conduc-
    tance regulator. *See* CFTR protein
Cytomegalovirus infection
  posttransplant, 164–165
  in transplant recipient, 158–159

D

Daily activities
  during hospital stay, 126
  during IV treatment, 127
Daily life, 179–185
Dating, 240–241
Daycare, 181
De-Tuss, 314
Death, 261–267
  adults and, 258–259
  carbon dioxide, 261–262
  causes, 261
  comfort, 262, 264, 265
  family reactions, 266
  myths, 263–265
    choking, 263
    fighting vs. rest, 264–265
    hospital vs. home, 264
    pain, 264–265
    predictions, 263–264
  oxygen, 261–262
  patients' concerns, 265–266
Decadron, 315
Declomycin, 315
Decongestant, 304
Deep breathing. *See* Thoracic expansion
Dehiscence, 290
Delatestryl, 315
Deliver 2.0 Liquid, 118t
Deltasone, 315
Demazin, 315
Demeclocycline, 315
Demerol, 315
Denial, 218
Depo-Testosterone, 315
Despair, 218
Dexamethasone, 315, 317
Dextromethorphan, 315
Dextrose, intravenous antibiotic adminis-
    tration, 128
Diabetes, 78, 82–83, 246
  in adults, 246–247
  in teenage years, 233
Diagnosis. *See* Cystic fibrosis, diagnosis
Dianabol, 315
Diaphragm, 23, 290
Diarrhea, 103–104
  bloody, 86
Dicloxacillin sodium, 295, 315
Diet supplement, 310
Dietary fiber, 307–308, 315
Dietary guidelines, 110t–111t
  high-calorie diet. *See* High-calorie
    diet
  low-fat diet, 104
Dieticians, hospital-based, 132
Digestion, 76, 290
Digestive enzymes, 76, 179, 180, 306–307,
    315, 318
  normal functioning, 75–77
  replacement, 81–82, 179, 180
Digestive system, medication, 306–310
Digital clubbing, 64–65

testing for CF, as indication for, 14
treatment, 65
Digitalis, 305–306, 315
Digitoxin, 315
Digoxin, 315, 317
Dilation, bronchiole, 30
bronchus, 30
Dilaudid, 315
Dimetane, 315
Dimetapp, 315
DIGS. *See* Distal intestinal obstruction
syndrome
Diphenhydramine hydrochloride, 89, 312,
315
Disability, determination of, 255–256
Disability insurance, 253
Disodium cromoglycate, 315
Distal intestinal obstruction syndrome,
84–85, 85, 91
in adulthood, 246
causes, 84–85
stomachaches, 91
symptoms, 85
in teenage years, 232
treatment, 85
Diuretics, 63, 305, 315
DNA, 203
DNase, 41, 301
teenage use, 229
Docusate sodium, 314
Donatussin, 315
Donor, 142, 290
Donor card, 147
Donor organ
living related donation, 154
removal, 142
Dorcol, 315
Doxycycline, 315
Drainage, 38–39
postural. *See* Postural drainage
segmental bronchial. *See* Flutter
technique
self-segmental bronchial, 328–332
Drinking, college students, 254
Dristan, 316
Drug glossary, 311–320
Ductus deferens, 98, 234, 247
Duodenum, role in digestion, 77

Dynapen, 316
Dyphylline, 316, 317

E

E-Mycin, 316
Ear oximeter, 70
EBV infection. *See* Epstein-Barr virus
infection
ECG, in hospital, 130
Echocardiograms, in hospital, 130
Ectasia, 290
Edema, 105
Education
adults, 253–255
family, 220–221
friends, 220–221
options for, 241–242
parents. *See* Parent education
research into, 276
EES, 316
Electrical charges, nasal, 2
Electrocardiogram, in hospital, 130
Electrolyte, 109
Elixicon, 316
Elixophyllin, 316
EMLA cream, 127, 302, 316
Emotional reaction, 217–219
clinic visit, 223
counseling, 222–223
daily living, 179
to death, 266
to diagnosis, 218
to difficult baby, 220
grandparents, 220–221
Employment, 255–256. *See also*
Unemployment
and health insurance, 253
when changing or leaving jobs,
251–252
job application, 256
Endotracheal tube, for transplant recipient,
167
Enema, 308
Ensure, 316
Ensure Liquid, 118t
Ensure Plus Liquid, 118t
Ensure Pudding, 118t
Entolase, 316

Entolase-HP, 316
Enzyme supplement, 91–92, 103
Enzymes, 290. *See also* Digestive enzymes
  enteric-coated, 306
  fibrosing colonopathy with higher
    doses, 81
  inability to secrete in CF, 78–82,
    103–104
  iron-deficiency, anemia and, 106
  pancreatic insufficiency, 78–82
  replacement, 81–82, 91–92, 103
  skipping, 91–92
  supplement, 91–92, 103
  in teenage years, 232
  types, 306
Ephedrine, 316
Epinephrine, 311, 316, 319
Epstein-Barr virus infection, in transplant
    recipient, 158, 159
Erythrocin, 316
Erythromycin, 297, 316, 318
Esophagitis, 87
Esophagus, 87–89, 290
  chest pain, 64
  inflammation, 87
  role in digestion, 76–77
Essential fatty acid, 79
Essential fatty acid deficiency, 105
Ethacrynic acid, 316
Exacerbation, pulmonary. *See* Pulmonary
    exacerbation
Exercise, 22–23, 40, 182, 187–201,
    334
  aerobic, 188
  anaerobic, 187
  and airway clearance, 40, 191, 334
  heart rate, 188
  in heat
    with CF, 192
    without CF, 188
  heat training
    with CF, 193–194
    without CF, 190
  in hospital, 129
  muscle, 189
  pacing yourself, 195–196
  pulse, 188
  at school, 182

  single session
    with CF, 190–191
    without CF, 187–188
  sweat, 192
  in teenage years, 228
Exercise-induced asthma, 191
Exercise programs
  activity type, 195
  bicycling, 199–200
  with CF, 192–193
  drink, 196
  food, 196
  guidelines, 194–195
  injuries, 196
  medical advice, 194
  medications, 196
  pacing yourself, 195–196
  running, 196–198
  swimming, 198–199
  time allotment, 194–195
  without CF, 189–190
Exercise test, 70–71
Exercise tolerance
  with CF, 192
  research into, 276
  without CF, 189
Exhalation, 21, 23–24
  forcible, 40
Expectorant, 303
Extractors, oxygen, 139

F
Family, 217–224
  marriage and, 256–258
  stress, 217–219, 220–221
  teenagers in, 235–240
Family history, 14
Fantasies, of hospitalized child, 125
Fat, 76, 79, 104, 110t
  low-fat diet, 104
Fat mass, 102
Fat-soluble vitamins, 79, 106–108
  supplemental, 106
Fatty acid, 105
Fatty liver, 89–90
Fecal fat test, pancreatic insufficiency,
    79–80
Fellowships, 290

CFF training awards, 283–284
  subspecialty, 131
Fertilization, *in vitro*, 247
FEV. *See* Forced expired volume
Fiber, 307, 316
Fibrosing colonopathy, 81, 82, 86
Fibrosis, 290
Financial resources, 222, 223
Finger clubbing, 64–65
  testing for CF, as indication for, 14
  treatment, 65
Fitness, 192–193
FK506. *See* Tacrolimus
Flaring, 24, 290, 291
Fleet enema, 316
Flow-volume curve, 67–68
Flu, 36
  amantadine for, 46
  flu virus, 36
  stomach flu, 92
Fluid secretion, from healthy bronchial
    cells, 3–4
Fluoroscopy, in bronchoscopy, 171
Fluoxymesterone, 316
Flutter technique, 332–333
  college students, 254
Flutter valve, 39
  posttransplant, 172
Folding, CFTR protein, 8
Forced expiration, 40, 333
Forced expired volume, 66–70
  disadvantages, 66
Forced vital capacity, 66
  disadvantages, 66
Formula, infant feeding, 109
Fortaz, 316
Friends
  with CF, 239
  reactions of, 238–239
  sickness of, 239–240
  visit from, 182
  without CF, 238
Fruit, 110t
Fundoplication, 89
Fungus, 36, 226
  growth in lung, 226
Furosemide, 305, 316, 317
FVC. *See* Forced vital capacity

G

G-tube, 119, 138
  complications, 139
  disadvantages, 138
Gallbladder, 91
Gallstones, 82, 91, 246
  abdominal pain, 91
  in adults, 246
Gammaglobulin, 26
Gantrisin, 316
Garamycin, 316
Gas delivery, 21–22
Gas exchange, 21–22, 290
Gastroenteritis, 92
  abdominal pain, 92
Gastroesophageal reflux, 32, 64, 78,
    87–89, 190, 291
  causes, 88
  chest pain, 64
  pulmonary problems, 88
  tobacco smoke, 88
  treatment, 88–89
  vomiting, 87
Gastrografin enema, 84, 308
Gastrointestinal system, 75–92
  adults, 245–247
  future therapy, 278
  medication, 305–310
  teenagers, 232–233
  testing for CF, indications for, 14
Gastrointestinal tract anatomy, 76
  normal, 75–77
Gastrostomy, 119, 138, 290
  advantages, 138
  complications, 139
  disadvantages, 138
Gaviscon, 316
GE reflux. *See* Gastroesophageal reflux
Gelsolin, future treatment with, 278
Gelusil, 316
Gene testing, 16–17
Gene therapy
  centers for, 282
  research into, 275–276
Gene(s), 203–206
  cystic fibrosis. *See* CF gene
  dominant, 204
  recessive, 204

Genetic diseases, 10
Genetics, 203–216
  basic scientific research, 270
  CF gene survival, 9–11
Gentamicin, 296, 312, 316
Geocillin, 316
Geographical location, 184–185
Geopen, 316
Gibson-Cooke sweat test, 95–96
Glossary of Drugs, 311–320
Glossary of Terms, 289–292
Glucose, 82–83, 233
Glycerol, cell growth and, 9
GoLYTELY, 232, 309, 316
Graft, 290
Grandparents, emotional reactions of,
    220–221
Granulation tissue, 139
GREAT STRIDES walk, 281
Grief
  at birth, 218
  at death, 266
Grieving response, 218
Growth chart, 101–102, 112f
Growth stimulant, 309–310
Guaifenesin, 316, 319
Gym class, 182
Gynecologic problem, abdominal pain, 92

H
Haemophilus influenzae, 35
Halotestin, 316
Head circumference, 102
Health insurance, 253
  during unemployment, 252
  when changing or leaving jobs, 251–252
Health services, college-based, 254
Hearing test, 130
Heart, 1, 22
  cor pulmonale, 62–63
  medication, 304–306
  right ventricle, 63
Heart failure, 62–63, 290
  treatment, 63
Heart-lung machine, 153
Heart-lung transplantation, 62. *See also*
    Lung transplantation
  history, 143

  procedure specifics, 152–153
Heart rate
  exercise, 188
  resting, 189–190
  target, 192–193
Heartburn, 64, 87
Heat, 188
Heat training
  with CF, 193–194
  without CF, 190
Height, 102
Helium dilution method, 68
Helplessness, 218
Hemoglobin, 22
  iron in, 105
Hemoptysis, 52–53, 232, 290
  bronchial artery embolization, 54–55
  bronchoscopy, 54
  causes, 52–53
  disadvantages, 54
  massive, 52
  significance, 52–53
  surgical treatment, 54–55
  treatment, 53–65
  vitamin K, 54
Hep-Lock, 290, 316
Heparin, 316
  intravenous antibiotic administration,
    128
Heparin lock, 316
Hetacillin, 317
Hexadrol, 317
Hickman catheter, 134, 135
High-calorie diet
  recipes, 335–342
  supplements, 118, 118t
High-calorie recipes, 335–342
Histamine, 304
History of CF, 343
Home care, 219–220
  beginning therapy, 219–220
Homework, 182
Hormone, 309–310
Hospitalization, 121–139
  admission procedures, 123–124
  annual rate, 121
  daily life, 124–125
    activity, 125–126

clothing, 125
  infection control, 126–127
  school work, 126
home care learning during, 132
personnel encountered, 130–132
  consultants, 131–132
  nurses and patient care assistants, 130
  physicians, 130–131
  other health professionals, 132
preparation for, 122–123
purpose, 121
treatments and tests, 127–130. *See also*
    specific treatments and tests
  aspects, 129
  blood tests, 130
  continued in the home, 132–139. *See*
    also Central lines; Intravenous (IV)
    treatments, home-based
  intravenous antibiotics, 127–129
  other, 130
Hospitals
  regional CF treatment centers,
      345–427
    United States, 345–390
    worldwide, 429–433
  teaching hospitals, 123–124
Hot weather, exercise
  with CF, 192
  without CF, 188
Huff technique, 40
  college students, 254
  in teenage years, 227–228
Hycodan, 317
Hycotuss, 317
Hydrocodone bitartrate, 317
Hydrocortisone, 317
Hydromorphone hydrochloride, 315
Hyper, defined, 291
Hyperalimentation, 291
Hypersplenism, 90
Hypertrophic pulmonary osteoarthropathy,
    65
  treatment, 65
Hypertrophy, right ventricular, 63
Hypo, defined, 291
Hypoalbuminemia, 104–105
  treatment, 105
Hypoelectrolytemia, 109

Hypomagnesemia, 108–109
  causes, 108
  diagnosis, 108
  signs of deficiency, 108
  sources, 108
  treatment, 108–109

I

iacfa Newsletter, 260
Ibuprofen, 44, 65, 231
ICF(M)A, 433
Ileum, 83–84
Ilozyme, 317
Imipenem, 298, 317, 319
Immune system, 1
Immunoglobulin, 26–27
Immunoreactive trypsin, 16, 80–81
Immunosuppression, 291
Immunosuppressive drugs, 155–159
  side effects, 158, 159–160
Imuran. *See* Azathioprine
in vitro fertilization, 247
"Inactive" status, on transplant list,
    150–151
Infant
  breast *vs.* bottle feeding, 109, 257
  hospitalization of, 124–125
Infant bronchiolitis, 34
  cold, 181
Infection
  airway
    causes, 6–7
    research into, 272–273
  basic scientific research, 271–272
  of bronchi, 29–31
  bronchial. *See* Pulmonary exacerbation
  bronchiole, 29–31
  as central line complication, 137
  following lung transplantation
    early, 163–164
    late, 164–165
  following organ transplant, 158–159
  inflammation and. *See* Inflammation
  intestinal, 103–104
  lower respiratory tract, 34–36
  lung, pleura, 63
  as lung transplant contraindication,
    150–151

Infection *(contd.)*
    protection against, 26–27
    respiratory tract, 33–36
    sinus, 32
    of urinary tract, 92
    vaginal, 249
    vs. colonization, 34
Infection control, during hospitalization,
        126–127
Infertility, male, 14
Inflammation
    airway, research into, 274
    bronchiole, 29–31
    bronchus, 29–31, 30f
    controlling in teenage years, 231–232
    described, 226–227
Influenza, 36
    amantadine for, 46
    stomach flu, 92
Influenza virus, 36
Infusaport system, 134–135, 135, 136,
        137
Inhalation, 21, 23, 24
Inhalation challenge test, 70
Inhalers, 42–43
    antiinflammatory, 231
    metered dose, 42
Insulin, 83, 233
Insurance
    health, 251–252
        during unemployment, 252
        when changing or leaving jobs,
            251–252
    social security disability, 253
Intal. *See* Cromolyn
Intercostal muscles, 24
Intern, 131, 291
Internal medicine, 291
International Cystic Fibrosis
        (Mucoviscidosis) Association, 433
Internist, 131, 291
Intestinal infections, 103–104
Intestine, 83–86. *See also* Large intestine;
        Small intestine
Intravenous (IV) treatments, 49, 127–129
    antibiotic types used, 128
    effectiveness, 128–129
    home-based

    in adulthood, 250
    long lines, 134–135. *See also* Central
        lines
    medical responsibility, 133–134
    prolonged use, 133–134, 134–137.
        See also Central lines
    vs. hospital-based, 133
    length of course, 129
    placement, 127–128
    shelf-life of solutions, 128
Intravenous nutrition, 120
Intussusception, 78, 85–86, 91
    abdominal pain, 91
Iodinated glycerol, 318
Iontophoresis, 95–96
Ipecac, 317
Iron deficiency, 105–106
IRT. *See* Immunoreactive trypsin
Isoetharine hydrochloride, 313, 317
Isoproterenol, 317
Isuprel, 317
IV. *See* Intravenous (IV) treatment

J

J-tube, 119, 138–139
    advantages, 139
    complications, 139
    disadvantages, 139
Jaundice, 90
Jejunostomy, 119, 138–139, 291
    advantages, 139
    complications, 139
    disadvantages, 139
Jejunum, 291
Jevity Liquid, 118t
Job application, 256
Jogging, 189
Joint problem, 64–65

K

Kanamycin, 296, 317
Kantrex, 317
Keflex, 317
Keflin, 317
Kefzol, 317
Kidneys, 1
Kindercal Liquid, 118t
Knee pain, 65

L

Lactose, 76
  abdominal pain, 92
  intolerance, 92
Lactulose, 309, 314, 317
Lanophyllin, 317
Lanoxin, 317
Laparoscopic fundoplication, 89
Large intestine, 77
Larotid, 317
Larynx, 20, 291
Lasix, 305, 317
Lavage, 60
  bronchoalveolar, 168, 169, 289
    complications, 171
Ledercillin, 317
Leg pain, 65
Life span, 2–3
Lincocin, 317
Lincomycin, 317
Linoleic acid, 105
Linolenic acid, 105
Lipase, 76, 77
Lipasorb Liquid, 118t
List, for patients awaiting donor organs.
    See Transplant list
Liver, 89–91
  future therapy, 278
  medications, 309
  preservation after harvesting, 147
  role in digestion, 77
Liver biopsy, 177
Liver cirrhosis, 78, 90
  incidence, 78
Liver disease, 247
  in adults, 247
Liver function tests, posttransplant, 177
Liver transplantation, 91
  availability, 143
  care following, 177–178
  complications, 176–177
  contraindications, 175
  history, 142
  indications, 174–175
  prognosis, 178
  technique, 175–176
  transplant list for, 175
"Living related" lobar transplantation, 154

Lobar transplantation, "living related," 154
Lobe, 20, 291
  segments, 20
Long lines. *See* Central lines
Low-fat diet, 104
Lower airway, adult, 244–245
Lower respiratory tract, 29–32
  colonization, 34
  infection, causes, 35
  infections, 34–36
Lufyllin, 317
Lumen, 291
Lung disease, complications in teenage years,
  231–232
Lung transplantation, 59
  availability, 143
  complications, 160–166
    early, 160–164
    late, 164–166
  contraindications, 144–145
  indications, 144
  "living related" lobar, 154
  procedure specifics, 152–154
  prognosis, 172–173
  sequential single, 153
  technique, 151–152
Lung volume, 68–69
  body box, 69
  helium dilution method, 68
  residual volume, 69
  tests, 68–69
  total lung capacity, 68–69
Lung(s), xv, 29–32
  adults, 244–245
  antibiotics, 293–294
  blockage, xv
  cleansing of, xvii
  collapsed, 55–59, 232. *See also*
    Pneumothorax, Atelectasis
  damage, xv
  defenses of, 24–27
  disease progression, 31
  drainage, xv
  future therapy, 278
  hyperinflated, 72
  infection, xv
    causes, 35
    protection against, 26–27

Lungs *(contd.)*
    medication, 293–303
    preservation after harvesting, 147
    teenagers, 226–232
    treatment, 37–52
    worsened, treatment, 47–52
Lymphocyte, 291
Lymphocyte-specific drugs, organ trans-
        plants, 156
Lymphoma, in transplant recipient, 159

M
Maalox, 317
Macroduct sweat collection system, 96
Maganins, future drugs from, 278
Magnacal Liquid, 118t
Magnesium, 108–109
Malabsorption
    of magnesium, 108
    pancreatic insufficiency, 80
    signs of, 103
Malnutrition, causes, 102–104
    enzyme deficiency, 103–104
    inadequate caloric intake, 104
    increased caloric needs, 104
Marax, 317
Marriage, 256–257
    and family, 256–258
Matthews Award, Dr. Leroy, 284
Maxair, 317
Maximum voluntary ventilation, 66
    compared with ventilation during
        exercise
        with CF, 191
        without CF, 189
Mealtimes, 180
Measles, 46
Mechanical percussor/vibrator, 38, 39
    advantages, 38, 39
Mechanical ventilation, 34
    respiratory failure, 62
Meconium ileus, 78, 83–84
    incidence, 78
    symptoms, 83–84
    treatment, 84
Meconium ileus equivalent. *See* Distal
        intestinal obstruction syndrome
Meconium peritonitis, 78, 84

Media, culture, 73
Medical care, 37
    in adulthood, 250–251
    in teenage years, 234–235
    transplant recipient
        liver, 177–178
        lung, 167–172
Medical history, hospital admission,
        123–124
Medical intern, 124, 131
Medical issues. *See also* Medical care
    in adulthood, 244–249
        gastrointestinal system, 245–247
        overall health, 249–250
        reproductive system, 247–249
        respiratory system, 244–245
    in teenage years, 226–234
        gastrointestinal system, 232–233
        lungs, 226–232
        reproductive system, 233–234
        sweat glands, 233
Medical resident, 124, 131
Medical specialty, 292
Medical students, 124, 131
Medical training, stages, 130
Medications, 293–320. *See also specific
        drugs*
    administration methods, 293
    allergy, 304
        allergy shot, 304
    anti-rejection drugs, 310–311
    anticonstipation, 307–308
    antireflux drugs, 307
    digestive system, 305–310
    gastrointestinal system, 305–310
    glossary, 311–320
    heart, 305–306
    in hospital, 129
    liver, 309
    lungs, 293–294
    by mouth (PO), 293
    by muscle (IM), 293
    parent responsibility, 180–181
    patient responsibility, 180–181
    polyp, 303
    respiratory system, 293–303
    side effects, 293
    sinus, 303

upper airway, 303–304
by vein (IV), 293
Medihaler-EPI, 317
Medihaler-1SO, 317
Mediport system, 134–135, 135, 136, 137
  in adulthood, 250
Meglumine diatrizoate, 316
Menstrual periods, 248
Mental retardation, xv
MESA technique, 247
Metaproterenol sulfate (Metaprel), 42, 311, 317
Metered-dose inhaler, 42
Methacycline, 317
Methandrostenolone, 315
Methanesulfonate, 320
Methicillin sulfate, 294, 317
Methyltestosterone, 317
Metoclopramide, 89, 317, 319
Mezlin, 317
Mezlocillin, 295, 317
Microsurgical epididymal sperm aspiration, 247
Milk of magnesia, 318
Mineral oil, 308
Minocin, 318
Minocycline, 318
Morphine, for low oxygen levels, 263
Mouth, 24
  role in digestion, 76–77
Mucociliary clearance, 163–164
Mucociliary escalator, 24, 25–26, 291
Mucolytics, 300–301, 318
Mucomyst, 41, 301, 318
  teenage use, 229
Mucous, defined, 291
Mucous plug, 63
Mucus, 1–2, 25
  blood, 52
  breaking up, 40–41
  defined, 291
Mucus-thinning agents
  future treatments, 278
  research into, 274–275
  teenage use, 229
Muscle mass, evaluation of, 102
Muscles, 21

bronchial, 21
  exercise, 189
  respiratory, 23–24
    accessory, 21
  strained, 63
Mutations, CF gene and CFTR protein, 7–8
MVV. *See* Maximum voluntary ventilation
Mycostatin, 318
Mylanta, 318
Mylicon, 309, 318

N
Nafcil, 318
Nafcillin sodium, 294, 318
Naldecon, 318
Narrowing, airway, following lung transplantation, 164, 166
Nasal flaring, 24, 290, 291
Nasal PD, 2, 17
Nasal polyp, 27, 28–29
  medication, 303
  polypectomy, 28–29
  removal, 28–29
  significance, 28
  steroid spray, 28
  treatment, 28
Nasalide, 303
Nasogastric tube, 119, 137–138, 291
  advantage, 138
  disadvantages, 137–138
National Institutes of Health
  CFF partnership, 285–286
  research grants, 285–286
Nebcin, 318
Nebulizer, 42, 43, 291
Nedocromil, 232, 300, 318
Neomycin, 296, 318
Neo-Synephrine, 303, 318
Nervous system, xv
Netilmicin, 296, 318
NETWORK newsletter, 260
Neutrophils, 31
Newborn, screening of, 16
Newsletters, 260
NG tube, 119, 137–138, 291
  advantage, 138
  disadvantage, 137–138

Nissen fundoplication, 89
Noncompliance, as lung transplant
    contraindication, 145
Nose, 24, 28–29
  adults, 244
  electrical charges in, 2
Novahistine, 318
Nurses, 130–131
Nutren 1.5 Liquid, 118t
Nutrition, 101–120
  evaluation, 101–102
  high-calorie recipes, 335–342
  importance, 102
  intravenous, 120
Nutritional supplement, 118, 118t
  intravenous nutrition, 118–120
Nutritional treatment, 109, 110t–111t
  basic, 109, 110t–111t
  dietary guidelines, 110t–111t
  high calorie nutritional supplements,
    118, 118t
  in hospital, 130
  tube feedings, 118–120, 137–139
    problems with, 119–120
Nutritionists, hospital-based, 132
Nystatin, 318

O

Obstruction of airway. *See* Airway
  obstruction
OKT3, transplant rejection therapy, 162,
  165, 311
Omeprazole, 82, 307, 318
Omnipen, 318
Open thoracotomy, 58
OPOs. *See* Organ Procurement
  Organizations
ORCC. *See* Outwardly rectifying chloride
  channel
Organ donation, 267
  for research, 267
Organ donor. *See* Donor
Organ failure, following lung
  transplantation, 161
Organ Procurement Organizations, 148
Organ recipient, 142
Organ support, 147
Organidin, 318

Organs
  donation of, 267
    for research, 267
  harvesting and preservation, 146–148
  potential recipients of, 148
  transplantation of. *See*
    Transplantation
Osteoarthropathy, 65
  treatment, 65
Outwardly rectifying chloride channel, 3
Overnight visit, 182
OVRs. *See* Vocational rehabilitation
  programs
Oxacillin, 294, 318
Oximetry, 70
Oxtriphylline, 312, 314, 318
Oxygen, 20, 22, 61, 301–303
  addiction, 302–303
  administration method, 301–302
  amount needed, 302
  breathing control, 22–23
  death, 261–262
  during exercise, 191
  gas delivery, 21–22
  gas transfer, 21–22
  low levels, 22, 61, 262–263
  respiratory failure, 22, 61
  side effects, 302
  treatment, 61–62
Oxygen concentrators, 139
Oxygen-delivery systems, 139
  for adults, 250
Oxygen extractors, 139
Oxymetazoline hydrochloride, 311
Oxytetracycline, 318, 320

P

PABA, 80
Pain, 264–265
  abdominal, 91–92
  bone or joint, 65
  chest. *See* Chest pain
  control in transplant recipient, 167
Pancreas, xv, 6, 78–82
  insufficiency. *See* Pancreatic
    insufficiency
  role in digestion, 77
Pancrease, 318

Pancreatic enzyme replacement, 81–82
  enteric coated, 81–82
Pancreatic insufficiency, 78–82
  bowel movement, 79–80
  diagnosis, 79–81
    Chymex test, 80
  treatment, 81–82
Pancreatin, 318, 320
Pancreatitis, 78, 82
  abdominal pain, 91
Pancreatitis-associated protein, 80
Pancrelipase, 315, 317, 318
Panmycin, 318
Pansinusitis, X-ray, 27
PAP, 80
Papase, 318
Parainfluenza virus, 36
Parent education, 218–219
  emotional reaction, 217–219
  marriage stress, 218
  treatment approach, 221
Parenteral nutrition, 120
  total, 291
Parents
  attitude development, 221
  education of. *See* Parent education
  role during hospitalization of child,
    124–125
  teenage issues and, 235–236
Partial thromboplastin time test, 108
Patient care assistants, 130–131
Patient survival, 37
PD. *See* Potential difference
Peak, 291
Pediamycin, 318
Pediasure Liquid, 118t
Pediazole, 318
Penicillin G benzathine, 313
Penicillin G procaine, 317
Penicillin V potassium, 313
Penicillin(s), 294–295, 312, 318, 320
Pen-Vee-K, 318
PEP mask, 39, 333
  teenage use, 228
Pepsin, 77
Peptamen Liquid, 118t
Peptidase, 77
Percussion, 60

  and drainage, 38–39
Percussor vest, 38
Percutaneously inserted central catheters,
    134, 135
  placement, 135
PFTs. *See* Pulmonary function tests
Phenylephrine hydrochloride, 317, 318
Physical education, 182
Physical therapists, hospital-based, 132
Physicians, 131–132
  consultants, 131
  intern, 131
  patient education of, 123, 131–132
  resident, 131
  subspecialty (fellow), 131
PICC lines, 134, 135
  placement, 135
Pilocarpine iontophoresis, 95–96
Piperacillin sodium, 295, 318
Pipracil, 318
Pirbuterol, 318
Plethysmograph, total body, 69
Pleura, 63
  infection, 63
  inflammation, 63
  in lung transplantation, 152
Pleurabrasion, 58
Pleural space, in lung transplantation,
    152
Pleurectomy, 58
Pleurisy, 63
Pleuritis, 63
Pleurodesis, 58
Pneumococcus vaccine, 45
Pneumonia, 34–35
Pneumonia vaccine, 45
Pneumothorax, 55–59, 63, 71, 232, 291
  bronchiole, 56
  bronchus, 56
  causes, 56
  scoring, 57
  signs, 57
  treatment, 57–59
  X-ray, 57
Pneumovax, 318
Poly-Histine, 319
Polycillin, 319
Polycose, 319

Polycose Powder, 118t
Polymox, 319
Polymyxin-B, 319
Polymyxin-E, 319
Polyp, 27, 28–29
  medication, 303
  polypectomy, 28–29
  removal, 28–29
  significance, 28–29
  steroid spray, 28
  treatment, 28–29
Polypectomy, 28–29
Portacath system, 134–135, 135, 136, 137
  in adulthood, 250
Portosystemic shunt, 91
Postmortem exam, 267
Posttransplant lymphoproliferative disease,
    in transplant recipient, 159
Postural drainage, 38
  Flutter technique, 332–333
  in hospital, 129
  infants, 321–324
  self-segmental bronchial drainage,
      328–332
  table for, 39
  techniques, 321–333
  in teenage years, 227–228
  toddlers, 324–327
Potential difference, 60
  nasal, 2, 17
Prealbumin, 107
Prednisolone, 319
Prednisone, 43, 231, 315, 319
  organ transplants, 158
  side effects, 43–44, 160
Pregnancy, risk of, 241, 248, 257
Pregnancy rate
  female CF patient, 248
  in vitro fertilization and, 248
Prenatal testing, 236
Preschool children, hospitalization of, 125
Preservation, harvested organ, 147
Prilosec, 319
Primaxin, 319
Principen, 319
Prognosis, 2–3
Prograf, organ transplants, 158
Prolastin, future treatments with, 278

Propulsid, 319
Prostaphlin, 319
Protein, 76, 110t
  regulating transmembrane conductance.
      See CFTR protein
Prothrombin time test, 108
Proventil, 319
Prunes, 319
Pseudomonas, 35, 36. See also Burkholde-
    ria cepacia
  airway infection, 145–146
  antibiotic resistance, 51
  as lung transplant contraindication, 145
  posttransplant complication, 163, 164
Pseudomonas aeruginosa, 35
  infection control for hospitalized child,
      126
Pseudomonas cepacia. See Burkholderia
    cepacia
Psychologic stress, 63, 92
  abdominal pain, 92
Psychological issues
  adjustment, research into, 276
  in adulthood, 258
  in teenage years, 235–240
    attitude and body image, 236–238
    friends, 238–240
    parents, 235–236
    siblings, 236
PT. See Chest physical therapy
PT test, 108
PTLD. See Posttransplant lymphoproli-
    ferative disease
PTT test, 108
Puberty, delayed development, 98
Pulmocare Liquid, 118t
Pulmonary capillary, 21–22
Pulmonary exacerbation, 29–31, 47–52,
    63, 180, 291
  aerosol antibiotics, 48–49
  chest pain, 63
  early treatment, 48
  intravenous antibiotics, 49
  minimizing in teenage years, 229–230
  oral antibiotics, 48
  symptoms, 47–48, 63
  in teenage years, 229–230
  treatments, 48–49, 50f

Pulmonary function tests, 66–70
  determining antibiotic treatment length, 129
  in hospital, 130
  posttransplant, 162, 168, 169
  in teenage years, 230–231
  uses of, 66
Pulmonology, 291
Pulmozyme. *See* DNase
Pulse, exercise, 188
Pulse oximeter, 170
Pulseox, 170
Pulseoximeter, 70

Q

Quality of life issues, 286
Quibron, 319
Quiet breathing. *See* Breathing control
Quinolones, 297, 319

R

Racquet sports, 195–196
Rales, lung, 230
Ranitidine, 82, 89, 306, 319
Reactive airways, 69
"Reasonable accommodation," 256
Recessive disorder, 204
Recipes, high-calorie, 335–342
Recipient, 291. *See also* Organ recipient
Rectal prolapse, 78, 86–87
  causes, 86
  treatment, 87
Rectum, 86–87
Reflux. *See* Gastroesophageal reflux
Reglan, 307, 319
Regulation, CFTR mutations, 8
Rehabilitation programs, vocational, 254–255
Rejection, 291
  following lung transplantation
    diagnosis, 162
    early, 162
    late, 165
    treatment, 162
Relative contraindications, lung transplantation, 144, 145
Relief
  at CF diagnosis, 218

at death, 266
Reproductive system, 98–99
  adult
    birth control and, 248–249
    female, 248
    male, 247–248
    vaginal yeast infections, 249
  delayed development, 98–99
  female, 98
  male, 98
  teenagers, 233–234
Research, xvii–xviii
  basic scientific
    CF tissue, 272
    genetics, 270
    infection, 271–272
    salt transport and CFTR function, 271
  clinical studies, 272
    airway fluid composition, 273–274
    airway infection, 272–273
    airway inflammation, 274
    gene therapy, 275–276
    mucus-thinning agents, 274–275
  divisions, 270
  education, 276
  exercise tolerance, 276
  future treatments, 278–279
  organ donation for, 267
  psychological adjustment, 276
Research ethics
  investigator's responsibilities, 278
  patient's responsibilities, 278
Research grants, 282–283
Resident, 292
  medical, 131
Residual volume, 69
Resistance, to antibiotics, 50–52, 74
Resistant, 292
Resource Plus Liquid, 118t
Respalor Liquid, 118t
Respiratory failure, 22, 61–62, 292
  carbon dioxide, 22, 61
  causes, 22, 61
    mechanical ventilator, 62
Respiratory syncytial virus, 36
  ribavirin, 46
Respiratory system. *See also* Lungs
  adults, 244

Respiratory system (contd.)
  in teenage years, 226–232
  testing for CF, indications for, 14
Respiratory therapists, hospital-based, 132
Respiratory tract, 19–74, 27–36
  anatomy, 20–27
  function, 20–27
  infections, 33–36
  lower. See Lower respiratory tract; Lungs
  medication, 293–303
  respiratory muscles, 23–24
  upper. See Upper respiratory tract
Rest, scheduling time for, 250
Retinol, 105
Retinol-binding protein, 107
Retracting, 24, 292
Retrograde amnesia, 170
Rhinovirus, 36
Rib
  broken, 63
  bruised, 63
Ribavirin, 319, 320
  respiratory syncytial virus, 46
Rickets, 107
Right ventricular hypertrophy, 63
Robitussin, 319
Rondec, 319
Rowing, 195–196
Running
  clothes, 196–197
  equipment, 196
  safety, 197–198
  starting, 197

S

Sadness, at death, 266
Saline, 292, 319
  intravenous antibiotic administration,
    128
Salmeterol, 42
Salt, 1. See also Sodium
  movement across cell membranes, 2–4
Salt loss, 97
Salt supplement, 97
Salt transport, basic scientific research,
    271
Salty sweat, 1
  testing for CF, as indication for, 14

Scandishake Liquid, 118t
School, 181–182
School-aged children, hospitalization of,
    125
School work, for hospitalized child, 126
Sclerotherapy, 91
Screening tests, newborn, 16
Second-hand smoke, 37, 183, 238
  college students, 254
Secretion, from healthy bronchial cells,
    3–4
Sedation, 292
  during bronchoscopy, 170
  of transplant recipient, 167
Segment, 292
Segmental bronchial drainage. See Flutter
    technique
Selenium, xix
Self-fulfilling prophesies, 237
Self segmental bronchial drainage,
    328–332
Semen analysis, 247
Senekot, 308, 319
Senna, 319
Sensitive, defined, 292
Sensitivity, 72–74
Sequential single lung transplantation, 153
Sex
  adults, 257–258
  teenagers, 241
Sexual intercourse, 258
Sexually transmitted diseases, 241
Shock, 218
Shortness of breath, 57
  assessing need for treatment, 230
Shunt, 91
Shwachman, Harry, Cystic Fibrosis
    Clinical Investigation Award, 283
Siblings, 221–222
  reaction to death, 266
  tension between, 236
Sickle cell disease, 10
Sidestream smoke, 37, 183, 238
  college students, 254
Silain, 309, 319
Simethicone, 309, 317
Sinuses, 27
  adult, 244

medication, 303
treatment, 27
X-ray, 27
Sinusitis, 32
Skating, 195–196
Skiing, cross-country, 195–196
Skinfold measurements, 102
Slo-Phyllin Gyrocaps, 319
Small intestine, role in digestion, 77
Smoking, 24, 25, 32, 88, 183, 238, 254
Social security disability insurance, 252
Social worker
    help for new parents, 222
    hospital-based, 132
Sodium, 1, 3–4, 93–97
    CFTR protein, 4–5
    heat training, 193–194
    infant, 97
    replacement during hot weather, 97
Sodium chloride, 319
Sodium methicillin, 314, 319
Somophyllin, 319
Soy milk, 105
Specialty, 292
Spectrobid, 319
Sperm, 98
    epididymal aspiration, 247
Sperm count, 234
Spirometry, 66–68
    flow-volume curve, 67–68
    forced expired volume in I second, 66
        disadvantages, 66
    forced vital capacity, 66
        disadvantages, 66
    maximum voluntary ventilation, 66
        disadvantages, 66
Spironolactone, 305, 312, 319
Sports, 182
Sputum, 31, 292
Stanozolol, 320
"Staph," 35
    posttransplant complication, 163, 164
Staphcillin, 319
Staphylococcus, 35
    as lung transplant contraindication, 145
Staphylococcus aureus, infection control
        for hospitalized child, 126
Starch, 76

Stenosis, 292
    airway, following lung transplantation,
        164, 166
Sterility, in males, 234, 247
Sternal bowing, 72
Steroid spray, 303
Steroids, 43–44, 299–300, 309, 310, 319
    See also Corticosteroids
    anabolic, 309
    inhalers, 231–232
    organ transplants, 158
    side effects, 160
Stoma, 292
Stomach, 89
    increased acid, 89
    pain. *See* Abdominal pain
    role in digestion, 76–77, 77
Stomach ache, 91–92. *See also* Abdominal
    pain
Stomach flu, 92
    abdominal pain, 92
Stress
    family, 217–219, 220–221, 222–223
    psychologic, 64, 92
    transplant-associated, 166–167
Subspecialties, 131
    CFF training awards, 283–284
Sucrose, 76
Sugar, 83, 233
Sulfa drugs, 295
Sulfamethoxazole, 295, 319
Sulfatrim, 319
Sulfisoxazole, 295, 316
Summer camp, 184
Sunlight, 107
Superior vena cava, 134
Surgery
    inflammation created by, 58
    intussusception, 86
    meconium ileus, 84
    meconium ileus equivalent, 85
    meconium peritonitis, 84
    pneumothorax, 57–59
    for pneumothorax, 57–59
    for varices, 91
Sus-Phrine, 319
Sustacal Liquid, 118t, 319
Sustacal Plus Liquid, 118t, 319

Sustacal Pudding, 118t, 319
Sustaire, 320
Sweat
  collection methods, 15
  exercise, 192
Sweat abnormality, 94–95
Sweat glands, 1, 6, 93–97
  normal sweat, 93–94
  teenagers, 233
Sweat test(s), 1–2, 15–16, 95–96
  problems, 96–97
  reliability, 15
Swimming
  equipment, 198
  learning, 199
  location, 198
  safety, 198–199
  starting, 199

T
Tacrolimus, 310
  organ transplants, 158
  side effects, 160
Tagamet, 306, 320
Tazidime, 320
Teaching hospitals, 123–124
Tedral, 320
Teenagers, 225–226. *See also* Adolescence
  care issues, 234–235
  career direction, 242
  dating, marriage, and family, 240–241
  education, 241–242
  hospitalization of, 125
  medical issues, 226–234
    gastrointestinal system, 232–233
    lungs, 226–232
    reproductive system, 233–234
    sweat glands, 233
  psychological and family issues, 235–240
    attitude and body image, 236–238
    friends, 238–240
    parents, 235–236
    siblings, 236
Tegopen, 320
Tendon
  pulled, 63
  strained, 63
Tennis, 195–196

Terbutaline sulfate, 313, 320
Terramycin, 320
Testicular torsion, 92
Testionate, 320
Testosterone, 315, 320
Tetra-BID, 320
Tetracycline, 297, 318, 320
Theo-Dur, 320
Theobid, 320
Theolate, 320
Theophyl, 320
Theophylline, 42–43, 299, 316, 320
Theospan, 320
Therapeutic trial, 80
Therapists, physical and respiratory, 132
Thiazides, 305
Thoracic expansion, 40, 333
Thoracoscope, 57, 58–59
Thoracotomy, 58
Thymosin beta-4, future treatments with, 278
Ticarcillin, 295, 320
Tilade. *See* Nedocromil
Timentin, 295, 320
TIPS, 91
Tobacco smoke, 24, 25, 32, 88, 183, 238, 254
Tobramycin sulfate, 296, 318, 320
Toddlers, hospitalization of, 125
Tornalate, 320
Torsion, testicular, 92
Total body plethysmograph, 69
Total lung capacity, 68–69
Toxicity, 292
TPN (total parenteral nutrition), 291
Trachea, 20, 292
Tracheostomy, 292
Trait
  cystic fibrosis, 10–11
  sickle, 10
Transbronchial biopsy, posttransplant, 162, 168, 169–170
Transfusion, 90
Transjugular intrahepatic portosystemic shunting, 91
Transplant list
  "active" and "inactive" status, 150–151
  for lung transplants, 149

organ harvesting and preservation, 146–148
potential recipients on, 148
waiting on, 149–150
Transplantation
anti-rejection drugs, 310–311
care following, 167–172
decision-making, 173–174
defined, 142
future of, 178
history, 142
indications and predictions, 143
liver. *See* Liver transplantation
lung. *See* Lung transplantation
organ harvesting for, 146–148
problems associated with, 154–160
lung transplants. *See* Lung transplantation
organ rejection, 155–159. *See also* Immunosuppressive drugs
psychological, social, and financial, 166–167
surgical, 159
transplant list, 146–148
potential recipients on, 148
Travel, 183–184
Treatment(s). *See also specific treatments*
aerosol, in hospital, 129
assessing need in teenage years, 230–231
future, research into, 277–278
intravenous antibiotic administration. *See* Intravenous (IV) treatments
lungs, 37–52
obstruction, 38–44
parent responsibility, 180–181
patient responsibility, 180–181
Triamcinolone, 299, 320
Triamcinolone acetonide, 312
Triaminic, 320
Trimethoprim, 320
Trimethoprim-sulfamethoxazole, 295, 312
Trough, 292
Trypsin, 77, 80–81
Tube feedings, 118–120
problems with, 119–120
Tussionex, 320
Tuss-Ornade, 320

U
Ulcer, 78, 89, 91
abdominal pain, 91
Ultrase, 320
Unemployment, 252–253
health insurance, 252
social security disability insurance, 252
United Network for Organ Sharing (UNOS), 148
Upper airway
adult, 244
medications, 303–304
Upper respiratory tract, 27–29
infections, 33–34, 183
Urecholine, 89
Uridine triphosphate, future treatments with, 278
Urinary tract infection, 92
abdominal pain, 92
Ursodeoxycholic acid, 90, 309, 311
UTP. *See* Uridine triphosphate

V
Vaginal yeast infections, 249
Vancenase, 303, 320
Varices, 90–91
treatment, 90–91
Vas deferens, 98, 234, 247
Veetid B-Cillin, 320
Vegetable, 110t
Velosef, 320
Ventilation, assisted, 34
Ventilator, for transplant recipient, 167–168
Ventilatory muscles, 23–24
Ventolin, 320
Ventricle, 292
Vibramycin, 320
Viokase, 320
Viokase Powder, 320
Viokase Tablet, 320
Vipep, 320
Viral infections. *See also specific viruses*
lung, 226
in transplant recipient, 158–159
Virazole, 320
Virus, 36
lung infection, 226

Visit, by friend, 183
Vital, 320
Vital signs, 123
Vitamin A, 105, 309
    sources, 106–107
Vitamin D, 107, 309
    signs of deficiency, 107
    sources, 107
Vitamin E, 107, 309
    signs of deficiency, 107
    sources, 107
Vitamin K, 108, 309
    hemoptysis, 54
    sources, 108
Vitamins, 179, 309
    fat-soluble, 79, 106–108, 309
    supplemental, 106
Vivonex, 320
Vocational rehabilitation programs,
    254–255
Voice-box. *See* Larynx
Volleyball, 195–196
Vomiting, 76–77
    GE reflux, 87
    intussusception, 86
    pancreatitis, 82

W
Walking, 195–196
Water, movement across cell membranes,
    2–4
Wedging, in bronchoscopy, 171
Weight, 101–102
Weight training, 189, 195–196
Wheezing, 32
White blood cell, 26
    functions, 26
Windpipe. *See* Trachea
Winstrol, 320
Wycillin, 320

X
X-ray
    atelectasis, 59, 60
    in hospital, 130
    pansinusitis, 27
    pneumothorax, 57
    sinus, 27

Y
Yeast infections, vaginal, 249

Z
Zantac, 306, 320
ZIG (zoster immune globulin), 46
Zinc, 107
Zone of inhibition, 73
Zoster immune globulin, 46
Zosyn, 295
Zymase, 320